MODERN ADVANCES IN CATARACT SURGERY

CONTRIBUTORS

JOAQUIN BARRAQUER, M.D.

Director, Instituto Barraquer, Barcelona, Spain

F. PHINIZY CALHOUN, JR., M.D.

Professor of Ophthalmology, Chairman of the Department and Director of Montgomery Laboratory of Ocular Pathology (Emory), Atlanta, Georgia

WOLFGANG HÖPPING, M.D.

Facharzt für Augenkrankheiten, Essen, Germany

TADEUSZ KRWAWICZ, M.D.

Professor of Ophthalmology, Director of Ophthalmological Clinic, Medical Academy, Lublin, Poland

GERD MEYER-SCHWICKERATH, M.D.

Professor of Ophthalmology, University of Bonn, Head of the Eye Department, Municipal Eye Clinic, Essen, Germany

BENEDETTO STRAMPELLI, M.D.

Chief of Ophthalmology, Reunited Hospitals, Docent in Ophthalmology, Eye Clinics and University of Rome, Italy

Modern Advances in Cataract Surgery

EDITOR R. M. Fasanella, M.D.

Diplomate, American Board of Ophthalmology; Associate Clinical Professor of Ophthalmology, Yale University School of Medicine; Diplomate, Pan American Congress of Ophthalmology; Fellow, American Academy of Ophthalmology and Otolaryngology; Member, Association for Research in Ophthalmology; Member, New York Society for Clinical Ophthalmology

ASSOCIATE EDITOR Barbara J. Matthews

DRAWINGS Robert Bray Wingate, A.B., M.S.

J. B. LIPPINCOTT COMPANY

PHILADELPHIA AND MONTREAL

Distributed in Great Britain by
Pitman Medical Publishing Co., Limited, London

Library of Congress Catalog Card No. 63-12498

Printed in the United States of America

This book is dedicated not to a single individual
but to all those persons who have made it possible.

It is dedicated to my patients, especially one, A.B.;
it is dedicated to my teachers, especially E.B.S. and E.M.A.;
it is dedicated to my staff, especially B.J.M.
and to my family, especially P.

Preface

In the last few years certain changes have taken place in surgery of the cataract. Drugs like alpha-chymotrypsin to cause zonulolysis and urea and mannitol in treating cases complicated by glaucoma have proved to be valuable assets in the successful outcome of procedures related to cataract extraction. Nystatin and amphotericin B* have played an increasingly useful role in cases with fungal disease. New instruments such as the light coagulator and the operating microscope have been designed to facilitate the technic of cataract surgery. New sutures and needles have been introduced which ensure easier and better wound closures. The practice of removing both cataracts in a patient during one hospital admission is not new and is gaining popularity in certain areas of the United States, although generally it is not favored.

Nevertheless, while these new trends have removed some problems formerly presented in cataract surgery, they are not foolproof. Constant re-evaluation is needed to avoid the pitfalls which will be met in all advances. For example, if alpha-chymotrypsin is improperly used, it may lead to complications such as wound separation; likewise, the light coagulator can cause damage to the cornea and the retina if it is handled improperly.

* Nystatin and amphotericin B as antifungoidal agents in ocular infection.

This book is meant to be practical and is written for the practicing ophthalmic surgeon. Because the literature is so voluminous and because critical evaluation is necessary in view of overzealous statements, an attempt has been made to interpret for the busy practitioner the various authoritative views which are justifiable in the present state of our knowledge. Based on practical experience an attempt also has been made to delineate the various steps that should be taken in cataract surgery. Not all of the old procedures have been abandoned or replaced. There is still room for the employment of such procedures in certain specific conditions. But in almost every case, the material is based on questions that have actually been asked at lectures and meetings. These have been regrouped to fit the sequence of cataract surgery steps. In addition, some problems for which there are no definitive solutions at this time have been included. Also included are articles by Phinizy Calhoun, Joaquin Barraquer, Benedetto Strampelli and Wolfgang Höpping and G. Meyer-Schwickerath. Also introduced is the work of T. Krwawicz, who, by his method of extracting intumescent lenses by the application of low temperature, offers a new approach which may make possible a greater number of intracapsular extractions.

The compiling of this book has been made possible by the work of many people in this field and by those with whom we have exchanged ideas. It is almost impossible to list all of them but we fully realize that any value that this book may have rests on the fact that we have been associated with these people.

R. M. FASANELLA

Acknowledgments

A surgeon turned writer cannot be objective enough to detect his own faults and, as is customary, must rely on his friends to read his material with a critical eye. I owe a debt of thanks to my busy colleagues who sacrificed their time to review portions of this book. Grateful acknowledgment is hereby made to Dr. H. Saul Sugar for his help with Glaucoma and Cataracts; to Dr. Frederick C. Cordes for his generous assistance with Congenital Cataracts; to Dr. Wilfred Fry who was kind enough to review Corneal Dystrophy and Cataracts; to Dr. Morton Rosenthal for his assistance with Myopia and Detachment; and to Dr. Louis Nahum who was of great help editorially.

I am particularly grateful to Drs. Ramon Castroviejo and Algernon Reese who aided me with many portions of this book and to Drs. Edmund B. Spaeth and Andrew S. Wong for reading every page of the manuscript and for furnishing me with their valuable criticism and counsel.

The following were of great assistance in the preparation of the manuscript: Miss Mary Czuckery, Mr. Anthony Fontana, Mrs. Mary Hibson, Dr. R. Cordero Moreno, Dr. H. Van Den Beld C., Dr. José Barraquer, Dr. Enrique Ariza H., Dr. U. M. Carbajal, Dr. Louis Girard, Dr. W. A. J. VanHeuvan and Dr. Jerome Freedman.

I have been fortunate in having the services of the well-known illustrator, Mr. Robert Bray Wingate, A.B., M.S., who has had extensive experience in ophthalmic art at the Ocular Research Unit of Walter Reed General Hospital, Washington, D. C.

Finally, I am indebted to the Storz Instrument Company for providing the instrument plates and to the numerous authors and publishers who granted permission for the use of their materials in this book.

R. M. F.

Contents

Introduction—The Use of Alpha-Chymotrypsin

A milestone in cataract surgery was the report of the Committee on the Use of alpha-Chymotrypsin which was presented at the 64th Annual Session of the American Academy of Ophthalmology and Otolaryngology, October 11-16, 1959, in Chicago. Here a national survey on the facility of cataract extraction and on operative and immediate postoperative complications with the use of the enzyme is best summarized in the introduction and summary by Derrick Vail, M.D., the Chairman of the Committee.*

We have heard from Dr. Schwartz that this enzyme isolated by Kunitz and Northrop has been available since 1933. It is a protein and thus is capable of producing an allergic reaction in the eye in sensitized individuals. Clinically, however, this seems to be more of a theoretical than a practical consideration, although such a possibility must be borne in mind and cases of allergic reactions following systemic use have been reported. Alpha-chymotrypsin is a proteolytic enzyme, having a specificity of action at certain peptide bonds, but it is capable of hydrolyzing other bonds such as esters, amides, hydroxyamides, hydrazides, and even carbon-carbon bonds. The optimum pH for maximum velocity of hydrolysis of protein and synthetic substrates by alpha-chymotrypsin is usually between 7 and 9.

Certain enhancers and inhibitors of the enzyme have been discovered. Among the enhancers is calcium chloride, sometimes used in the vehicle for ophthalmic use. It should be borne in mind that while calcium chloride may enhance the effect of the enzyme, it also may prolong its activity. Further investigation of this point must be carried out.

Among the inhibitors are DFP and beta-phenyl-proprionic acid. What, if any, practical use will develop from this information is hard to see at this stage of our knowledge.

Dr. von Sallmann helped us very much when he reported that he was unable to produce an allergic reaction in animals experimentally sensitized to this enzyme by installation or by injection subconjunctivally, or in the anterior chamber, or in the vitreous. This evidence supports wide clinical impressions.

His studies on the effect of this substance on the corneal endothelium are of great importance to us. His illustrations show these effects beautifully. However, we are told that the injection of a 0.9 per cent solution of sodium chloride by itself will produce the same type of injury, although to a lesser degree. In other words the addition of alpha-chymotrypsin is a slight increment in potential damage to the endothelial cells. This is important in considering the question of the cause of striate keratitis, which is found more frequently when alpha-chymotrypsin is used than otherwise.

However, when the enzyme reaches into the corneal stroma through extensively damaged endothelium, a heavy opacity results. Such opacities also occur with a 0.9 per cent solution of sodium chloride. The corneal changes are of a transient nature as a rule, and Dr. von Sallmann concludes that it was

* Vail, Derrick: Report of the Committee on the Use of alpha-Chymotrypsin in Ophthalmology, Summary, Trans. Am. Acad. Ophthal. Otolaryng. *64*:54, 1960.

improbable that a specific enzymatic action was the cause of the lesion. Using a different technic, which may or may not be a factor, David Shoch and his co-workers found no evidence of endothelial damage in the eyes of twenty-four rabbits. This discrepancy in the findings needs to be resolved.

Finally, Dr. von Sallmann confirms the histologic findings of the St. Louis workers, Ley, Holmberg and Yamashita, who showed by electromicroscopic studies that the zonule fibers are fragmented by the action of the enzyme.

Dr. Maumenee gives us a horrifying picture of what happens when the retina is placed in a solution containing 150 units of alpha-chymotrypsin. However, this concentration and the duration of exposure exceed, by far, the same factors when alpha-chymotrypsin is employed in cataract surgery.

Maumenee's report shows that the supporting structure of the retina is more sensitive to the enzyme than is the rest of the retinal tissue. This damage occurs when alpha-chymotrypsin is injected into the vitreous of an experimental animal. This may have some clinical importance in suggesting that the enzyme should not be used in cases of fluid vitreous or subluxated lens, or where the hyaloid membrane is not intact.

Dr. Troutman's report involved an enormous amount of analytic work on the questionnaires and is still somewhat incomplete. However, enough facts have been gathered to warrant the following conclusions:

1. The incidence of striate keratitis is greater when the enzyme is employed. We believe that this is due largely to mechanical injury to the endothelium by instruments, either forceps or erisophake (about equal incidence). The marked decrease in the depth of the anterior chamber consequent to the forward dislocation of the lens means much less room for manipulation and a greater chance for rubbing or scraping of the endothelium of the cornea than otherwise. The deleterious action of a solution, either of saline solution or alpha-chymotrypsin, upon the corneal endothelium must be considered a part of this problem. The preparation of the solution and the vehicle used may also play a part. As yet we don't know.

2. A 1:10,000 dilution is as effective as a 1:5000 dilution. This finding conflicts with the experience of Barraquer and needs further investigation.

3. Great care must be devoted to the preparation of a fresh solution, the technic and instrumentation of its injection into the posterior chamber, and its removal by irrigation of the anterior chamber two minutes after injection.

4. A very high percentage of surgeons "felt" that the facility of extracting the lens was enhanced by use of the enzyme. This clinical impression was beautifully supported by the double blind study conducted by Dr. Schwartz.

5. One of the most important findings of this statistical study is the marked decrease in the number of ruptured capsules that occurred when the enzyme was employed in the operation on one eye, when compared with the incidence of ruptured capsules that occurred in the other eye of the same individuals when the enzyme was not used. In other words, the use of the enzyme means fewer ruptured capsules.

6. While we cannot be sure, because of the difficulty in getting figures in a comparable control series, we believe that the complications that occur during the operation or during the healing postoperative stage are no greater or no less whether the enzyme is used or not. The one and major exception to this statement is the finding that 0.2 per cent of the total cases had posterior luxation of the lens, a most serious complication, although known to occur rarely in cases in which the enzyme was not used. The figures Dr. Troutman has given us regarding the presentation of vitreous and the actual loss of vitreous seem high, and they probably are, but we do not know what the percentages would be in an up-to-date comparable control series. Theoretically, at any rate, we should expect a higher percentage of loss of vitreous when the enzyme is used, considering that we are dealing with a dislocated lens.

7. Is the incidence of absent or shallow chambers greater when the enzyme is used? This was a difficult question to answer. Much depends on the technic of the operation, i.e., type of incision, whether multiple sutures were used, and so on. Our figures do show an increase of such cases, especially in the

lower age group. Reports in the literature on the use of alpha-chymotrypsin indicate that the wound healing is not retarded, and catgut sutures do not dissolve. More facts are needed.

8. Barraquer and others have mentioned the occasional case in which edema of the conjunctival flap has occurred. Our studies give us no information on this point. Barraquer believes that this is due to (a) incision too far in the cornea and (b) lack of proper wound closure.

9. It is possible that the round pupil operation has fewer complications than result from complete iridectomy. More study along this line is needed.

10. This report cannot tell us anything of the late effects of the use of alpha-chymotrypsin; the time is too short. A further report on this series a year or so from now should be made. We know from Dr. Maumenee's experimental studies that the retina can be damaged by the enzyme when it is injected into the vitreous. We don't know whether the pars ciliaris retinae is injured under the conditions of cataract surgery by seepage of the enzyme into Petit's canal. If it is, a higher incidence of aphakic retinal detachment might be expected. If it isn't, a lower incidence might occur, because the mechanical pull of the zonular fibers is abolished during the operation.

11. Modifications of our present technic and new instrumentation devised to assist us in the removal of the lens in view of the altered conditions because of zonulolysis will undoubtedly occur.

On the basis of the information obtained from this and a partial survey of the growing literature, your Committee recommends that alpha-chymotrypsin should not be used in the surgery of the lens in the following conditions:

1. Cases in which the patient is under twenty years of age.
2. Cases of endothelial dystrophy.
3. Cases of subluxated lenses.
4. Cases of traumatic cataract, especially when vitreous is presented.

Finally, we beg you to remain conservative in your actions regarding the use of zonulolysis until we know much more about it. . . .

With the passage of time, the initial wave of enthusiasm and the hope that this drug might help cataract surgery in all age groups have proved to be overly optimistic, but new vistas in intraocular surgery have been opened up. There are, of course, problems and obstacles ahead, but it has been said that the "impossible takes just a little longer." Fortunately, to explore that small sphere called the eye, there are pioneers such as Ridley, Meyer-Schwickerath and Barraquer.

1

Preoperative Considerations

PREOPERATIVE EVALUATION OF CATARACT PATIENTS

Many of the rules and the considerations that applied previously in the preoperative evaluation of cataract patients are still applicable today. Primarily, the surgeon must remember that to the patient, at this time, his eye operation is the most important thing in life. Despite the speed of the modern world, it is still very wise for even the busiest ophthalmic surgeon to take the time to talk with and "get the feel of" the patient. This also allows the patient to get to know his surgeon.

Regardless of any progress that we have made in ophthalmology, if the cataract extraction does not help the patient to see better, even though it may have been executed beautifully, the patient will not be happy. And, after all, it is the result that counts. Progress still has not eliminated the problem patient who on the first examination is found to have far-advanced cataracts, making it nearly impossible to evaluate the function of the eyes. When the involvement is bilateral, the problem is doubly serious. When possible, a preoperative prognosis today will help to soften the blow tomorrow.

Unfortunately, when the cataract is mature, most of the tests used to determine the status of the retina are subjective. Light projection is still very useful, but it is seldom that a patient with a macular degeneration cannot pass the color test. Although the accuracy of the electroretinogram in determining retinal status is somewhat limited, its precision is improving, and it can give us some clues about the status of the retina, including the macular area. Examination at the slit lamp is important and may help the surgeon to anticipate some of the problems that may be encountered at surgery. Similarly, when indicated, gonioscopy and outflow studies are useful.

Before surgery, for maximum co-operation on the part of the patient, it is always wise to give the patient a general idea of the steps involved in cataract surgery. At this time, I find it wise to spend time explaining to the patient and a responsible member of his family some of the details of postoperative problems, including at least a brief story on the adjustment to aphakia. Since I have not yet found any completely satisfactory way of explaining the optical problems of lens removal in the patient with a monocular cataract, I try to make comparisons which I can only hope the patient will understand. I try never to operate on these patients at an early stage. Realizing that the patient and his relatives are often too excited or confused by my explanation at the time, in all cataract cases I dictate a letter to the referring physician in their presence, repeating the over-all findings and the prognosis. Occasionally, I find it helpful to read all or parts of this letter to the patient postoperatively if he again

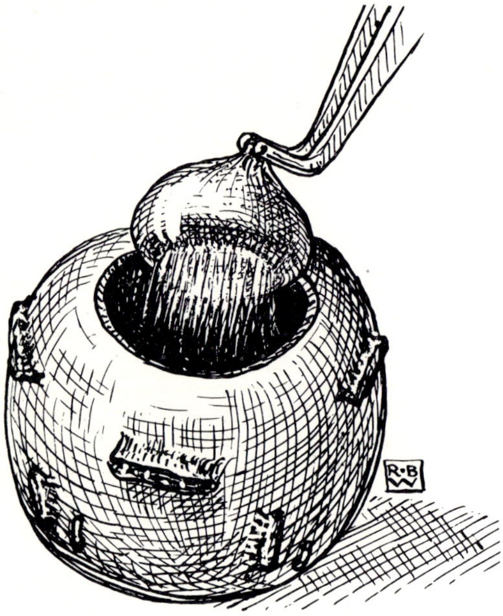

FIG. 1. A drawing of an experimental cataract demonstrating adhesion of the lens to the hyaloid. (Modified from Reese, A. B., and Wadsworth, J. A.: Am. J. Ophthal. *46*:495)

needs an explanation such as that related to the monocular cataract or to senile macular changes. Furthermore, I have some member of my staff repeat this entire explanation at a more leisurely pace. In addition, the patient is given a written explanation of what we have told him that he may read at home.

On the day of admission to the hospital we make a point of seeing the patient and his family briefly in our office, quickly reviewing the problem and sending a note to the hospital. This includes a plan of operation and whether it is to be done under local or general anesthesia, noting carefully any medical problems, especially allergies, and any drugs that the patient is using. Our hospital provides patients with a beautifully illustrated brochure to acquaint them with what to expect in the hospital.

An example of part of the story told to the patient with a monocular cataract is as follows.

Monocular Cataract

You have excellent vision in one eye and a cataract giving you very poor vision in the other eye. This we call the one eye or the monocular cataract problem. Normally, we never operate cases like yours unless the vision in your good eye, with correction, drops to 20/40 or less. That is, when with your glasses, you can see out of your best eye only about to the middle of the eye chart. If we do operate, you will be most unhappy because following the surgery, in order for you to see well, the eye that has been operated on needs a heavy magnifying lens, whereas your good eye requires no lens or your old lens. Therefore, the two eyes will normally not fuse or work together. I like to compare this with the problem of trying to team a small pony with a large work horse—they just don't seem to work together well.

If, however, the lens in the eye with the cataract becomes ripe or overripe, we have no choice but to operate on that eye because many serious problems can set in. I like to compare this situation with a bad or a rotten apple in a basket causing damage to the rest of the good apples in the same basket. In the case of the eye, the lens can swell; the capsule or outer shell of the cataract can rupture, and many serious complications will follow.

After removing a ripe cataract in one eye, you can continue, if you are wearing glasses, to wear your own old glasses or we can fit you with a contact lens in front of the operated eye. With a contact lens, the two eyes can often work together. However, many people cannot learn to wear contact lenses for one reason or another. For those who will not tolerate a contact lens, waiting until the other eye shows a drop in vision is required before a cataract glass is prescribed for the operated eye. This may be a long time or never in your lifetime. At that time, if you use the operated eye, you will be happier to use the cataract glass in front of the operated eye than to see out of the unoperated eye.

Because I know that this is difficult to understand I am giving you a little pamphlet that I have written describing to you some of the things that you should know about cataracts, cataract surgery and getting used to wearing your glasses following surgery. You can read it more leisurely and ask my nurse or my secretary to answer your questions. If they cannot do so, I will be very happy to try to answer them for you.

I know that Dr. Edmund Spaeth disagrees with my views on monocular cataracts and says that *all* monocular cataracts should be removed. In a personal communication, he stated that he felt that

The longer one delays with monocular cataract surgery the more does convergence and the possibility for binocular vision with contact lenses recede. Then when the second cataract must be done there is *no* chance for binocularity—there may even be a constant diplopia. Early monocular cataract surgery with subsequent contact lenses is a *basic* procedure.

LIGAMENTUM HYALOIDEO-CAPSULARE

Ligamentum hyaloideo-capsulare is sometimes referred to as adhesions of the lens capsule to the hyaloid membrane. (Today these are the "fashionable" terms to use in speaking of vitreous loss.)

Up until recently there has been very little in the literature on the part played by adhesions between the anterior hyaloid membrane and the lens capsule (Fig. 1). Wieger first described the normal adhesion of the lens capsule to the hyaloid membrane and gave it the name "ligamentum hyaloideo-capsulare"[5] (Fig. 2). Reese and Wadsworth helped to crystallize much of our thinking in regard to this adhesion. They felt that "this adhesion between the posterior lens capsule and the anterior hyaloid occurs sufficiently in degree and frequency to be reckoned with in performing intracapsular cataract extractions."[5] In the past when the adhesion syndrome had been encountered at the time of cataract extraction, it was frequently misinterpreted as tough zonules. This was further emphasized by the work of the Barraquers on the use of alpha-chymotrypsin. Even though the zonules were broken with alpha-chymotrypsin, very often vitreous would present because of adhesions of the lens capsule to the hyaloid membrane (Fig. 3). These problems were noted especially in children, less frequently in adults.

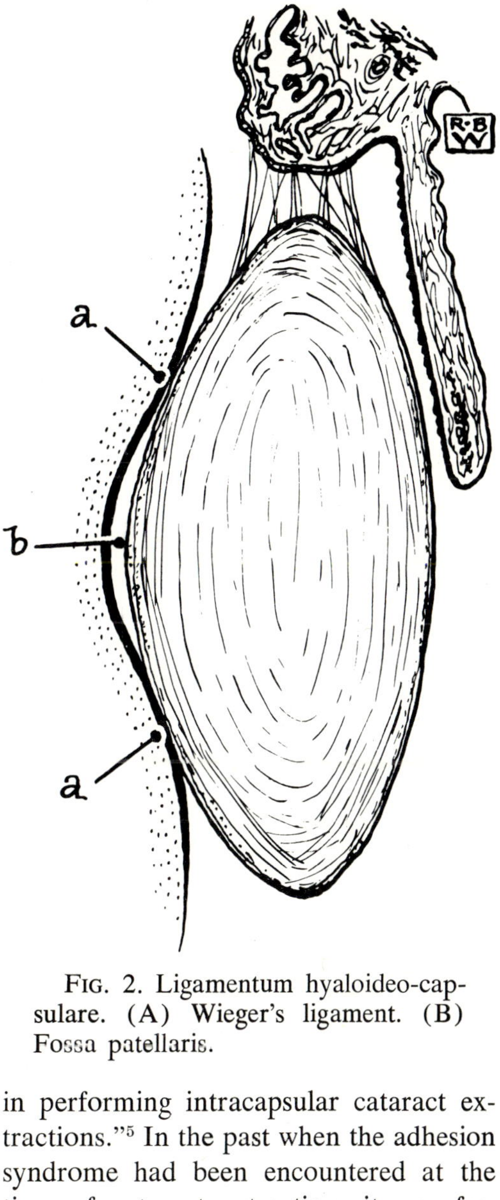

FIG. 2. Ligamentum hyaloideo-capsulare. (A) Wieger's ligament. (B) Fossa patellaris.

There are four main causes of adhesions between the lens capsule and the hyaloid membrane:

1. Capillary attraction in the retrolental fossa (fossa patellaris, Fig. 2, b). There is less attraction in adults (Fig. 4).
2. The ligamentum hyaloideo-capsulare (Fig. 5)
3. Embryonic fibers such as remnants of the hyaloid or the tunica vasculosa lentis (Fig. 6)

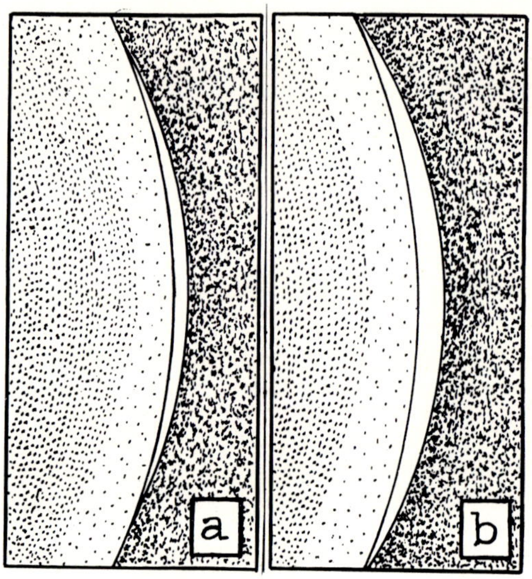

FIG. 4. (A) Retrolental space in an adult. (B) Retrolental space in an elderly person. (Modified from Arruga, H.: Ocular Surgery, Barcelona, Salvat Editores, S. A.)

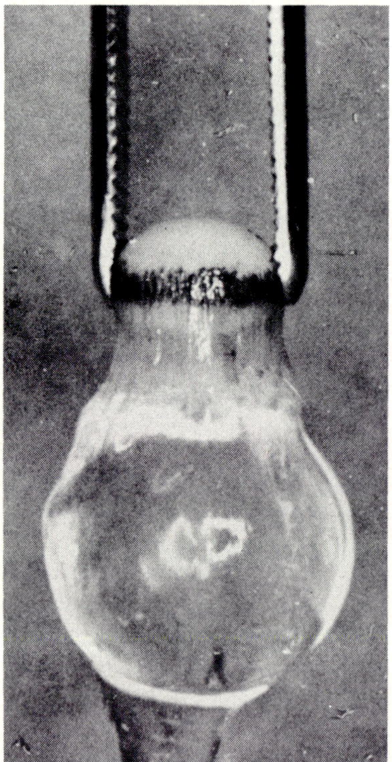

FIG. 3. Adhesion of the hyaloid membrane of the posterior surface of the lens. The external tunics have been removed from a supposedly normal human eye. The intact vitreous body dangles from the lens, which is grasped with forceps. (Dr. A. B. Reese)

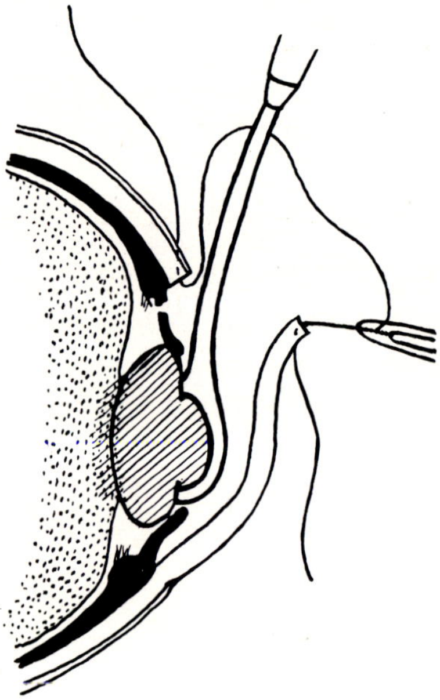

FIG. 5. Schematic representation of adhesion secondary to a ligamentum hyaloideo-capsulare. (Modified from Guillaumat, Louis, *et al.*: Traitement Chirurgical des Affections Oculaires, Paris, France, Gustav Doin)

4. Trauma or inflammation

Clinically, the site of this ligamentum can sometimes be seen as an opaque ring on the vitreous face (Fig. 7). Following trauma and inflammation a pigmented ring sometimes can be noted on the posterior lens capsule.

The diagnosis of these adhesions is based on:

1. The feel of resistance when the zonules are broken and the lens cannot be removed easily. This can be noted especially after alpha-chymotrypsin has broken the zonules.

2. Direct visualization with or without the aid of an operating loupe

Clinically, the results of these adhesions are: (1) the capsule can rupture; (2) vitreous can be lost; or (3) a detachment can follow.

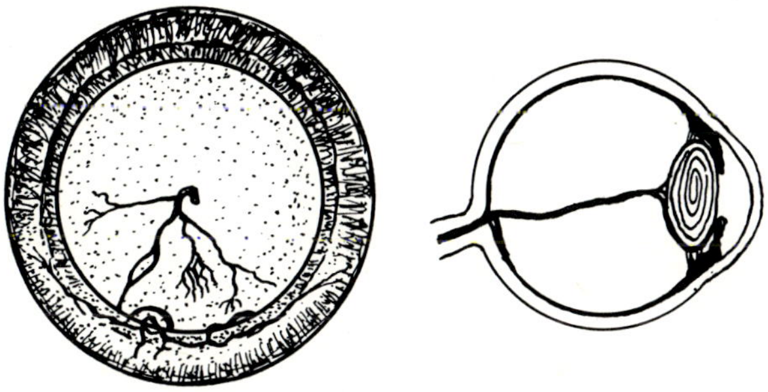

FIG. 6. Persistence of blood vessels of tunica vasculosa lentis. (Modified from Cordes, F. *in* Haik, G. [ed.]: Symposium on Diseases and Surgery of the Lens, St. Louis, Mosby)

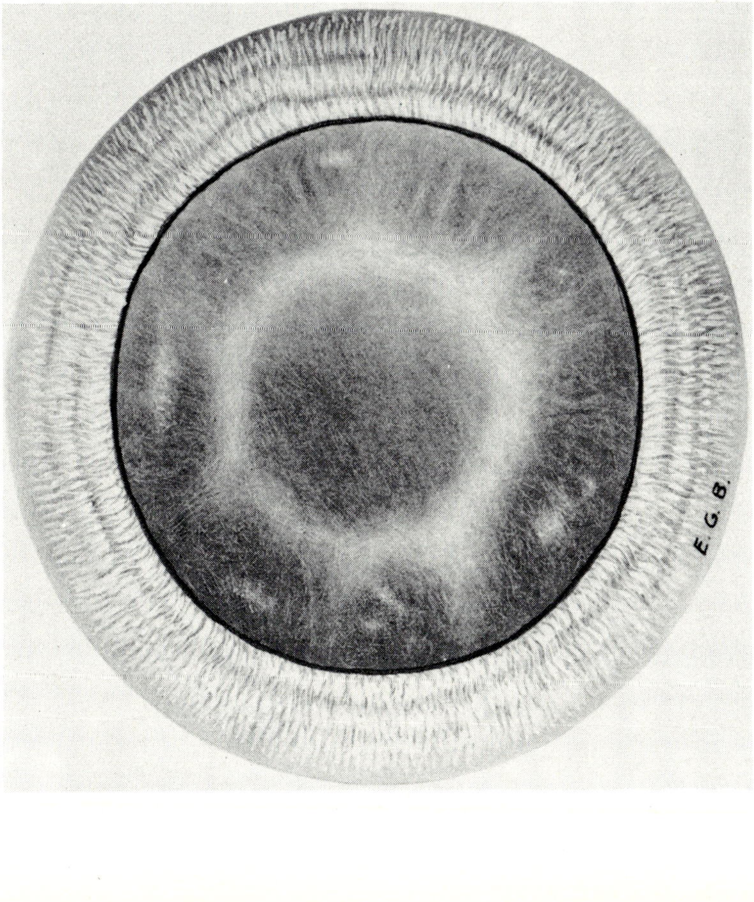

FIG. 7. Clinical appearance of the ligamentum hyaloideo-capsulare. At the time of the extraction of a supposedly uncomplicated cataract, the lens and the hyaloid were so firmly adherent that no separation could be accomplished even though the lens was lifted partly out of the eye. An extracapsular extraction was done, and the ring seen postoperatively (shown above) was interpreted to be the site of the ligament. The lens in the fellow eye behaved similarly and showed a comparable ring after extraction. (Dr. A. B. Reese)

Surgical Treatment

No complete solution has been evolved yet as to what can be done when one is faced with the problem of posterior lenticular adhesions. Perhaps because of the greater area of pull, an erisophake is better than a capsule forceps. However, there are some prominent American eye surgeons who feel that the capsule forceps should be used, especially with the use of alpha-chymotrypsin.

These adhesions cannot always be anticipated preoperatively. Following trauma or inflammation, some surgeons feel that a planned extracapsular is the operation of choice. Others feel that following inflammation a planned intracapsular should be done. If the zonules are broken and one encounters resistance when attempting a planned intracapsular extraction, one can change to an extracapsular extraction.

There has always been a great deal of disagreement as to whether a sliding or a tumbling technic is better. In adhesions of the lens capsule to the hyaloid membrane, the problem is the same. Barraquer has used both technics in these cases but still has problems of vitreous presentation. He favors the erisophake, but, of course, alpha-chymotrypsin has no effect on posterior lenticular adhesions even though it weakens the zonules. For hard or flat lenses, he favors sliding.[1]

Those who advocate a sliding technic present the following arguments:

1. There is a clear view of the problem.
2. One can, in this situation, more easily shift to a more complete extracapsular extraction if the need arises.
3. The edge of the sclera or the iris can be used in shearing off the vitreous adhesions.

Those who advocate a tumbling procedure feel that the cornea can act as a shield pushing the vitreous back. Reese says:

> . . . lesser degrees of the adhesion syndrome can be overcome if the surgeon is patient and does not try to make a precipitous delivery thus allowing time for the peeling away of the capsule from the hyaloid. This separation of the two structures is better accomplished with an erisophake than with forceps because with an erisophake one can completely evert the lens [Fig. 8]. A slow and complete eversion of the lens by rotation of the face of the erisophake in the process of delivery facilitates the peeling away of the two adherent structures. This cannot be accomplished as well with forceps because with forceps the lens cannot be everted sufficiently without making the capsule so taut that it ruptures.[4]

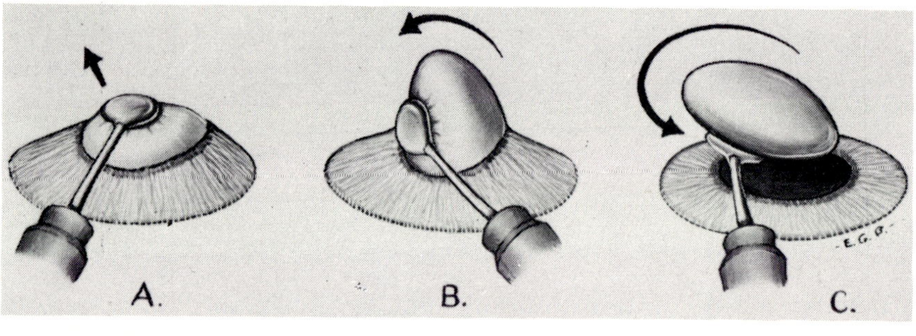

FIG. 8. Complete eversion of the lens with the erisophake. After rupture of the zonules below, the eversion of the lens helps to separate the hyaloid and the lens when there is an adhesion of the two surfaces. (Dr. A. B. Reese)

Sometimes a spoon or a muscle hook through the cornea can be wedged between the hyaloid and the capsule to break these adhesions gently (Fig. 9). However, this does not always occur.

Turning and twisting the lens in a rotary movement with the erisophake as many as 10 or 15 times is one method of breaking these adhesions. Others favor the direct approach using a snare, scissors, a muscle hook or a spatula. In this situation, I do not know a perfect solution at present, but I will use the erisophake in a rotary movement, followed by a tumbling procedure using pressure exerted through the cornea to break these lens-vitreous adhesions.

Summary

The causes of adhesions between the lens capsule and the hyaloid membrane are: (1) capillary attraction; (2) ligamentum hyaloideo-capsulare; (3) embryonic fibers (hyaloid or tunica vasculosis); and (4) trauma or inflammation.

The operator can see the adhesions with or without the aid of an operating loupe. If he cannot see them, sometimes he can feel the resistance when the zonules are broken and the lens cannot be removed easily.

The results of these adhesions are: (1) capsule ruptures; (2) vitreous presentation or loss; and (3) detachments.

The surgical treatment consists of a planned extracapsular extraction. Most American surgeons use the capsule forceps instead of the erisophake. Those in favor of sliding argue that: (1) there is a clear view of the problem; (2) one may shift to an extracapsular extraction more easily if the need arises; and (3) the sclera may be used for shearing.

In tumbling, the cornea may be tucked behind the lens, thereby breaking the adhesions. Another approach is a rotary movement of the lens with the capsule forceps or the erisophake. The last approach is more direct. Some favor using a snare, scissors, a hook or a spatula to break the adhesions.

INFECTIONS

There are no real "modern advances" with regard to infection or the control of infection. I routinely prescribe fresh sodium sulfacetamide drops to be used locally the day before and the day of surgery. When an eye is clinically congested or inflamed, and in all one-eyed patients, bacteriologic studies and antibiotic sensitivities are determined. A negative eye smear is not sufficient. Should the culture prove to be positive, appropriate antibiotics should be given until cultures are negative.

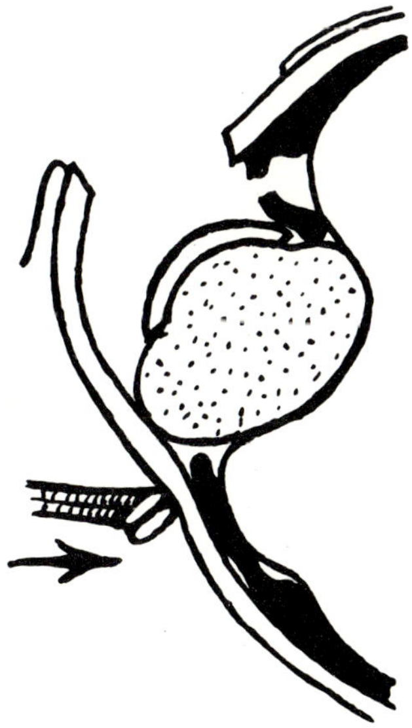

FIG. 9. Breaking of adhesions by pressure through the cornea using the erisophake for tumbling (Modified from Barraquer, Joaquin: An. Inst. Barraquer *2*:63, No. 1)

Preoperative Cultures and Antibiotics

Although I do not routinely take cultures preoperatively or order systemic antibiotics preoperatively or postoperatively, I agree that there may be justification of this procedure in:

(a) one-eyed patients, (b) extensive operative procedures, (c) patients with so-called "weak ocular tissues" (such as high myopia, congenital nystagmus and retinal degeneration), (d) multiple operations, especially if performed within a short period of time, (e) operations on the contralateral eye during a single confinement, (f) subsequent to some extracapsular extraction (since the lens material can favor bacterial growth), (g) patients with serious metabolic disease such as diabetes or serious neoplastic disease, especially if the patient has received potent anticancer drugs or irradiation, (h) elderly or feeble individuals showing suboptimal nutrition and poor general health.[3]

There are surgeons who feel that if cultures are indicated for *any* type of case, they are indicated for *all* intraocular operations.

Some put a great deal of faith in cultures; however, a great deal depends on the way cultures are taken and by whom. Also, it must be remembered that this is not a guarantee against infection. If cultures are done, they should be done at least 1 *week* before surgery—not 1 day. Furthermore, internists point out that the routine use of antibiotics preoperatively helps to establish resistant strains of organisms. Cases of eye infection have followed routine subconjunctival injections of antibiotics given immediately after surgery.

Fungal Infections and Steroids

Since fungal infections are more prevalent with their use, when possible one should avoid steroids. Merthiolate and sodium sulfacetamide are good antifungal drugs and can be used safely for prophylaxis.

Choice of Operation

Since lens cortex is an ideal medium for the growth of organisms, the surgeon must consider this possibility when determining his choice of operation, especially in children. In this respect, discissions in infants and young adults can be followed by severe intraocular infection because of the large amount of lens matter left behind. This type of problem has been reported after Wheeler discissions. In many cases the source of the infection is the patient's own organisms.

Tear Passageways

Tear passageways are irrigated routinely in all my patients at least a few weeks prior to cataract surgery. It is always my policy to correct any defect noted in the nasolacrimal system prior to intraocular surgery. I know of some very fine surgeons who use as their only test the application of pressure over the tear sac to determine whether this area is clean or potentially infected. If there is only a minimal amount of discharge in this area, they are satisfied with cauterizing the tear puncta, using an antibiotic, and then proceeding with the cataract surgery. Under these circumstances I would consider it safer to take cultures and do sensitivity studies before going ahead with the surgery. However, if I have noted a frank discharge from the tear passageways, a dacryocystorhinostomy is done before the cataract surgery. (In the very old patient, I still feel that a dacryocystectomy is justifiable.)

By irrigating the tear passageways preoperatively, besides gaining knowledge of a potential area of infection adjacent to the eye proper, I also learn how the patient will react under local anesthesia during the actual lens extraction. If the patient cannot tolerate irrigation of a normal passageway, he is probably a good candidate for supplemental intravenous anesthesia or even complete general anesthesia.

In the operating room, I still use Post's solution for the sterilization of sharps. I have not used gas sterilization with beta-propiolactone. To date, I have had only two questionable infections in my own cases of intraocular surgery.

Other Prophylactic Considerations

A very high percentage of eye infections come from sources other than the patient's own eye—doctors, nurses, other hospital personnel and even eye medications may be responsible. Among the modern trends that may reduce eye infections in the operating room are newer methods of draping, new masks, more frequent changes of gloves and masks, air conditioners and more careful sterilization. The skin around the eyes and even the lids are covered by drapes. Masks of plastic material are considered safer than those of cloth, but, of course, these should be changed between cases. After prepping the eye, new gloves should be used. Rubber bulbs such as those used on the erisophake and irrigating syringes should be autoclaved with water rather than air inside the bulbs. If the surgeon plans to inject air into the anterior chamber at the time of surgery, it is safer to fill the syringe with air and then to autoclave it. (As yet I have not encountered a need for this last procedure in our operating room.)

The massage of the lids following retrobulbar anesthesia creates more secretions, but bacterial cultures taken before and after massage fortunately have shown no real difference.

Excessive trauma is an important factor in intraocular infection. Infection is seen more frequently following extracapsular extractions than following intracapsular extractions. Today with the use of retrobulbar anesthesia, hyaluronidase and massage, there are softer eyes and a greater temptation to do more manipulation. One should avoid this excessive trauma. It is a wise rule to do as little as possible in cataract surgery.

SURGERY OF BINOCULAR CATARACTS DURING ONE HOSPITAL ADMISSION

After considering the question of infection, this seems to be an appropriate time to question the advisability of operating both cataracts in a patient during one hospital admission. This practice is becoming more popular in this country.

It is well known that this practice is followed in some countries such as India where cataracts are very common and access to an ophthalmic surgeon is most difficult.

In this country the sky-rocketing cost of hospitalization is the chief justification for operating on both cataracts in one hospital admission. Most surgeons do not follow this practice, but, although they are in the minority, there are a few fine surgeons who will operate on both eyes in one admission. A very few will do both eyes during the same trip to the operating room. Most will wait for 2 to 4 days before operating on the second eye. Certainly, if one is going to do a second eye, waiting 4 days is better than waiting 2 days.

For many reasons, some of which are obvious, I personally would not want both of the cataracts operated on myself or on some member of my family. Nor would I want any cataract surgery performed as an office procedure. (This includes needling of a secondary cataract because I have known of cases in which eyes have been lost following this procedure.) This is a rule that I always apply to any anticipated surgery for my patients; it is one which is most rewarding.

Several years ago I had three patients who insisted on having both cataracts operated on the same trip to the operating room. In all three, their reasoning seemed justified by the specific circumstances. One was an elderly lady who said that she lived alone and was financially unable to prolong her hospitalization. (Actually, finances played little or no part in this case.)

The second lady, a nurse's sister, came from a great distance and did not want to make a second trip at a later date.

The third lady pleaded financial problems (in this case there were some); far more importantly, there were multiple medical problems. Among these problems was a history of repeated episodes of drug addiction necessitating prolonged periods for cure.

At first, I told each of these patients that I absolutely would not operate both cataracts on one admission, stressing the fear of possible infection in both eyes as my main reason. After much give and take, I compromised and said that I would wait 2 days before doing the second eye in each patient.

The first lady, who claimed finances as her chief reason for wanting both eyes operated, had most uneventful intracapsular cataract extractions and an uneventful hospital stay. However, her convalescence at home was not so easy. Three weeks after surgery, because of poor adjustment to her trial aphakic correction, she fell down the steps of her home, broke both wrists and seriously damaged one eye.

The second lady, the nurse's sister, looked fine 2 days after intracapsular extractions but on the 3rd day (now 1 day after extraction of the second cataract) she developed a film over the vitreous face of the first eye. The most probable cause was infection related to the flare-up of a sinus condition on the same side. Hospitalization was greatly prolonged because of the need for massive doses of antibiotics. Fortunately, 1 year later, after an opening was made over the vitreous face and drugs were given for a secondary glaucoma that had set in, her vision was 20/40 with correction in this eye. It is indeed fortunate that the same problems did not affect the second eye (20/20 with correction). Had I waited 4 days rather than 2 before surgery on the second eye, perhaps the clinical signs of trouble in the first eye would have become more manifest.

(Recently my feelings regarding the possibility of infection when the second eye is operated on during the same admission, even with an interval of a week between operations, have been confirmed by others who report that the frequency of infection is many times greater when both eyes are operated on during the same hospital admission.[2])

The third lady, who had so many medical problems, including drug addiction, did splendidly until the 3rd day following surgery on the second eye. At this time she became disoriented and developed bleeding into both anterior chambers. Fortunately this cleared rapidly, but, although she finally developed 20/20 vision in both eyes 3 months postoperatively, the period of anxiety was most trying for all concerned.

In summary, I do not recommend cataract surgery on both eyes during the same hospital admission. If it must be done, waiting a period of 4 days between the first and the second eye is the minimal interval that I would advise.

REFERENCES

1. Barraquer, Joaquin: Personal communication.
2. Givner, Isadore: Symposium; complications of cataract surgery, Lecture before New York Eye and Ear Infirmary Alumni Association, April 11, 1962.
3. Leopold, I. H., and Apt, L.: Postoperative intraocular infections, Am. J. Ophthal. *50*:1225, 1960.
4. Reese, A. B.: An appraisal of the current trend in cataract surgery, Montgomery Lecture, Ireland, 1962.
5. Reese, A. B., and Wadsworth, J. A.: The adhesions of the lens capsule to the hyaloid membrane and its relation to the intracapsular extraction, Am. J. Ophthal. *46*:495, 1958.

2

Operative Considerations

ANESTHESIA

The tendency to use tranquilizers in conjunction with other preoperative anesthetics is increasing, and more favorable reports are appearing in the literature. Reduction in postoperative nausea and vomiting has been attributed to the use of these tranquilizers. Normally I use meperidine hydrochloride (Demerol) and the barbiturates in adult patients. Previously, I used chloral hydrate in patients over the age of 50, since it was felt that this drug was tolerated better by older patients. However, nausea and vomiting seemed to occur more frequently, possibly because of the gastric irritation on an empty stomach even though a capsule is used to avoid the sometimes unpleasant taste. Therefore, I reverted to the use of Seconal and Nembutal and now note less vomiting. However, with the barbiturates, there may be a slight increase of confusion in the senile patient. The use of chloral hydrate suppositories is a suggested alternative that I have not used as yet.[27] I no longer use promethazine (Phenergan) either intramuscularly or intravenously; on several occasions when it was used, an alarming drop of blood pressure was noted at the time of surgery. During the procedure our local anesthesia is often supplemented with meperidine hydrochloride (Demerol) and intravenous Seconal or Nembutal given slowly by the anesthetist. Oxygen given under the drape has been most helpful. Recently it has been stressed that the administration of oxygen, not a barbiturate, is a rational therapy for a systemic toxic reaction from a local anesthetic.[27] Some investigators feel that succinylcholine should be used as a relaxant in this situation.[30] Our Anesthesia Department still favors a barbiturate and oxygen. For intraocular surgery, I, too, would favor the barbiturates and oxygen.

As for the reduction of postoperative nausea and vomiting by the use of specific antiemetics and tranquilizers, it should be asked, "What part do the somnifacient qualities of this or that drug play?"

It is noted in the operating room that patients who have exhibited nausea and even vomiting can be controlled well after a supplemental intravenous barbiturate and/or oxygen. When these drugs are given adequately, the patient should be calm and relaxed.

General Anesthesia

Barraquer points out that general anesthesia has become more popular for ocular surgery, especially because of the introduction of endotracheal intubation which provides an airway without impeding the operative field. He feels that with modern preoperative medications and complete excellent control of the patient there is an elimination of sudden variations of intraocular pressure which may occur with local anesthesia.[7] I was most impressed with the perfect anesthesia that I saw in his clinic. Although I rarely use a complete general anesthesia for cataract surgery in adults, I feel more secure if I add a complete local block.

Local Anesthesia

At present I favor 2 per cent Xylocaine, usually without Adrenalin but supplemented by hyaluronidase. I always include a retrobulbar injection and do not use the blunt needle recommended by Atkinson for this injection.[4] Retrobulbar anesthesia in children is felt to increase the intraocular pressure by increasing the orbital volume.[9]

Dr. Reese and Dr. Ira Jones point out that they

have not used any form of retrobulbar injection for two years in the belief that such injections do not help in reducing the vitreous pressure. On the contrary, they more often than is realized promote vitreous pressure by producing hematomas of the extraocular muscles. Such a hematoma, and thus vitreous pressure, is appreciated by the fact that the iris tends to override the scissors or the blade of the knife at the time of the section, the iris tends to prolapse after the section, or the wound edges tend to gape somewhat or do not lie in apposition. In such instances, very slight exophthalmos may be present but undetected unless looked for. Also, in the postoperative course slight ecchymosis under the conjunctiva or the skin of the lid may be additional evidence. We find that a subconjunctival injection of cocaine at four places around the limbus and a van Lint, O'Brien or Atkinson lid injection are adequate. In the two years' regimen of no retrobulbar injection, we have encountered less vitreous pressure than previously, as evidenced by either a flat or concave vitreous face during surgery, and also by the fact that to the best of our knowledge, no vitreous has been pushed out of the eye during the operation.[26]

A recent questionnaire in regard to preferences concerning anesthesia in adult intraocular surgery indicates that while the trend in England seems to be toward more general anesthesia, this is probably not so in the United States. Xylocaine 2 per cent is still the local anesthesia of choice. Most combine this with hyaluronidase. Curare is used routinely by a small percentage of those surveyed, and one quarter of the group use it in combination with local anesthesia. Thus it appears that while many men use a technic that is just a little different, most seem to get the same end-results.[18]

Just as good eye surgery requires a good eye surgeon, good anesthesia depends on a good anesthetist. With good anesthesia anxiety is lessened or alleviated and, as Dr. Atkinson stated, "There is more trouble with too much sedation than too little."[5]

Ophthalmologists who work in a general hospital often are not as fortunate in terms of anesthesia for their patients as are ophthalmologists in a specialty hospital. As a rule, in a general hospital the anesthetists fear or avoid especially those cases involving intraocular surgery.

One of the very fine papers presented at the Wills Conference in February, 1961, was given by Dr. Samuel Blank, Chief of Anesthesia at the Wills Eye Hospital for more than 15 years. During this period, Dr. Blank has given many lectures on this subject, including a yearly course at the annual meeting of the American Academy of Ophthalmology and Otolaryngology. His lecture on "Anesthetic Aids for Local Anesthesia" is reprinted here (with minor modifications) with his permission.

Anesthetic Aids for Local Anesthesia

In the past 15 years at Wills Eye Hospital, general anesthesia has become increasingly popular in ophthalmic procedures. The percentage has risen from approximately 20 per cent to almost 50 per cent. This increase has been due not only to advances in the field of general anesthesia, but also to the increased complexity of ophthalmic surgical procedures. Consequently, even though local anesthesia is still employed in over half of all eye operations, there has been an increasing demand for some supplementary sedation and tranquilization of the patient during the local procedure to simulate a state closely akin to general anesthesia.

The material to be presented is a brief review of our various experiences with technics and combinations of drugs used at Wills over the past decade.

Premedication for Local Anesthesia. The following drugs are used for premedication:

A. Barbiturates—most effective
   1. Pentobarbital (Nembutal)—100 mg. 2 and 1 hours orally preoperatively
   2. Secobarbital (Seconal)—100 mg. 2 and 1 hours orally preoperatively
   3. Phenobarbital—desirable for older age group, producing less agitation than do the shorter acting barbiturates; 60 to 120 mg. 6 and 2 hours preoperatively intramuscularly

B. Anticholinergics—atropine preferable, 0.4 mg. by hypodermic 45 minutes preoperatively. Scopolamine may cause agitation.

C. Opiates—morphine is best if tolerated. Test dose the day before surgery is valuable. Demerol may cause hypotension in sensitive patients.

We have been through the gamut of preoperative tranquilizers dating back to Thorazine, and gradually the use of these agents has diminished until at present we rely primarily on supplementing premedication with heavier sedation intravenously immediately prior to or during the procedure as required.

The dosages suggested are not hard and fast and must be modified according to the size, the age and the general physical state of the patient. Opiates are not really necessary prior to local anesthesia, and if any question exists regarding sensitivity, they should be omitted. Other agents may be used in specific cases. One in particular deserves mention—"the alcoholic." In this instance alcohol should be given by mouth preoperatively, or an intravenous infusion of 5 per cent alcohol should be started and continued during the procedure.

Supplemental Agents. The drugs and agents that have been and are still being used here at Wills to supplement local anesthesia during surgery include the following:

A. Barbiturates intravenously
   1. Seconal Sodium—50 to 100 mg.

B. Opiates intravenously
   1. Morphine—8 mg.; may repeat in robust patient
   2. Demerol—50 mg. (or less); hypotension may occur

C. Tranquilizers intravenously
   1. Phenothiazine derivatives
      a. Vesprin—5 to 12 mg. I.V.
      b. Phenergan—25 mg. I.V.
      c. Largon—10 to 20 mg. I.V.
   2. Vistaril—25 to 50 mg. I.V.

D. Inhalation agents with oxygen for analgesia
   1. Nitrous oxide
   2. Trilene

It would be possible to add to the list an equal number of effective agents, but no one drug to date has been the complete answer. We have given a generous trial to many, and right now one drug seems to be giving us the most help immediately at the operating table—Largon. Again it is not 100 per cent effective by itself and requires certain combinations as will be pointed out.

The advantages of Largon include the following:

1. Its action is almost immediate when it is given intravenously.

2. Confusion and agitation are minimal in the aged.

3. Respiratory depression is minimal.

4. Hypotension has been negligible to date.

5. It is relatively short acting (approximately 1 hour when given intravenously).

The disadvantages of the drug are similar to those of other phenothiazine derivatives, namely, occasional excessive depression due to potentiation of previously administered barbiturates and opiates, occasional confusion and excitation because of oversedation, and prolonged respiratory and circulatory depression postoperatively. Advice on combating these untoward reactions will be presented later.

Typical combinations of drugs as used at present at Wills are listed below. The drugs may be given consecutively through the same venipuncture but are not mixed in the same syringe.

1. Largon—20 mg. + Seconal Sodium 75 mg. I.V.

   May repeat in one hour.

   Do not give if patient is confused.

2. Largon—10 mg. +
   Seconal Sodium—50 mg. +
   Morphine Sulfate—8 mg.

   Combination is given intravenously, each drug being given separately.

   Repeat any or all in 1 hour for longer procedures. Oxygen should be supplemented. Caution is necessary with Largon, since, like most tranquilizers, it potentiates the action of barbiturates and opiates.

Side-reactions may occur with the above combinations or with any of the drugs listed previously.

Management of Side-Reactions. Some of the problems encountered and their management in general are as follows:

A. Respiratory depression
   1. Oxygen—with assistance if necessary.
   2. Opiate antagonist
      a. Lorfan Tartrate—1 mg. I.V.
      b. Nalline—5 to 10 mg. I.V.
   3. Barbiturate antagonist
      a. Ritalin—10 to 30 mg. I.V.

B. Circulatory depression
   1. "Vagal" reaction—hypotension, bradycardia
      a. Treatment—Atropine I.V. 0.2 to 0.4 mg.
      Vasopressor drugs
   2. Hypotension
      a. Intravenous fluids
      b. Vasopressor drugs—Wyamine, Vasoxyl, Levophed, etc.

An understanding of the reactions and the state of the patient under local anesthesia must be realized. For instance, a heavily sedated patient may become confused and agitated. An increase of more sedation will only make matters worse and seriously endanger the procedure and the patient. Oxygen in this case may help. Also, oversedation will cause hypoxia, and the resultant restlessness may be interpreted as insufficient sedation. The surgeon may call for more, and if it is given, the situation will worsen. The point to be made is that additional sedation should only be administered to a patient who is fully aware of his surroundings and is suffering from apprehension. Pain under local anesthesia is due to inadequate blocking, but sensitivity to pressure and discomfort can be controlled with opiates and combinations of drugs as outlined previously.

Not all confusion and excitation reactions are due to oversedation. One must always be on the lookout for adverse or toxic reactions to the local or the topical anesthetic agents.

Toxic Reactions to Local and Topical Anesthetic Drugs. Various types of local reactions encountered and some methods of their management are as follows.

Central Nervous System Stimulation

A. *Symptoms*
   1. Mild—talkative, dizzy, flushed, rapid pulse
   2. Moderate—restless, headache, nausea and vomiting, muscular twitching, blood pressure elevation
   3. Severe—all preceding signs, followed by convulsions, asphyxia and death

B. *Treatment*
   1. Thiopental sodium or secobarbital sodium I.V.
   2. Curare drugs intravenously
   3. Oxygen, endotracheal airway with artificial respiration

Central Nervous System Depression

A. *Signs and Symptoms*
   1. Drowsiness, analgesia, loss of consciousness
   2. Muscular relaxation and flaccidity
   3. Skin pale and moist
   4. Fall in blood pressure with weak, thready pulse
   5. Shallow respiration
   6. Death due to persistent hypotension and respiratory failure

B. *Treatment*
   1. Oxygen, airway with artificial respiration
   2. Intravenous fluids
   3. Vasopressor drugs intravenously—ephedrine, methedrine, Levophed

Peripheral Cardiovascular Collapse

A. Collapse due to direct action on heart or vascular bed—vasodilatation

B. Procaine may produce bradycardia and cardiac standstill or arrest.

C. Cocaine may produce ventricular tachycardia and ventricular fibrillation.

D. *Treatment*
   1. Artificial respiration with oxygen
   2. Intravenous fluids. Steroids
   3. Vasopressor drugs—Vasoxyl, Neo-Synephrine, Levophed.
   4. Cardiac massage if cardiac arrest occurs

In conclusion, all of the agents and the drugs mentioned are potent drugs, especially when used intravenously. A complete understanding of what they can do for or against your patient is necessary; above all, the surgeon and the anesthetist should be well versed in the recognition and the management of any adverse reaction.

CARDIAC ARREST: MANAGEMENT

Because general anesthesia is necessary for cataract surgery in children and occasionally in adults and since I, personally, have seen two cases of cardiac arrest, I feel that it is appropriate to add a description of the modern approach to this cause of sudden death that is often associated with anesthesia and surgery.

In the two cases I observed (in one of which I was assisting) open cardiac massage preserved life. On another occasion one of my former residents had to perform open cardiac massage himself during the sudden and unexpected cessation of circulation during surgery. A relatively simple eye procedure on a child under general anesthesia performed by a colleague ended tragically in the death of the patient. Still another close friend and colleague of mine was sued for not initiating the appropriate steps to combat cardiac arrest. Thus it is seen that the need for knowledge of the treatment of cardiac arrest is *real* and not just theoretic.

Cardiac arrest may occur as a primary cardiac collapse or secondary to failure of pulmonary ventilating function. While the final treatment of each case may vary, the immediate aim is prompt restoration and maintenance of the oxygenation system by artificial ventilation and artificial circulation.

The major requirement in cardiac resuscitation is rapid diagnosis followed by immediate reinstitution of the oxygenation system by artificial means. Only 3 to 5 minutes are available before irreversible brain damage occurs. Included in this brain damage is cortical blindness which has been reported to follow cardiac arrest in children.[39] Procrastination for absolute proof of the diagnosis is dangerous. Previously, the need for open cardiac massage added to this delay. Today there is no need for 100 per cent proof that arrest is present. With the use of external cardiac massage, delay is unnecessary.

Diagnosis

The diagnosis can be made by the *absence* of: (1) major pulses, (2) precordial heart beat, (3) pupil constriction, and (4) respirations.

Treatment

The initial steps in resuscitation from cardiac arrest are: (1) artificial pulmonary ventilation, and (2) artificial circulation.

Satisfactory ventilation of the lungs can be provided by the technic of mouth-to-mouth or mouth-to-nose breathing. Circulation of unoxygenated blood does not protect the central nervous system or oxygenate the myocardium. When an anesthetist is available and after the body has been oxygenated by this simple method of mouth-to-mouth breathing, tracheal intubation may be performed and oxygen administered by intermittent positive pressure through an endotracheal tube or a mask at a rate of 14 to 16 times per minute.

External Cardiac Massage

Simultaneously the surgeon must provide artificial circulation by closed-chest massage 60 to 80 times per minute until a carotid or a radial pulse is detected (Fig. 10, *left*).

Technic. In treating adults, the heel of the surgeon's transversely placed lower hand alone must touch the lower sternum (Fig. 10, *right*). Pressure of a second hand on top of this first hand must force the sternum inward 1½ to 2 inches. For older children, use of the heel of one hand is sufficient, and for infants only slight pressure on the lower sternum with one or two fingers is necessary.

Evidence of Effective Cardiac Massage. Treatment should continue until the patient's color improves and his pupils become constricted. When resuscitation is stopped for a few minutes, the pupils will often dilate. When the treatment is successful, a pulse in the carotid, the brachial or the femoral arteries is noted. Blood pressure should be in the range of 90 to 150 mm. Hg systolic. When the central nervous system is protected, as evidenced by these signs, then time is available to pursue other steps at a more leisurely pace. By this time the ophthalmologist should have the help of a team that is accustomed to dealing with this specific emergency.

Drug therapy, electrocardiograms, defibrillation if necessary, continued cardiovascular and pulmonary support or post-resuscitation therapy can follow.

Ancillary equipment such as a cardiac pacemaker and mechanical devices to replace the human hand in external cardiac massage are not likely to be the primary approach and are beyond the scope of this discussion.[17, 25]

DIGITAL MASSAGE

The optimal time for the application of digital pressure is 5 minutes[20]; some recommend 10 minutes. I no longer rely on tactile pressure to estimate intraocular pressure before proceeding with the actual surgery but use the tonometer at the end of 5 minutes in almost every case. Massage may be continued if the pressure is not low enough. Dr. Arruga has substituted a plastic bottle containing lead weights to secure a more uniform type of pressure. This is used instead of tactile pressure.[2] He points out that the ophthalmodynamometer also may be used to secure a more uniform type of pressure.

Ocular Hypotensive Agents

In addition to digital massage, ocular hypotony can be secured by acetazolamide (Diamox) or Diamox-like drugs and hypertonic urea. These drugs are especially useful where loss of vitreous is anticipated (urea, in particular, in children), "bull-necked" adults, patients with high myopia and cases with dislocated lenses or malignant glaucoma where lens extraction is indicated.[7]

Acetazolamide (Diamox) must be started several days prior to intraocular surgery if it is to be effective in lowering pressure in eyes that show no ocular hypertension.

Timing is important in the use of intravenous urea. The opening in the eye for cataract surgery must be made ½ hour after starting the urea; otherwise the ocular hypotension may cause difficulty in making a keratome incision[23] (see Incisions and Closures, p. 30, Glaucoma and Cataracts, p. 130).

LID RETRACTION

It is well known that the speculum can exert pressure on the globe. However, few realize that the same type of pressure can

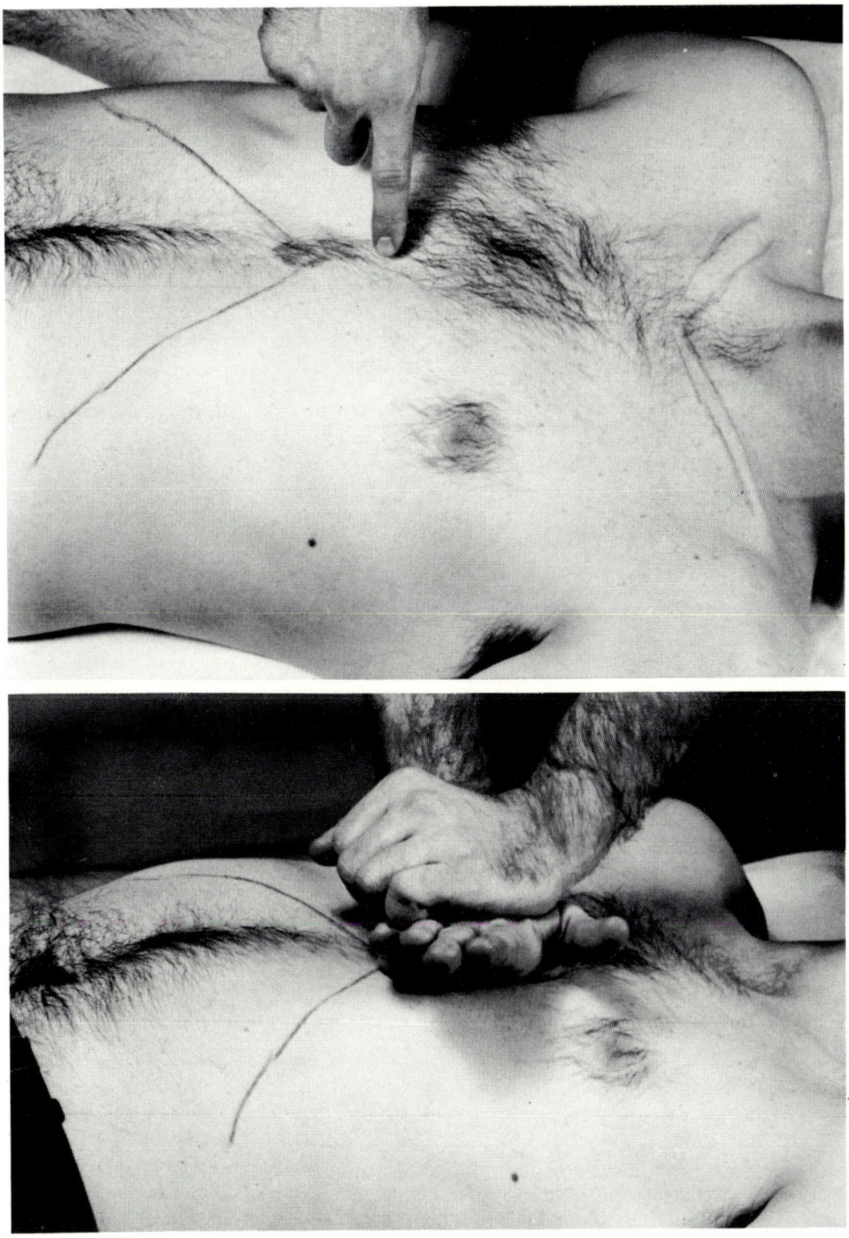

FIG. 10. (*Top*) Exact point of application of pressure for external cardiac massage if complications are to be avoided. Costal margins, clavicles, suprasternal notch and xiphoid are outlined. (*Bottom*) Method of applying external cardiac massage. Costal margins are outlined. Note that the heel of the transversely placed lower hand alone touches the lower sternum. Pressure must force the sternum inward 1½ to 2 inches. (Jude, J. R., Kouwenhoven, W. B., Ing, and Knickerbocker, G. G.: J.A.M.A. *178*:1063)

be exerted by lid clamps. I routinely use lid clamps of the Castroviejo type (Fig. 11, *left*) and have noted, especially in those eyes on which a canthotomy has not been performed, that by pulling on a certain one of the sutures holding on the lid clamp, the pressure can be increased prior to opening the eye. Therefore, I will perform a canthotomy or release the pressure on the lid clamp and the suture which caused the pressure to rise prior to opening the eye. Occasionally even with the canthotomy it is noted with the tonometer that the pressure is still high. In this case massage will be continued until the pressure as recorded on the tonometer drops to within normal limits.

Rather than a canthotomy, some use a lid clamp of the Castroviejo type on the lateral canthus. In a recent correspondence, Dr. Edmund Spaeth stated that he felt that

> With facial nerve block and retrobulbar anesthesia the lid clamps are quite unnecessary—in fact unwise. Use a good blepharostat. Canthotomy is unnecessary with adequate anesthesia. I have not done it in over 1000 cataract extractions.

A new, small light-weight blepharostat exerting little or no pressure on the globe has been designed by José Barraquer[7] (Fig. 11, *right*).

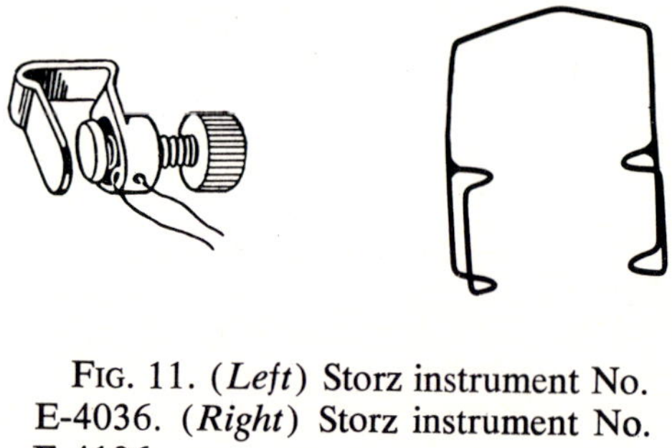

FIG. 11. (*Left*) Storz instrument No. E-4036. (*Right*) Storz instrument No. E-4106.

FLIERINGA-BONACCOLTO RING

It is now felt that ideally the Flieringa-Bonaccolto ring should be used routinely in all cataract surgery (Fig. 12). However, since vitreous is lost less frequently now and since it takes additional time to use the ring, it should be reserved for those cases in which one expects to lose vitreous. The ring is used ideally in patients with high myopia or where liquid vitreous is anticipated, also in protruding eyes and in persons who have a short "bull-neck." However, from a practical standpoint one should learn to use this ring on normal eyes.

As it is usually described, the ring is too small and is placed too far anteriorly. To prove this I have tested the intraocular pressure with an ordinary sized ring in place and by traction on the sutures before the eye is opened at surgery. Traction under these conditions elevates the intraocular pressure. Therefore, if the ring is used, it should be large and placed at the equator (Figs. 13 & 14). New methods of scleral support are being sought.[16] (See Congenital Cataracts, p. 115.)

Finally, since some 50 per cent of adult eyes contain liquid vitreous, it is difficult to say which eyes will need the ring.

From a practical standpoint it is easiest to anchor the ring through or under the 4 rectus muscles at the equator. Of course, one must avoid perforating the globe and causing a detachment. Bleeding from the muscles is possible but less serious.

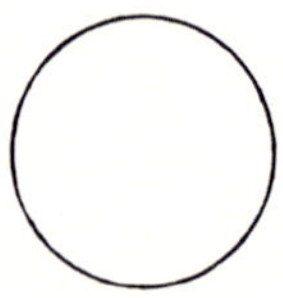

FIG. 12. Storz instrument No. E-4034.

FIG. 13. Flieringa-Bonaccolto ring in place. (Paton, R. T. *in* Fasanella, R. M. [ed.]: Management of Complications in Eye Surgery, Philadelphia, Saunders)

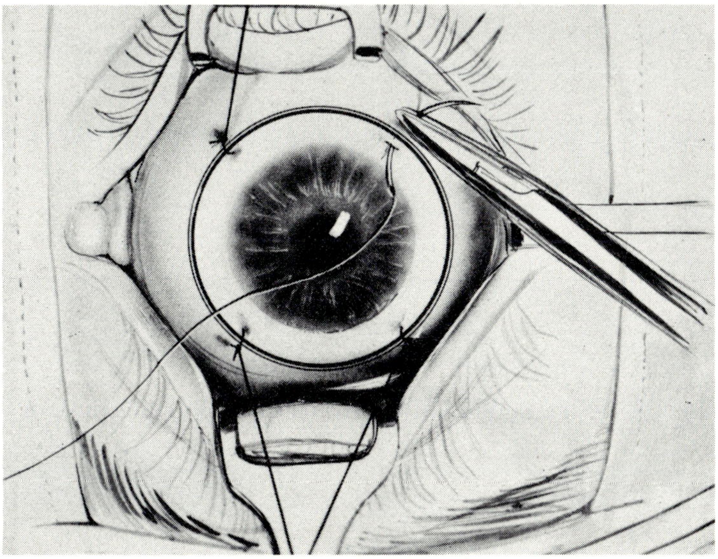

Ideally, the support of the ring would come from bites in the sclera at the level of the equator. Ordinarily the weight of 4 Kelley clamps to hold the sutures tied to the ring frees the hands of the assistant and the surgeon. If vitreous loss threatens or occurs, gentle traction by the operating team is indicated.

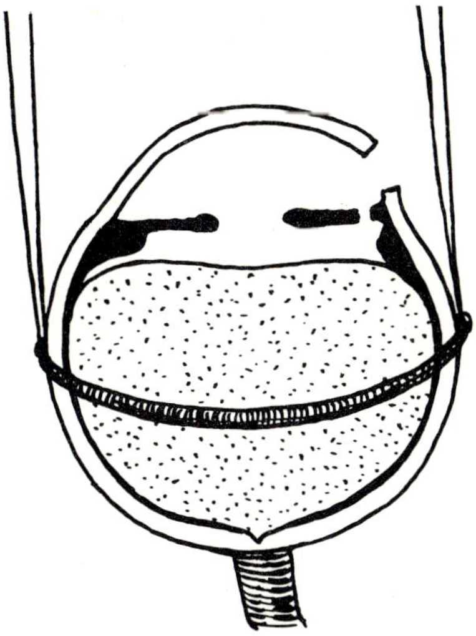

FIG. 14. Flieringa-Bonaccolto ring at the equator. (Modified from Barraquer, Joaquin: An. Inst. Barraquer *2*:63, No. 1, 1961)

INCISIONS AND CLOSURES

In 1959 an excellent report appeared which reviewed the history of incision and closure on 1,000 patients over a period of

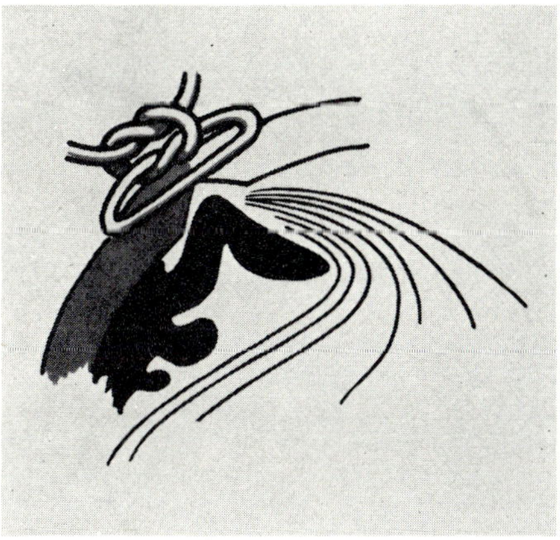

FIG. 15. Posterior gaping of the incision can be produced by a long superficial bite with a suture that is tied too tightly. Result: Incarceration of the iris or the vitreous, leading to persistent striate keratopathy, late fistulization or cystoid scar and vitreous traction bands. (Roper, K. L.: The Cataract Operation: A Study of Details, Am. Acad. Ophth. & Oto-laryng., 1961)

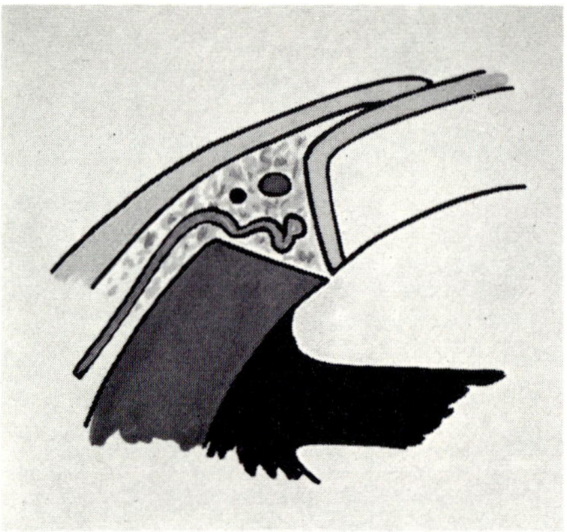

FIG. 16. Anterior gaping can result from inadequate bites or tying too loosely. This may result in lack of formation of the anterior chamber and minor ruptures of the wound with hyphema between the 4th and the 8th postoperative days. (Roper, K. L.: The Cataract Operation: A Study of Details, Am. Acad. Ophth. & Oto-laryng., 1961)

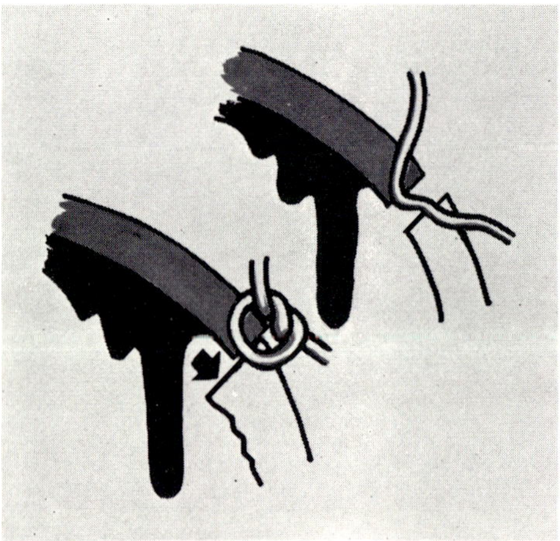

FIG. 17. Too shallow a corneal bite can lead to corneal edema or striate keratopathy when the aqueous enters the cut end of the stroma. Such persistent edema might lead to postoperative corneal dystrophy. (Roper, K. L.: The Cataract Operation: A Study of Details, Am. Acad. Ophth. & Oto-laryng., 1961)

5 years. In this group no hyphema of a degree sufficient to interfere with the outcome of the operation had occurred, no iris prolapse was encountered, and the

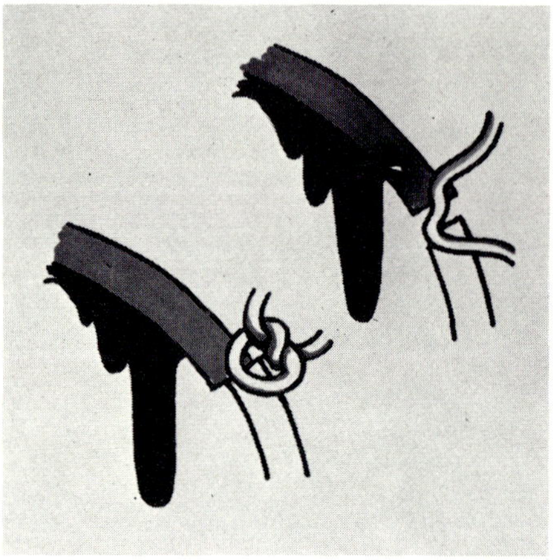

FIG. 18. Too shallow a scleral bite may predispose to a scleral ingrowth. (Roper, K. L.: The Cataract Operation: A Study of Details, Am. Acad. Ophth. & Oto-laryng., 1961)

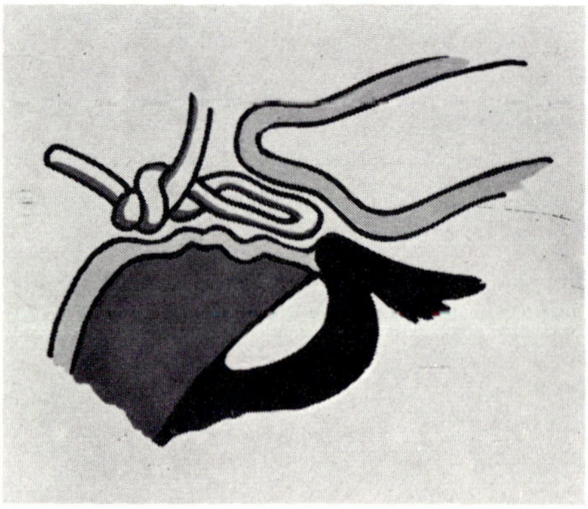

FIG. 19. Normal healing may be inhibited by the inclusion of extraneous material between the cut edges of the corneoscleral incision. Here iris is caught in the wound, resulting in an updrawn, eccentric pupil and making epithelial ingrowth a possibility. (Roper, K. L.: The Cataract Operation: A Study of Details, Am. Acad. Ophth. & Oto-laryng., 1961)

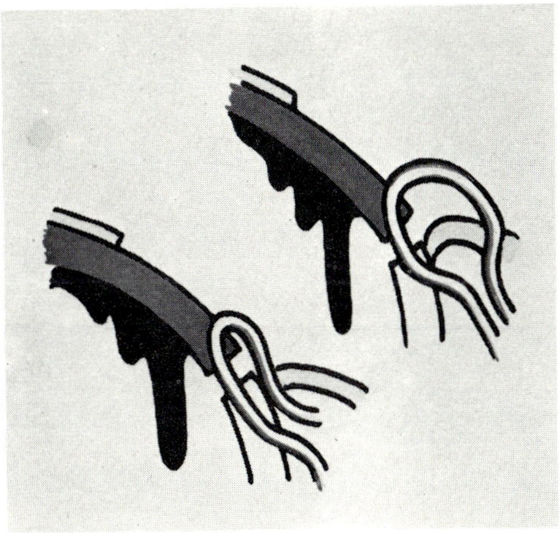

FIG. 20. The lower sketch shows the suture correctly placed through the base of the flap, while in the upper the suture is placed too far from the base. (Roper, K. L.: The Cataract Operation: A Study of Details, Am. Acad. Ophth. & Oto-laryng., 1961)

astigmatic error was minimal.[29] Some of the methods of incision and closure have become very complicated. It has been said that the ideal wound closure should: (1) provide firm approximation; (2) be preplaced; (3) furnish good apposition with sutures passing through the cut edges; (4) provide a good conjunctival flap to cover the incision; and (5) not be too complicated.[24] Roper has pointed out some of the problems related to wound healing. These are illustrated in Figures 15 to 22. Figure 23 shows the original type of McLean suture.

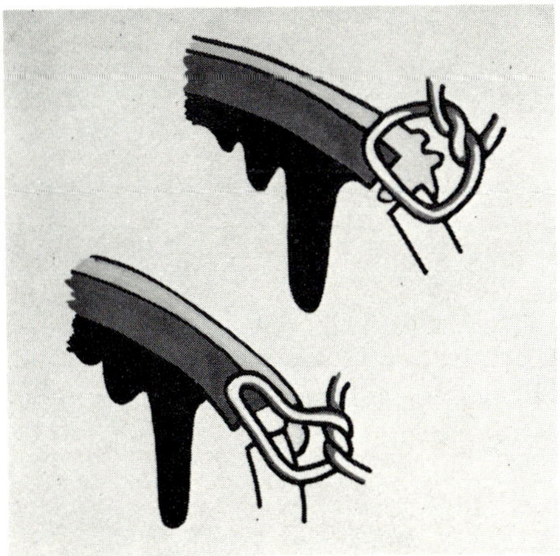

FIG. 21. Shows the sutures tied in the two instances shown in Figure 20. (Roper, K. L.: The Cataract Operation: A Study of Details, Am. Acad. Ophth. & Oto-laryng., 1961)

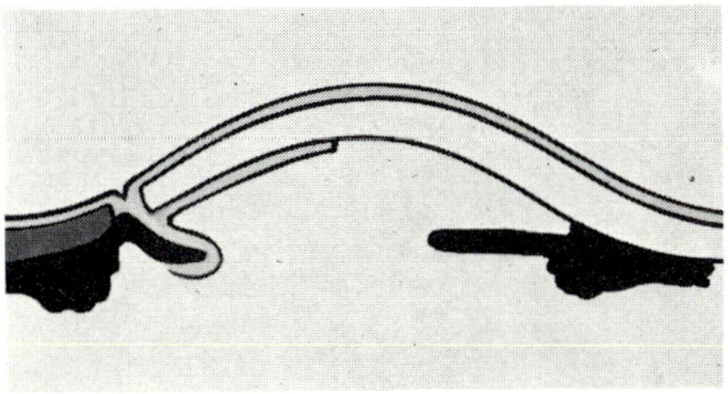

FIG. 22. When sutures are placed too deeply, sloughing, incarceration of the iris leading to a fistulous tract, epithelial ingrowth, etc., often result. (Roper, K. L.: The Cataract Operation: A Study of Details, Am. Acad. Ophth. & Oto-laryng., 1961)

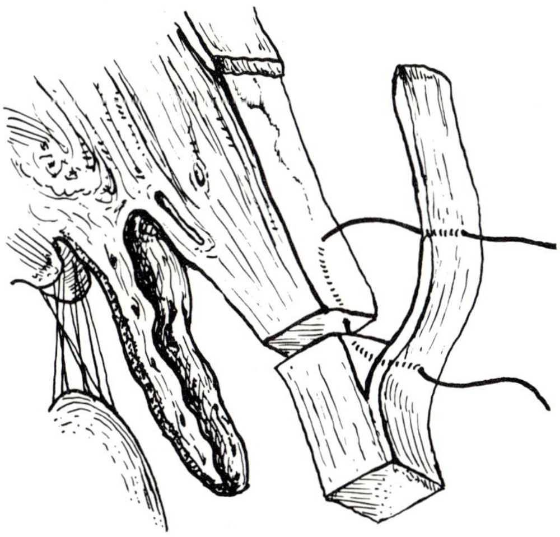

FIG. 23. Perpendicular incision covered by corneal flap with McLean type of suture in position. (Modified from Scheie, H. G.: A.M.A. Arch. Ophth. *61*:431)

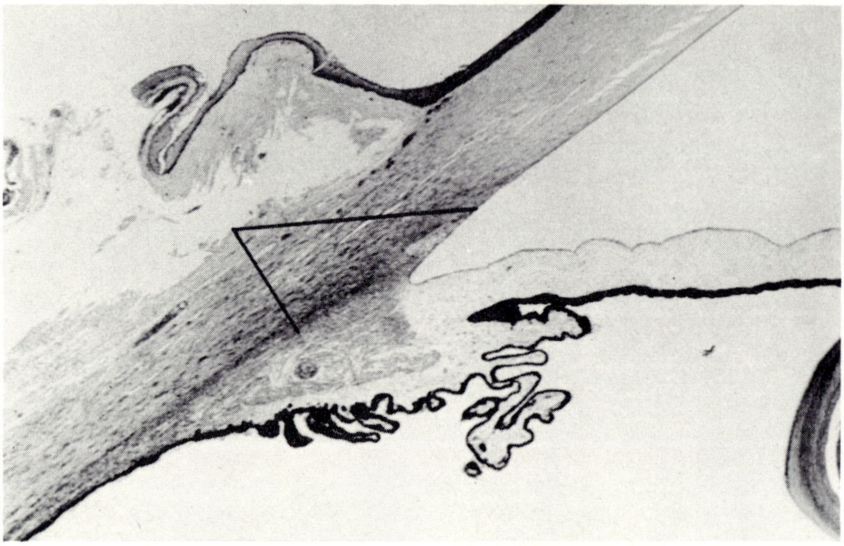

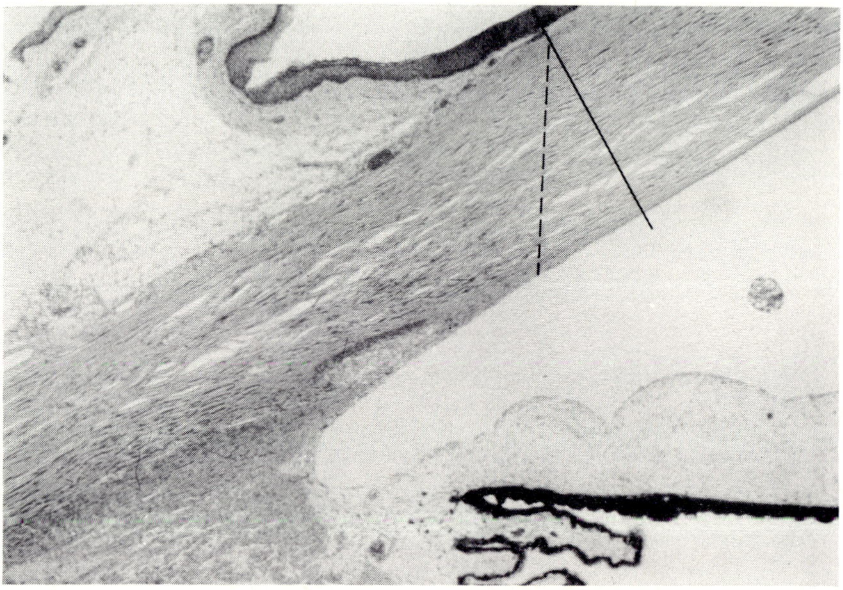

FIG. 24 (*Top*). An incision starting 1 to 2 mm. behind the posterior border of the limbus will enter the anterior chamber only if it is made parallel with the iris surface. The incision will enter the globe adjacent to the ciliary body if it is made perpendicular to the surface. (Swan, K. *in* Clark, W. (ed.): Symposium on Glaucoma, St. Louis, Mosby)

FIG. 25 (*Bottom*). The anterior border of the limbus (broken line) generally is parallel with the visual axis. An incision (solid line) begun at the anterior border of the superior limbus and made perpendicular to the surface will be entirely corneal and will enter the anterior chamber a considerable distance from the chamber angle. (Swan, K. *in* Clark, W. (ed.): Symposium on Glaucoma, St. Louis, Mosby)

Previously, a light held from the side in a darkened room was used to determine the landmark of the surgical limbus. However, the relatively sharp line of demarcation between the bluish semitransparent limbal stroma and the opaque white scleral fiber is even more accurate (Figs. 24-26).

Swan has pointed out that there is a scleral limbus and a corneal limbus.[34] Some use the term internal for the corneal limbus and external for the scleral limbus. The internal limbus may be from 1 to 3 mm. from the external limbus. Because the peripheral iridectomy should fall in the most desired spot, which is peripheral, it is important, especially in glaucoma, to make the opening incision over the scleral (external) limbus. When a peripheral iridectomy is not done in this area, it will not be truly peripheral and will account for more flat chambers.[34] If one uses the corneal (internal) limbus, that is, the area at which the conjunctiva seems to end, there is a greater tendency to have extracapsular extractions, especially since an incision of 180° will create a smaller opening with a corneolimbal type of incision than will one with the sclerolimbal type. In other words, with a corneal incision, a shelf will often develop which will make it difficult to remove the lens, especially if it is large. However, it must be pointed out that there are some very fine surgeons who use a pure corneal incision, at times with no conjunctival flap and even when they are using alpha-chymotrypsin.

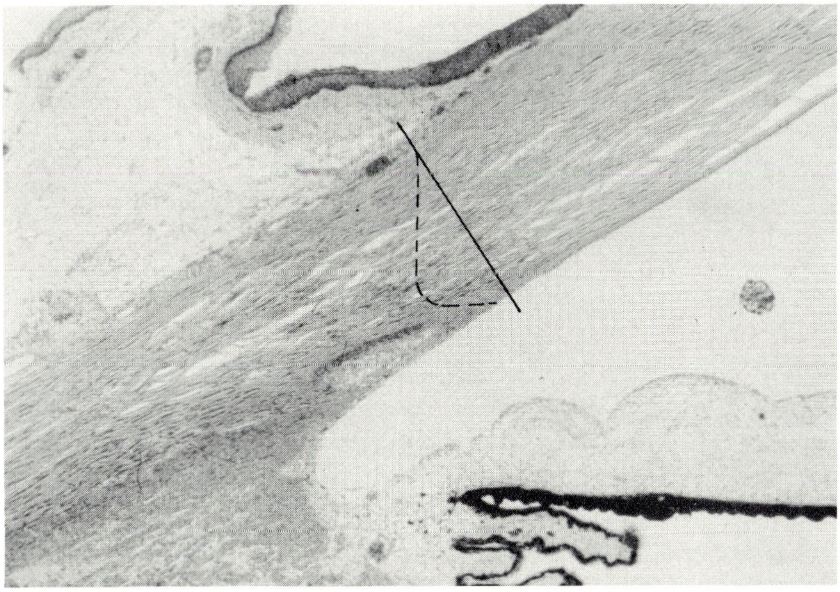

FIG. 26. The posterior border of the limbus (broken line) varies, but in most eyes an incision (solid line) started at the junction of semitransparent limbal stroma and opaque sclera will pass through the nonfunctioning part of the trabecula in front of Schlemm's canal and the deep scleral plexus to enter the anterior chamber at its narrowest part. (Swan, K. *in* Clark, W. (ed.): Symposium on Glaucoma, St. Louis, Mosby)

Position of Incision When Corneal Dystrophy, Diabetes and Bleeding Tendency Have Been Diagnosed Preoperatively

When corneal dystrophy has been diagnosed preoperatively, it is usually agreed that the ideal solution is a scleral type of incision. However, here, too, there are excellent surgeons who will not agree with this. In general, scleral incisions are indicated in the corneal dystrophy of Fuchs and most other corneal dystrophies. As a rule, although some surgeons use them almost as a matter of routine, a corneal site is indicated in diabetes, in blood diseases such as purpura, and where hemorrhages were noted in previous operations. Corneal incisions do not cause hemorrhage unless there is corneal vascularization.

Dr. Estrada, who favors a corneal incision without a conjunctival flap, finds no increase of striate keratitis even after the use of alpha-chymotrypsin. For cases showing dystrophy he will use a scleral incision done with an *ab externo* approach.[15]

Position of Incision for Cataract Following a Filtering Procedure

The ideal position for incision when a filtering procedure has been done prior to the cataract extraction is still a matter of great dispute. The lateral position of the keratome is one approach for those who use a keratome and especially for those

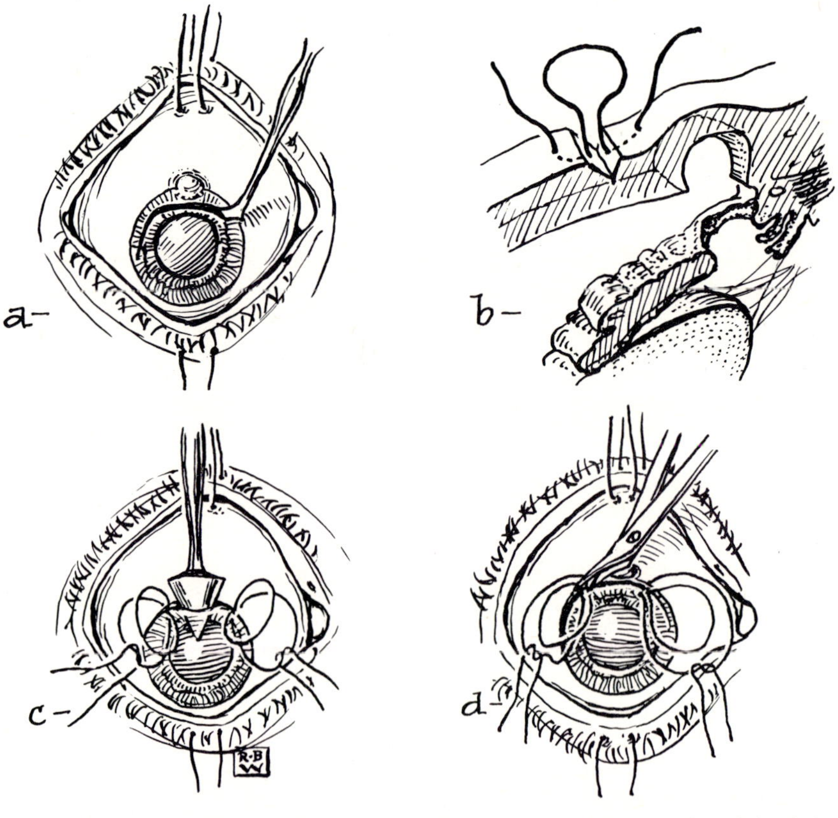

FIG. 27. Cataract extraction through the cornea anterior to the bleb of the antiglaucoma filtering operation. (Modified from Callahan, Alston: Surgery of the Eye: Diseases, Springfield, Ill., Thomas)

who prefer the slide technic. For those choosing to use the slide technic, there will be less chance of creating a shelf at the 12 o'clock position if the keratome incision is made laterally, starting at the 9 or the 3 o'clock position instead of at the 12 o'clock position. Any shelf that may have been created from the lateral position can be corrected as one approaches the 12 o'clock position. If the keratome incision is small, a shelf that has been created in this area can be rectified by using a gradual, rather than an abrupt, slope toward the desired side.

The lateral approach for entering the anterior chamber is not new. Many Spanish surgeons use it. For those surgeons who use the slide technic, a corneal shelf in the 12 o'clock position makes it more difficult to grasp the lens capsule at the equator and to deliver the lens.

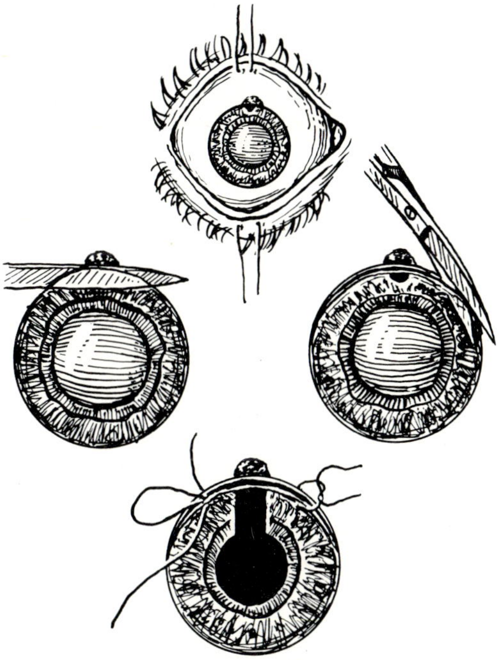

FIGURE 28
(Modified from Guillaumat, Louis, *et al.*: Traitement Chirurgical des Affections Oculaires, Paris, Doin)

Figures 27 and 28 show modifications of the incision in the presence of cataract, glaucoma and filtering blebs. If the filtering bleb is maintaining a normal ocular pressure, I will stay more corneal and avoid the bleb. If there is a tendency toward hypotony, I may occasionally make my incision through this bleb. Some surgeons feel that the bleb should be avoided at all times because of the danger of closing the filtering scar. Some feel that if the bleb is avoided, the cataract incision can be placed anywhere. Theoretically, there is probably less danger of closing the filtering scar if the incision is made below or away from the bleb or at the side.

Among those who favor making the incision from below are Dr. Berliner and Dr. Castroviejo. Dr. Berliner stated that in his hands in operating near the bleb he noted more dystrophy. In addition to making his incision from below (as a rule, patients with these problems usually have only one good eye), he will add a full iridectomy even though there may be a little more photophobia. Dr. Castroviejo said that in using a temporal incision he found that part of the incision came too close to the bleb, and he noted that in working to the side of the bleb or beneath it, he found more striate keratitis and more corneal edema. In operating near the bleb there was a tendency to make the pressure a little higher than it was prior to cataract extraction. Therefore, Dr. Castroviejo felt that one should not meddle with or operate anywhere near the bleb at any time. Dr. Castroviejo's present choice is an inferior approach. He will add a radial iridotomy in the 6 o'clock position. These eyes will show a V-shaped defect, but there will not be too much additional photophobia. His reason for doing this is that many of these patients have a rigid pupil due to atrophy of the iris, synechiae or the long use of miotics.[11]

The advantage of the incision being made anywhere other than above must be counterbalanced by the technical difficulties which may lead to other complications. The keratome incision is started in a lateral position, advancing to the area of the bleb. Since the wound is corneal, it must be larger than 180°.

I do not favor removing the lens from a lateral position or from the inferior position. Many surgeons disagree with this.

Actually, I feel that in most cases the glaucoma will remain controlled whether the lens is extracted from above, laterally or even below if the trephine, a sclerectomy and an iridencleisis wound are avoided. Through hard experience, I have learned that it is difficult to transfer this idea of a lateral or inferior incision to a resident assistant. Despite careful instructions, one of my senior residents became confused by this unusual position and instead of drawing the sutures taut as I was removing the lens, he spread the wound wide open with a subsequent loss of vitreous.

Figure 29 shows the combination of sclerectomy and iridectomy for glaucoma combined with extraction of a cataractous lens. The sclerectomy may be done with a punch (Fig. 30), scissors or cautery. There are those who favor simultaneous glaucoma and cataract surgery[21] (see p. 131). An iridencleisis may be combined with a lens extraction. Some recommend a cyclodialysis with a cataract extraction. In this case, the cyclodialysis may be done inferotemporally, followed by an injection

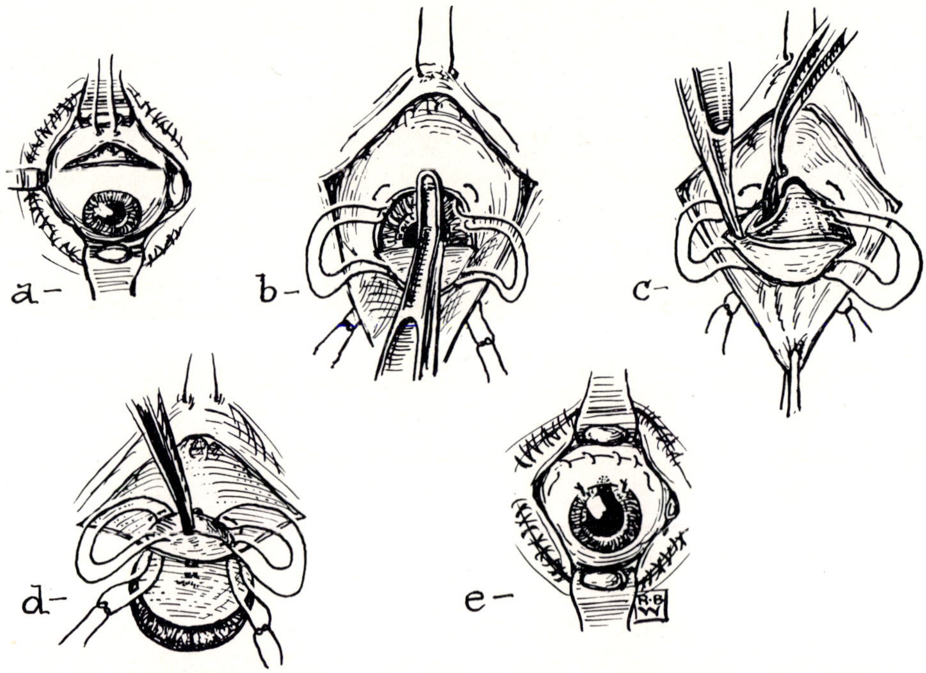

FIG. 29. Sclerectomy and iridectomy for glaucoma combined with extraction of cataractous lens. (Modified from Callahan, Alston: Surgery of the Eye: Diseases, Springfield, Ill., Thomas)

Plates 1 and 2

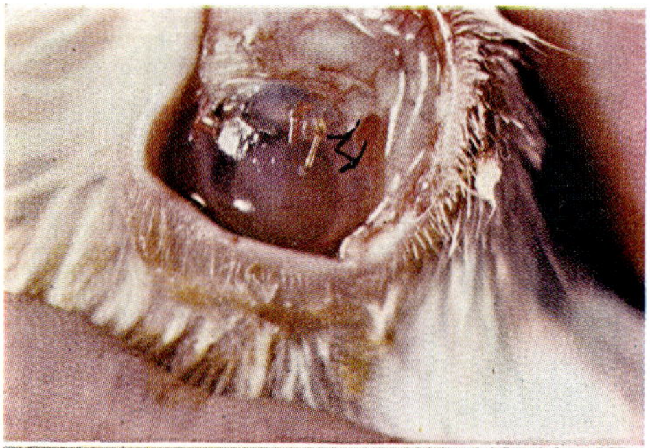

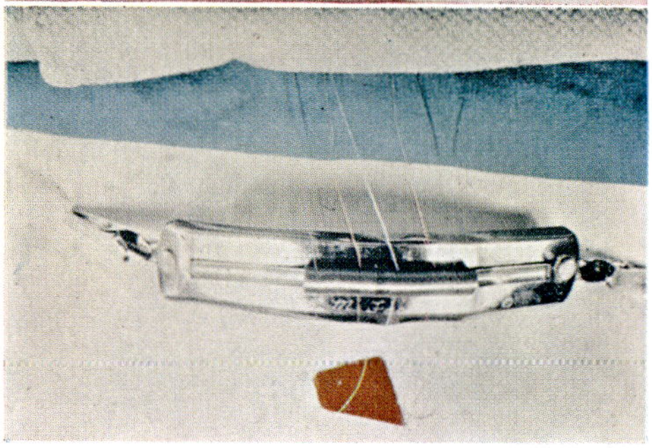

of air and closure of the conjunctiva. Then the cataract is removed in the usual way.[21] However, I agree with Berliner, Sugar and others who point out that the anterior chamber may remain flat for too long unless it is closed meticulously with a well-closed large conjunctival Tenon's flap. Berliner and Sugar feel, and I again agree, that a sclerectomy should be avoided to prevent delayed re-formation of the anterior chamber.[32] Depending on the outflow studies and the appearance of the angle with the gonioscope, and on whether or not the pressure can be brought down to within normal limits with the use of drops, I prefer not to combine the glaucoma operation with the cataract extraction.

In many borderline cases of glaucoma and cataract, nature itself provides microscopic filtering blebs which often cannot be grossly visualized in the wound.[19]

Hypotensive Measures for Extracting Cataracts in the Presence of Glaucoma

One should never open an eye that is hard. In addition, with the use of acetazolamide (Diamox), intravenous urea and massage, the pressure should not be elevated prior to opening the eye for glaucoma and cataract surgery. Some feel that in a nonglaucomatous eye, acetazolamide (Diamox) will not lower the intraocular pressure unless it is started 2 to 3 days prior to surgery. Some surgeons feel that Diamox will not lower intraocular pressure appreciably in children[9] (see p. 115). Urea seems to be an ideal osmotic agent. It has a low molecular weight and is nontoxic with poor ocular penetration, thus permitting the development of a high and sustained osmotic gradient. With this therapy even a glaucomatous crisis can be broken and the patient prepared for surgery.

Urea has only limited usefulness in patients with secondary glaucoma who demonstrate a turbid aqueous and damage to the blood-aqueous barrier. Thus, it may not be counted on to help appreciably in a case such as diabetic rubeosis with glaucoma.

Liver and brain damage are contraindications to the use of urea; however, it may be used safely—under the supervision of an internist—in renal and heart disease where caution is advisable. In renal disease, moderate elevation in B. U. N. (blood urea nitrogen) is not a contraindication to the use of urea, since the signs of uremia are not due to elevation of urea but to other toxic substances. Cardiac and hypertensive patients should be observed carefully during the infusion, and the rate of urea administration should be slower than is usual.[1] In regard to the reports that there have been some deaths for which urea was blamed, Dr. Galin felt that since patients can die from commonly used drugs such as aspirin or peni-

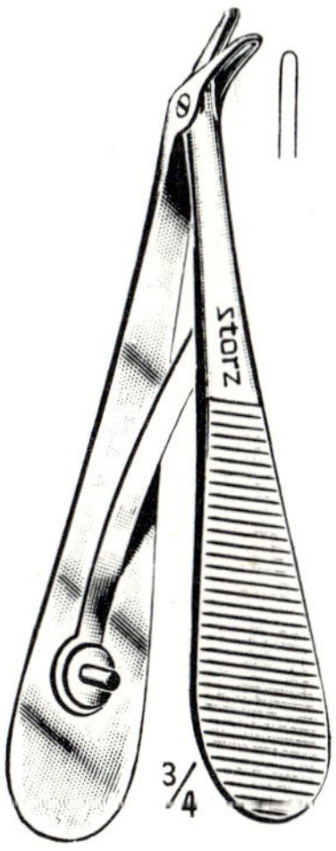

FIG. 30. Corneoscleral punch (Storz instrument No. E-2800).

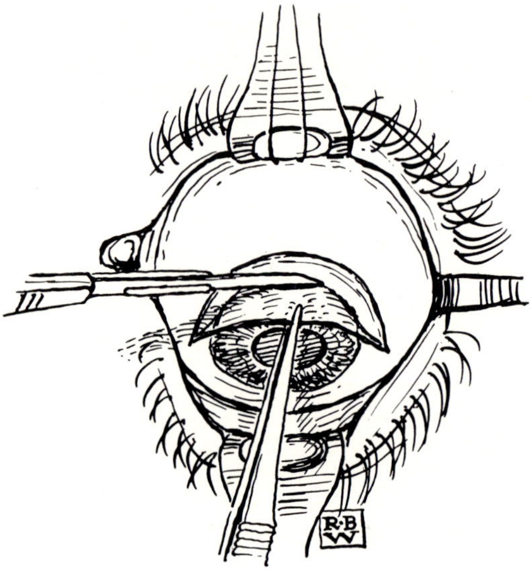

FIG. 31. The surgeon makes a trough in the limbus using a Bard-Parker No. 15 blade held vertical to the plane of the eye. (Modified from Paton, Katzin, & Stilwell: Atlas of Eye Surgery, New York, Blakiston)

cillin, the use of urea can be considered a calculated risk.

Actually, sometimes the eye can be too soft when urea is used prior to cataract extraction. In order to prevent this, the intravenous urea should be started ½ hour prior to the actual incision. It is difficult for the surgeon to make an opening into the anterior chamber in an eye that is too soft. One complication that should be anticipated is that urea will cause the patient's bladder to fill rapidly while he is under local anesthesia. A urinal in or near the operating room may be most helpful! I do not favor an indwelling catheter. Urea should be discarded if it has been exposed to air. Burning at the site of injection also should be anticipated, and one must be certain that the needle is well within the lumen of the vein. It is recommended that the lower extremities should not be used for infusion in older patients. Large veins should be selected for the injection because the possibility of venous thrombosis at the site of injection is lessened when these large veins are used. Novocain (procaine) injected into the site of the same needle will overcome the pain. Headaches that follow the use of urea can be attributed to a fall in the cerebrospinal fluid pressure and, like those seen after spinal taps, pass with bed rest and analgesics. Nausea and vomiting, mental confusion, disorientation and hyperthermia have been reported occasionally but are not contraindications to its use. Antiemetics may be of some help for nausea and vomiting. Intravenous pentobarbital can be used for the mental confusion. Hyperthermia is rare. These side-effects are annoying but not dangerous.[36] Mannitol may be used instead of urea.[39a]

CONSIDERATIONS RELATED TO TECHNIC

Figure 31 shows the technic for making a trough. Most surgeons use a Bard-Parker knife for making this trough. A fresh Bard-Parker knife should be used for each cataract extraction (Fig. 32, *left*). Others use a modified cystotome for making this groove (Fig. 32, *right*). If one perforates, the scissors or a cataract knife can be used for enlarging the corneal wound.

Figure 33 shows a corneoscleral inci-

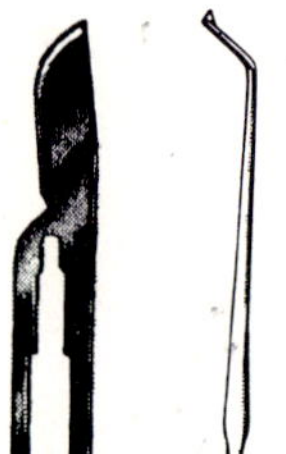

FIG. 32. (*Left*) Bard-Parker blade (Storz instrument No. E-336). (*Right*) Sclerotome, Atkinson (Storz instrument No. E-374).

sion with a preplaced modified type of McLean suture. Today the needles are sharp enough so that a groove need not be used.

Recently Dr. McLean said:

> I suspect that if when I started getting enthusiastic about preplaced sutures in the beginning of my cataract work, we would have had in those days needles, suture material and instruments such as we have today, I might never have done it! On the other hand, I still use that technic, I still like it and I feel that it has certain advantages.[22]

If a Verhoeff type of track suture is used and the anterior chamber is lost, the thread will usually close off the leak. I prefer postplaced sutures, as I find them less complex; however, I may use preplaced sutures in the superior nasal quadrant of the left eye in the patient with glaucoma or where trouble is anticipated.

Among the tricks used to apply sutures past the bridge of the nose are those of changing the hand used for carrying the needle, reaching over the head, reversing the direction of application of the bites, use of deeply bent needle carriers or changing the direction of the needles in the needle carrier. In this situation, there is no problem for operators who are ambidextrous. The late Dr. Weve once mentioned to me that a good eye surgeon must simulate a good boxer (i.e., "He must use his hands as well as his feet").

Most surgeons apply corneoscleral sutures from the cornea to the sclera by going over the nose. Going from the sclera to the cornea is helpful and in a sense is

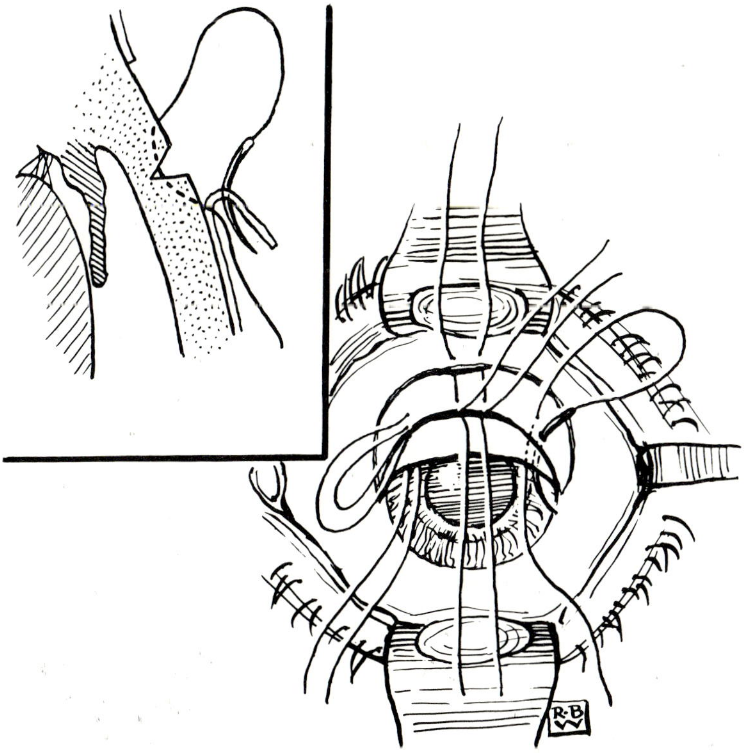

FIG. 33. Scheie corneoscleral closure with mattress suture at 12 o'clock and scleroconjunctival sutures at 10:30 and 1:30 o'clock. (Modified from Scheie, H. G.: A.M.A. Arch. Ophth. *61*:431)

comparable to a backhand stroke in tennis. Without having the needle cut its way out and without sacrificing a true radial bite, I like to change the direction of the needle in the carrier and pull the needle from the corneal to the scleral side. This method can be used for preplaced or postplaced bites. Today surgeons are making an opening into the eye with a prepared Gillette razor blade held with a variety of instruments (Fig. 34, *left*). Two of the advantages here are the assurance of a sharp blade at all times and the minimal cost. Another advantage is that the initial opening into the eye can be made exactly as desired (i.e., slanting or vertical in the position desired). Dr. Castroviejo feels that one of the main improvements in cataract surgery is an accurate incision in 100 per cent of cases. This is even more of an advantage in cataract surgery in the presence of glaucoma which already has been treated surgically. Although he feels that a Gillette razor blade—and even a keratome—is less elegant than a classic Von Graefe incision, the razor blade can be used to make the incision accurately wherever one wants it, including whatever plane one wants to place it in. As a rule, in cataract extraction, Dr. Castroviejo prefers to make his incision immediately behind the conjunctival flap, which makes it almost a corneal incision.[10]

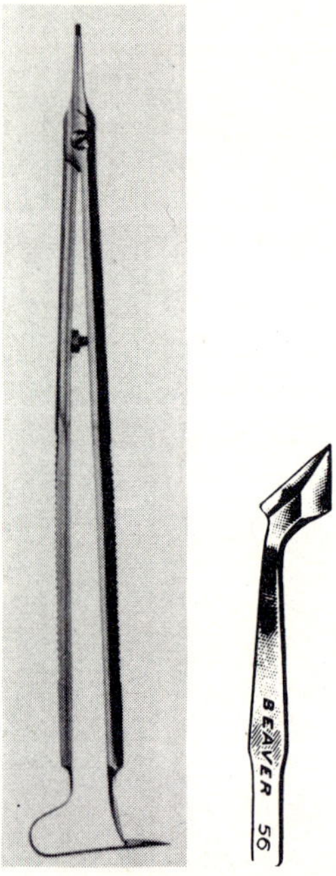

FIG. 34. (*Left*) Blade breaker (Storz instrument No. E-1077). (*Right*) Beaver blade (medium) (Storz instrument No. E-356).

In order to avoid the slight shelf created by the keratome, I prefer a sharp, replaceable keratome Beaver blade (Fig. 34, *right*) introduced from the temporal position of the eye (Fig. 35). The bevel or the vertical component can be created with scissors as the 12 o'clock position of the cornea is approached. An extra keratome should always be ready for use in case the first is defective.

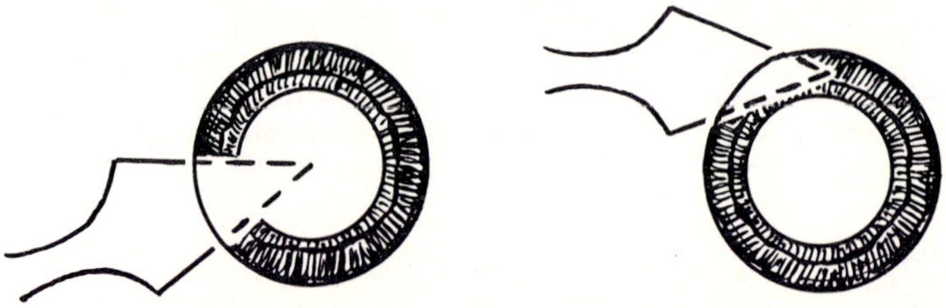

FIG. 35. Diagram illustrating the movements of the keratome for corneal section. (Modified from Arruga, H.: Ocular Surgery, Barcelona, Salvat Editores, S. A.)

I have often been asked which angle of cataract incision I prefer and why: "the slanting, the vertical or the mitred?" By vertical is meant the perpendicular type of corneal incision most often used in corneal transplants. By mitred, one means what is known as the stepped, "half-lap" or carpenter type of joint incision. This incision sometimes is also called a "three-step" procedure (Fig. 36). If one counts the conjunctival opening, it may be called the "four-step" procedure. A slanting incision is said to produce a greater area for wound healing. However, since the cornea is avascular, there is less hyphema in this type of incision. Those who favor the slanting incision, especially if it extends to the sclera, point out that the blood vessels in the sclera promote better wound healing. As a rule, most surgeons agree that a corneal incision is not to be used if one anticipates using alpha-chymotrypsin, since the number of wound disruptions is greater. The surgeon who uses alpha-chymotrypsin usually covers the corneoscleral edge with conjunctiva. Many surgeons now favor the mitred or "half-lap" type of incision. I find this more complex and unnecessary, preferring an incision that usually is slanted toward the scleral side and well covered with conjunctiva. I try to make a beveling of my incision that is gentle and well back at the limbus. It enables me to deliver the lens safely by either a tumbling or a sliding technic. This

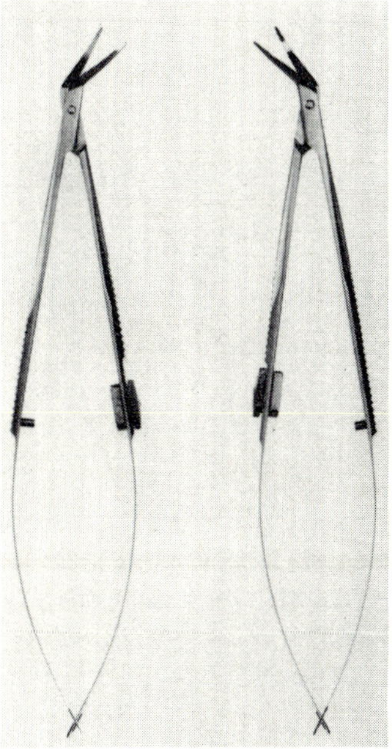

FIG. 37. New Troutman scissors (Storz instruments Nos. E-3306 and E-3307).

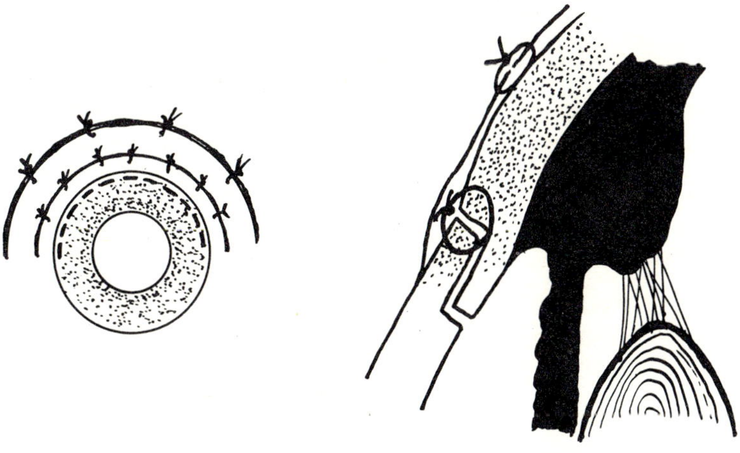

FIG. 36. Four-step closure. (Modified from Barraquer, Joaquin: An. Inst. Barraquer, vol. 2, No. 1, 1961)

type of incision is good for both a small and a large lens. Dr. Dunnington favors a slanting incision because he feels that it is easier to get accurate approximation with this type of incision. He concludes that "actually it doesn't really matter whether the incision is vertical or slanting."[13]

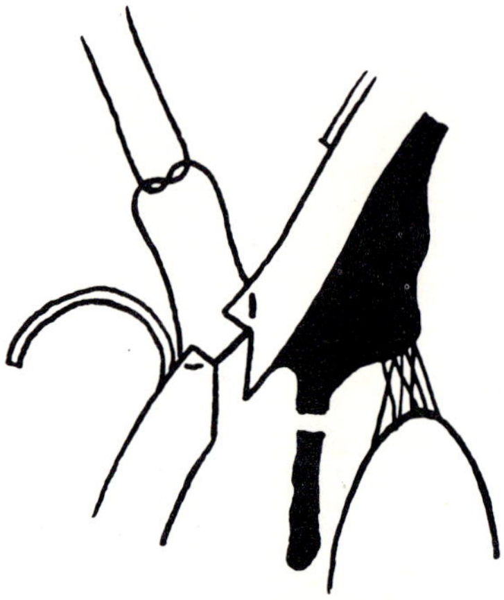

FIG. 38. A semibeveled cut. (Modified from Barraquer, José: An. Inst. Barraquer *3*:51, No. 1, 1962)

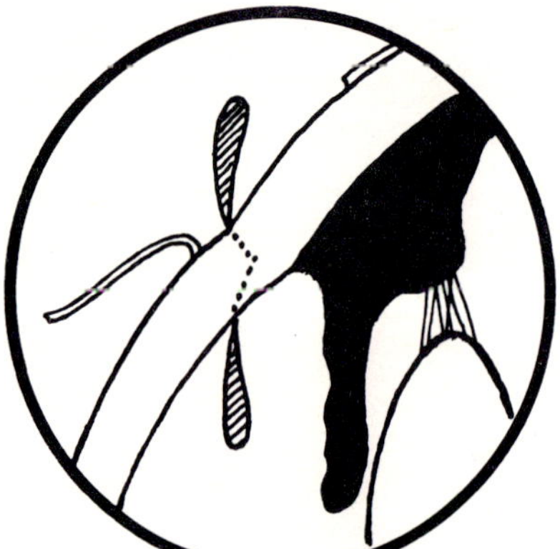

FIG. 39. The semibeveled cut that can be obtained with the new José Barraquer scissors (Storz instrument No. E-3280). This can be done in a single maneuver. (Modified from Barraquer, Joaquin: Trans. Am. Acad. Ophthal. Oto-laryng. *66*: 46)

For the step incision, new scissors designed by José Barraquer and by Troutman are recommended (Fig. 37). The José Barraquer scissors produce a semibeveled cut (Figs. 38 & 39). The blades are straight and flat and are designed to cut from right to left. A stop in the shank prevents complete closure of the blades if this is desired. Notching of the incision is minimal. I have used these scissors for my usual incision and for the "step" incision and find that when they are new their cutting quality is superb. Although a corneal curve is absent, the cuts are clean with little or no damage to the iris. The Troutman scissors are designed on a smaller scale than the Castroviejo scissors and allow better control when entering the anterior chamber and reduce contact with the iris and the corneal endothelium.

As a rule, I use the Castroviejo curved right and left scissors (Fig. 40). The curve of the blades follows the surgical limbus very beautifully. By inserting them

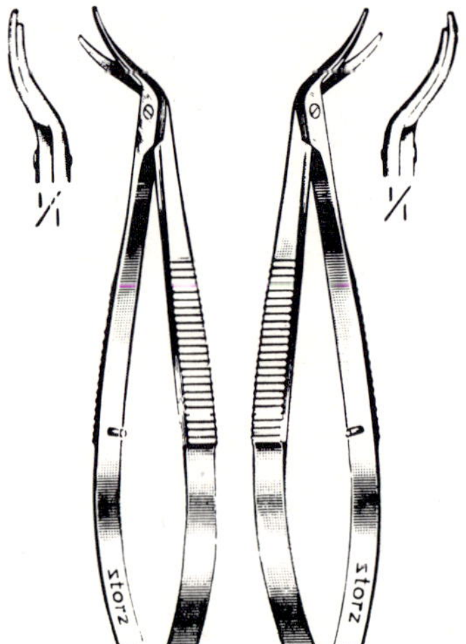

FIG. 40. Castroviejo corneal section scissors, right and left (Storz instruments Nos. E-3300 and E-3301).

in long steps rather than short steps, I have not seen any more notching of the wound. However, I may have brushed off some of the iris pigment, especially in the 9 and the 3 o'clock positions, producing an effect similar to that noted when one touches the wings of a butterfly. This is visible only with the biomicroscope and seems to cause no other damage. To date I have not cut the iris with these scissors. To prevent this pigment loss in the 3 or the 9 o'clock positions, I find that if my assistant holds the conjunctival flap with two flat Bonaccolto forceps (Fig. 41) I can obtain a better angle by resting the knuckles of the hand that is holding the spring-action scissors on my other hand. This maneuver, in addition to the assistant's help, permits me to introduce my inner blade for a greater distance, thus avoiding notching.

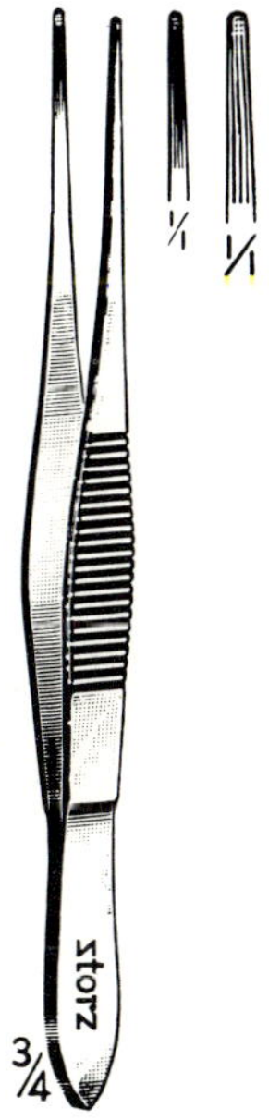

FIG. 41. Bonaccolto utility forceps (Storz instrument No. E-1906).

SIZE OF INCISION

As a rule, especially with the use of alpha-chymotrypsin and in dystrophies, the wound should be 180° to 200°. Incisions that are too anterior, especially corneal ones, can reduce the aperture needed to extract the cataract and should be larger than 180°. Incisions that are too posterior can injure the iris or the ciliary body or can cause anterior synechiae, etc.[8] Ideally, the incision should be made at the sclerolimbal junction where the bluish translucent limbus joins the white opaque fibers. If this is a "step" incision, this can be the same as that recommended in a peripheral iridectomy and just in front of the junction of the posterior border of the limbus and the sclera extending about halfway through the stroma. It can be split forward about ½ mm., the final incision being made perpendicularly into the anterior chamber.[35] A corneolimbal incision shortens the wound and favors a ledge. If the incision is short or corneal or has a ledge, there is a greater chance of performing an extracapsular extraction. A ledge shortens the incision and makes a slide technic more difficult. The use of an erisophake necessitates a larger incision than does a capsule forceps.

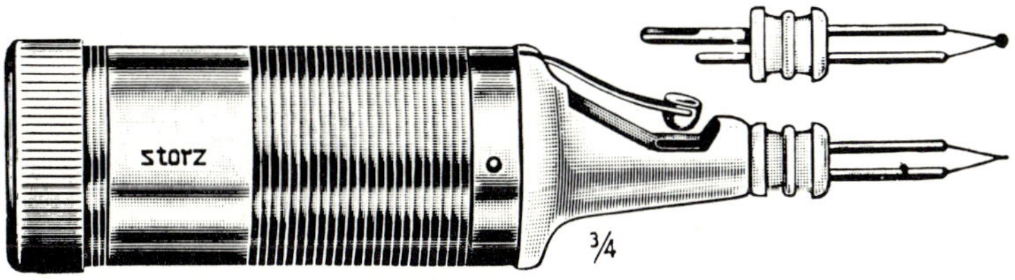

FIG. 42. Storz instrument No. E-915.

HEMOSTASIS

In reference to hemostasis during the production of a conjunctival flap or the incision of the cornea or the sclera, previously I used the Hildreth coagulator (Fig. 42) but was annoyed by the fact that it did not always work. However, the use of a new battery for each operation helped to partially solve this problem. The use of cotton for hemostasis is avoided, and irrigation is used instead. Cotton finds its way into the anterior chamber once it is opened.

The ideal technic is that described by Dr. Barraquer:

> Bleeding from small vessels is seen most easily when the operative field is frequently irrigated with artificial aqueous solution, excess fluid being removed by suction. Soaking of the drapes does not seem to predispose to sepsis any more than it does in neurosurgery. Application of a 2-2, 5 Volt galvanocautery through the irrigating solution produces coagulation of the vessels. Foot switch control is more convenient than manual control.[7]

It has been pointed out that the Barraquer cautery is effective even in a wet field.

My present preference for coagulation is the new Storz Geiger cautery as I find that it can be counted on to work. The needle and the handle are sterilized in the autoclave.

PROBLEMS RELATED TO SUTURE MATERIAL

The present trend seems again to be the use of chromic sutures. The removal of silk sutures can be almost as difficult as the placing of these sutures, and for this reason many feel that chromic sutures are ideal. For a while, I noticed that many surgeons were returning to the use of silk sutures. Some of the reasons for this may have been as follows:

1. At the time of surgery it is easier to place a silk suture in a certain position and to have it stay there. Also, as Dr. Estrada has pointed out, with the use of 8-0 silk sutures, even without a conjunctival flap, these can be kept in for as long as 3 or 4 months if a drop containing methylcellulose is used at least twice a day.[14]

2. There are many disadvantages to the use of chromic sutures at the operating table. These disadvantages fall into two categories:

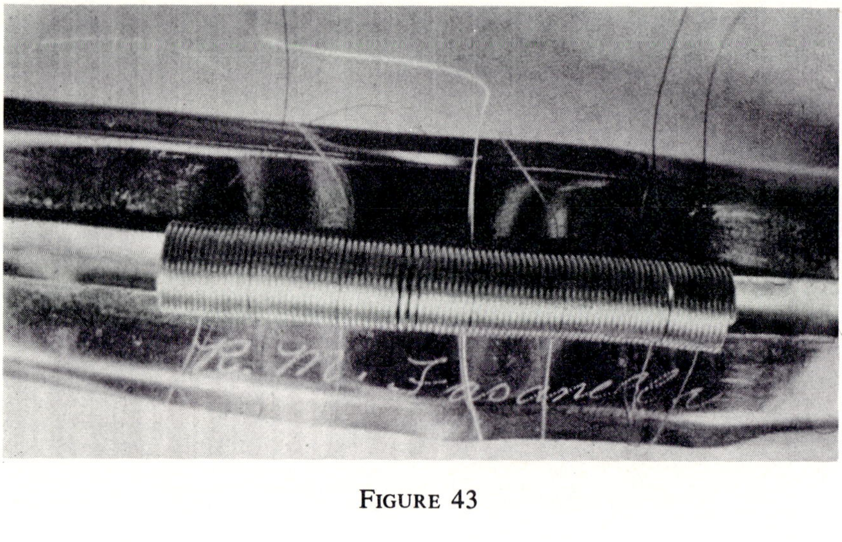

FIGURE 43

a. The difficulty, especially for older surgeons, of identifying the sutures, and

b. The stiffness of the sutures.

A black silk suture can be laid aside and will not encumber the process of extracting the lens.

Another trick which can be utilized in attempting to see and identify these sutures is to cut the suture short. Because of its stiffness, the chromic suture will often stand upright and can be identified more easily. However, if the surgeon uses this trick with a limbus flap, he must make sure that he has a good conjunctival flap to pull on in case vitreous should present.

The use of colored beads placed on the ends of chromic sutures has been suggested.

For quick identification of the sutures and for holding them in place, the use of a coiled spring is excellent. Despite the fact that the coil platform can be bent to curve with the shape of the head, this coil and platform still create a small hillock over which the surgeon has to work (Fig. 43).

If only one preplaced or postplaced suture is used, the problem of identifying sutures is minimal; however, this offers less security at the time. A knot on the end of the suture is of some help. Additional sutures can be placed and cut following the first suture; this will not lead

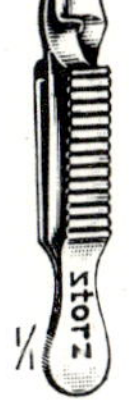

FIG. 44. Serrefine (Storz instrument No. E-3900).

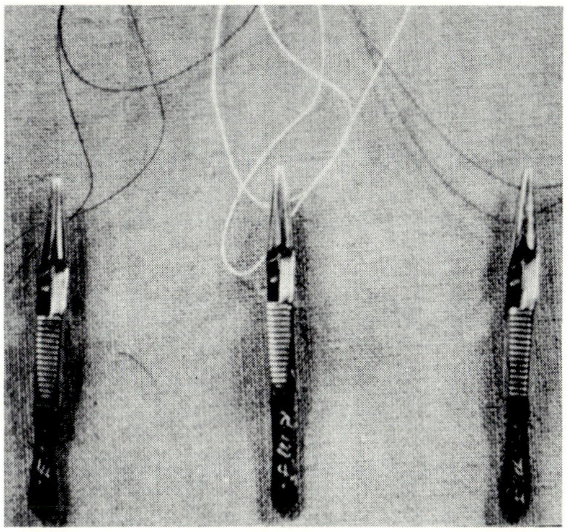

FIGURE 45

to problems of identification, but possibly the wound closure will be less exact.

Serrefines, or small bulldog clamps, have been used; however, most of these are too heavy, and they have a tendency to close the wound before the lens is delivered (Fig. 44). Lighter serrefines can be obtained in England and Europe, but even these may still pull the wound together (Fig. 45). Although these European serrefines are extremely light, they often have to be folded into the towel so that they do not lie in an awkward position or become twisted or difficult to identify. My present choice is an even lighter serrefine used in neurosurgery.

Various types of paper clips can be utilized for rapid identification of chromic sutures[40] (Fig. 46). One end of the paper clip can be sharpened and inserted in the head towel to prevent the sutures from twisting on themselves.

In an attempt to overcome the problem of identifying sutures at surgery, dyes have been incorporated into the sutures. Slight areas of infection around these sutures have been reported, especially when they were not covered by conjunctiva. Plate 1 shows a rabbit's eye. The colored sutures that are most visible in a rabbit eye are sometimes not as useful in a human eye because the iris background is different. Different colors can be identified against the drapes used in various operating rooms. For example, Plate 2 shows the sutures contrasting with a white background. The contrast against colored drapes also is shown, as is the contrast of the suture material on a red background (i.e., blood). Sutures that are easily visible under one set of conditions may not be seen so readily under other conditions.

As for the softness of chromic sutures, most surgeons are acquainted with the trick of wetting the folded towel in which the chromic sutures are placed. Some use glycerin to soften the sutures and dyes for ease of identification. However, when the sutures are placed on the cornea, they often become stiff again, and the dye may run. The most modern chromic sutures directly incorporate the qualities of softness and ease of identification that are found in silk sutures. These new sutures have finer and smaller needles for which finer needle holders should be used. Since the quality of chromic suture material can depend on the method of manufacturing and the particular batch, the rate of absorption of the suture material can vary. The factors that may play a part in the variability of the suture absorption are the patient's eye itself, whether chromic suture material has been used previously and systemic and local medications, notably the steroid group. Recently, Dr. Dunnington, who previously favored chromic suture material, turned to the use of plain catgut because the rate of absorption seemed to be more predictable and better tolerated by the patient.[13] My present choice is a 6-0 dark blue Ethicon chromic suture.

Number of Sutures

I personally prefer 5 to 6 sutures. There is a general tendency on the part of other surgeons to use this or even a greater number of sutures. This is especially true with the use of alpha-chymotrypsin. In these cases, if the wound edge is washed and the excess enzyme in the anterior chamber is irrigated out, there should be no more than the usual number of filtering wounds or flat chambers. If filtering blebs or flat chambers occur and the enzyme has been used correctly, other causes must be sought and the problem treated as though the enzyme had not been used. I feel that it is a rather simple matter to place 5 or 6 sutures. Some surgeons feel

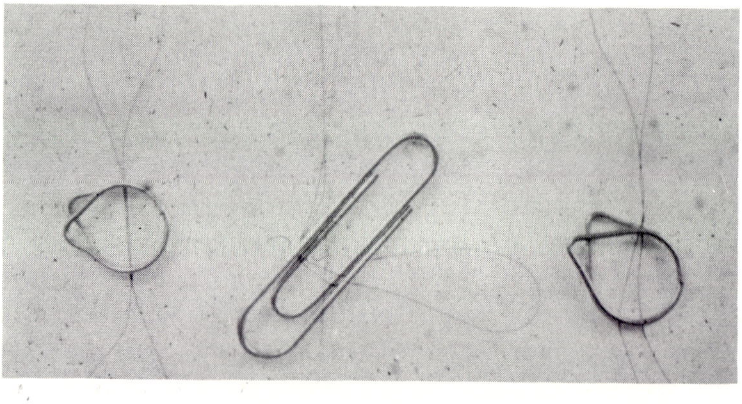

Figure 46

that 2 sutures and occasionally 3 are sufficient in most cases. It is important to place the sutures while enlarging the wound. If the entire wound is enlarged at one time, it is easy to displace the entire corneal surface to the right or to the left. If the first suture is placed after the keratome incision is made, more nearly accurate apposition is obtained—the smaller the keratome incision the greater the chance of placing the suture edge-to-edge. However, if the keratome incision is too small, it is difficult to enlarge the wound with scissors without cutting the suture or the iris. After the first suture is placed, which I usually make snug, occasionally I may tie one knot lightly. Then, I enlarge the wound slightly and place another suture. In this fashion a good tight closure can be obtained. For this reason, I do not use either a preplaced suture or a mitred incision, both of which I feel are a bit more difficult and, in my hands, unnecessary. I have rarely had flat chambers or any postoperative wound disruption after adopting this technic. Excellent surgeons are still using 2 sutures, or 3, and many of them use a preplaced McLean type of suture. It is the feeling of these surgeons that if only a few sutures are used it is especially important that these sutures be accurately placed and that they should be removed immediately and replaced if there is any question regarding the accuracy of their placement. This they feel is the important point in avoiding complications. However, I feel that well-placed multiple sutures are indicated in order to prevent a flat chamber, iris prolapse and late wound disruption, especially with the use of alpha-chymotrypsin. It is my feeling that it is better to use too many than too few sutures. I agree with Dr. Joaquin Barraquer who says that "because the globe is soft and quiet, thanks to modern anesthesia, the correct application of postplaced sutures does not present any problem."[7]

I have used the 8-0 virgin silk dyed with methylene blue as recommended by Barraquer. One must have a fine instrument to tie these fine sutures and to carry the needle. With the nursing shortage, I cannot always count on assistance in threading the 4 mm. Grieshaber corneal needles. Occasionally I have had to remove them, even though most of them are so inert that they may remain buried subconjunctivally indefinitely. If these sutures must be removed, the use of fluorescein to dye them makes the sutures more visible. The Zeiss operating microscope or the slit lamp offer greater magnification for their removal.

SURGERY OF THE IRIS

Round Pupils vs. Full Iridectomies

The advent of alpha-chymotrypsin has effected no essential changes in the surgery of the iris in cataract extractions. In the early days of its use, there were a large number of iris prolapses reported, but now these are being prevented by better technic, including adequate lavage of the excess alpha-chymotrypsin from the wound edge and the anterior chamber. Furthermore, careful incision and closure with additional sutures have helped to prevent iris prolapse (see Chap. 6).

Round Pupils. Today the majority of surgeons prefer the round pupil because they feel that it is more natural and physiologic. Most surgeons feel that the round pupil should be used in all uncomplicated cataracts except in children. Some say that it should be used in all patients under 50 where the pupil dilates easily and fully; others set no age limit. *Cosmetically,* the round pupil is indicated in those eyes which are prominent or exophthalmic and the lid does not cover the cornea well. It should be used when the other eye has a round pupil and when the patient desires it. Patients with monocular cataracts with a normal second eye are good candidates for a round pupil. *Optically,* it is felt that there is better vision, especially where contact lenses are used. There is less photophobia. As far as *safety* during the operation is concerned, it is said that the round pupil is the best immediate protection against vitreous herniation. Iridectomies (and iridotomies to a lesser extent) help to prevent iris prolapse and glaucoma. Preservation of the pupil enhances the action of miotics if they are needed postoperatively.

Full Iridectomy. Those in favor of a complete iridectomy (sometimes called full or sector) say that all patients, especially those with complications and especially those patients of 50 or over, should have a full iridectomy. It is indicated where the pupil does not dilate easily and well. In the older patient when the pupil does not dilate well, it is wise to do a full iridectomy. As time passes, many of the pupils that dilate partially will dilate even more poorly, and, therefore, the larger opening is preferred. Some feel that it should be used in all congenital cataracts and in all subluxated or luxated lenses.[6] Iridectomy is important in children because of the many serious complications that can occur, especially postoperatively. This is discussed more fully in Chapter 4 under "Congenital Cataracts." *Cosmetically,* a full iridectomy is less appealing, although it is not so bad in elderly patients where the lid aperture becomes narrower with age. A full iridectomy is indicated if one has previously been performed in the other eye.

Optically, some feel that the acuity is not lessened appreciably. However, if the iridectomy is large, there is more photophobia. There is less postoperative "delayed" vitreous herniation and with this fewer macular and corneal changes if the vitreous touches the endothelium.

Safety is one of the greatest arguments in favor of a full iridectomy. It should be used in all patients with only one eye. It is indicated in high myopia, where there is a history of retinal detachment, in diabetics, where there were complications with the round pupil in the other eye and in cases of old uveitis where synechiae have been laid down. Where there has been an inflammation such as an iritis, there is less chance of the pupil becoming closed. For complicated cataracts a full iridectomy helps to prevent seclusion and occlusion of the pupil or reactivation of iridocyclitis.[6]

If the pupil becomes eccentric, small or bound down, or if there is a vitreous loss, the chances for managing detachment are far more favorable with a complete iridectomy. If a detachment occurs or is suspected, it is easier to visualize the holes through an iridectomy. In the patient with a high myopia in addition to an iridectomy at 12 o'clock, a vertical iridotomy at 6 o'clock is an excellent precautionary measure.

In diabetics it is felt that it is easier to wash pigment out if it is present after a full iridectomy. However, there are those who feel that the less one does to the iris the better, especially since there is a greater tendency for hemorrhage in addition to pigment loss (see p. 120). Almost everyone agrees that a full iridectomy should be done in cases of dystrophy or endothelial changes. A full iridectomy is a safety factor in glaucoma. Although a well-done peripheral iridectomy should suffice, it seems safer to do a full iridectomy in angle-closure glaucoma which is medically controlled preoperatively.

In open-angle glaucoma a full iridec-

FIGURE 47

(Modified from Guillaumat, Louis, *et al.*: Traitement Chirurgical des Affections Oculaires, Paris, Doin)

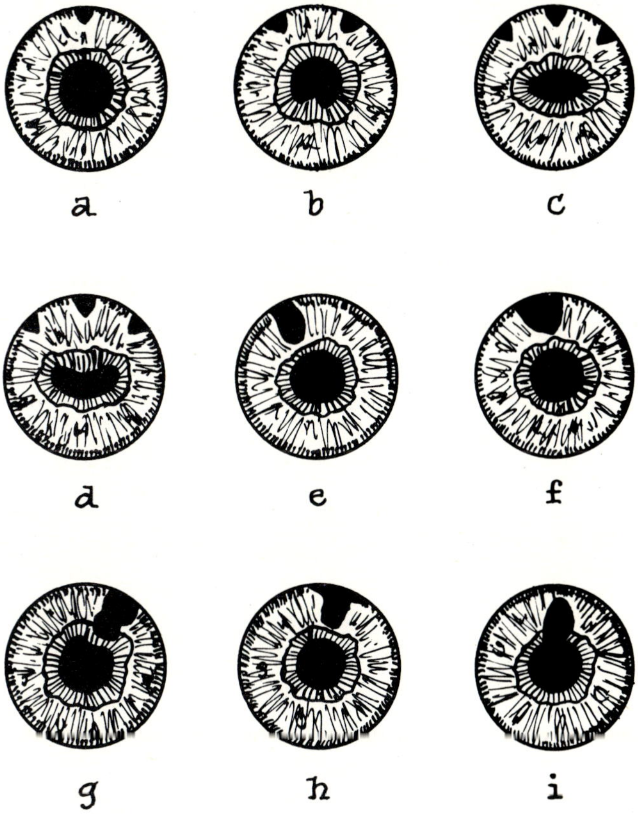

tomy theoretically has no immediate benefit. Many feel that a full iridectomy should be used in all suspicious or borderline cases of glaucoma or if at any time there has been a preoperative increase in pressure. There is less chance of causing pupillary and angle block with an iridectomy as a prophylactic procedure during cataract surgery for patients with or without glaucoma. Vitreous-block glaucoma occurs more frequently following round-pupil extraction.

In patients who have glaucoma controlled with drops, the addition of an iridectomy is often sufficient to control the elevated intraocular pressure. Very often no drops will be needed postoperatively. I do not feel that surgery, such as a filtering procedure, is necessary in many of these cases.

Dr. Edmund Spaeth feels that an iridectomy is indicated in all certain glaucoma cases and all possible glaucoma cases. He reminds us that not all hypertensive cases are glaucomas.

I am often reminded of Dr. Sugar's statement: ". . . iridectomies are better than iridotomies and two iridectomies are better than a single one."[33] He suggests that perhaps sector iridectomy might be wiser than peripheral iridectomy if pupil-block glaucoma alone is to be considered.

A great safety factor is the mechanical ease of removing the lens at the time of operation. Full iridectomies facilitate extraction of the lens. This should always be used where vitreous is either presented or suspected or where it follows cataract extraction. Under these circumstances it is felt by many that both the patient and the surgeon are happiest and just that much ahead when a full iridectomy has been

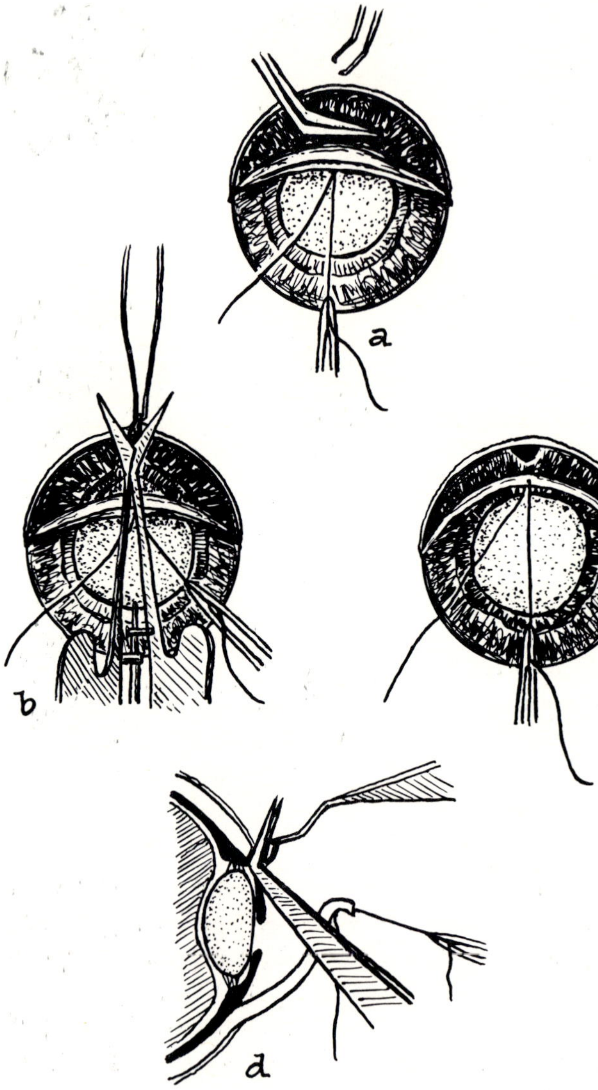

FIGURE 48

(Modified from Guillaumat, Louis, *et al.*: Traitement Chirurgical des Affections Oculaires, Paris, Doin)

performed. Full iridectomies are indicated in dislocated lenses. More hypermature lenses are delivered intracapsularly with a full iridectomy. If, on the incision, the iris prolapses and the lens and the iris present, full iridectomy is wisest. If the pupil is round in the "bull-necked" patient, there is a tendency for iris prolapse, even with multiple sutures.

Full iridectomy is indicated in most extracapsular types of extractions. In terms of safety, a full iridectomy means less exacting postoperative care. With a full iridectomy, there are fewer updrawn or eccentric pupils and fewer cases of mushroom or late vitreous herniation into the anterior chamber.

Technic for Round Pupil. As for iridectomies, one can consider two main types: a total or full iridectomy and those iridectomies and iridotomies associated with round pupils. Figure 47 shows various forms of peripheral iridectomies and iridotomies.

FIG. 49. Technic of peripheral iridectomy while an assistant raises the cornea. (Modified from Arruga, H.: Ocular Surgery, Barcelona, Salvat Editores, S. A.)

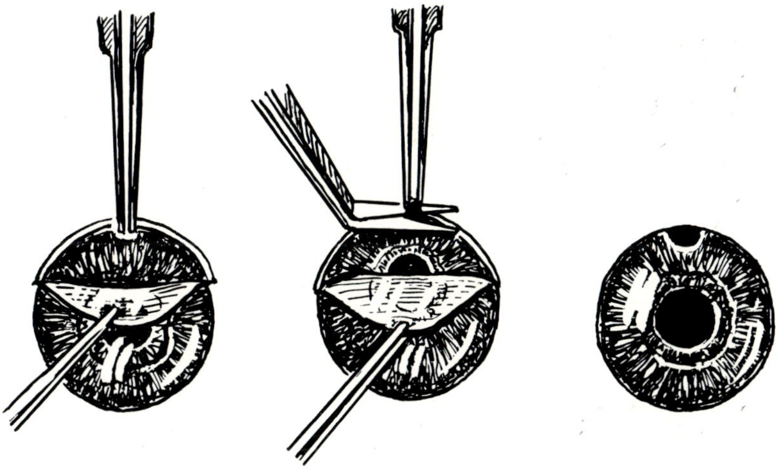

PERIPHERAL IRIDECTOMY. Figure 48 shows one method of doing a peripheral iridectomy, and Figure 49 shows the use of another forceps. I find that the Bonaccolto fine forceps which resembles a jeweler's forceps is excellent for performing very small iridectomies (Fig. 50, a). This forceps has now been modified by Storz and has a bend so that it is possible to support the hand on the patient's brow and perform a peripheral iridectomy exactly where one wants it (Fig. 50, b). The Barraquer-Katzin corneoscleral forceps is also excellent for iridectomies (Fig. 51). Dr. Estrada prefers a corneal incision and a peripheral iridectomy. To accomplish this he starts his corneal incision laterally and exaggerates the curve toward the scleral side in the area of 12 o'clock. This gives him access to the peripheral iris.

If one prefers to perform a round-pupil type of cataract extraction and if there is miosis with an inability of the pupil to dilate fully, at the time of surgery one must make a distinction between a taut sphincter due to muscle tension and one

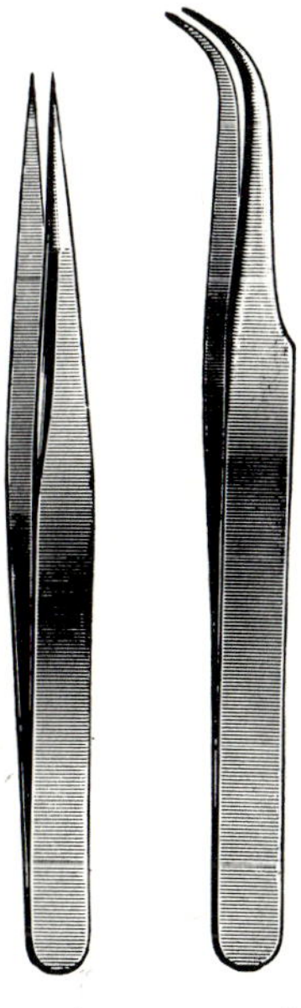

FIG. 50. Storz instrument No. E-1947.

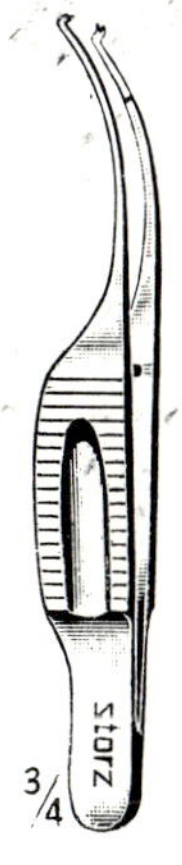

FIG. 51. Storz instrument No. E-3190.

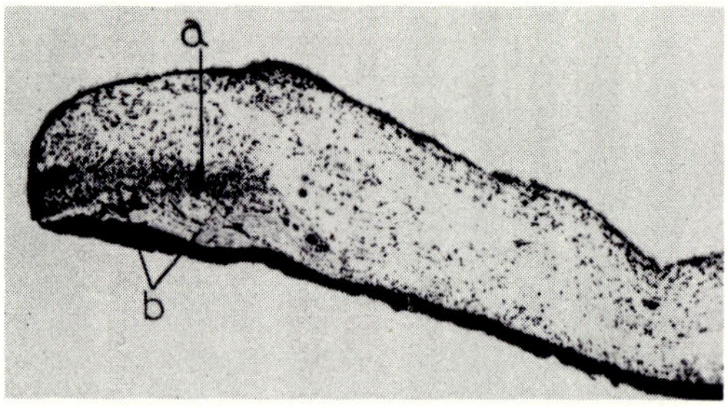

FIG. 52. Senile sclerosis of the pupil. (A) The sphincter muscle. (B) Acquired collagenous fibrous tissue between the sphincter muscle and the pigment epithelium. (Dr. A. B. Reese)

due to sclerosis. In regard to this situation, Dr. Reese says:

> As the round pupil is the rule now, there is more and more an appreciation of the fact that in quite elderly people the iris sphincter may be tight due to so-called sclerosis of the sphincter muscle. As a manifestation of senescence, a gradually increasing layer of collagenous fibrous tissue may interpose itself between the sphincter muscle and the pigment epithelium [Fig. 52]. This sclerosis at this site tends to cause miosis with an inability of the pupil to dilate fully. If at the time of the lens extraction, it is appreciated that the pupil is taut and will not relax due to sclerosis, a small radial incision through the pupillary margin will dilate the pupil adequately to permit the lens to pass through. Such a small nick in the sphincter still permits a postoperative round pupil. A taut sphincter muscle in the absence of sclerosis can be overcome at the time of the extraction by merely holding the lens against the pupillary area until the muscle relaxes. This principle of exerting pressure on a sphincter muscle to promote relaxation is employed elsewhere throughout the body whether it is in the cervix, the rectum or the eye. Therefore, a distinction should be made between a taut sphincter due to muscle tension, and a taut sphincter from sclerosis. The one can

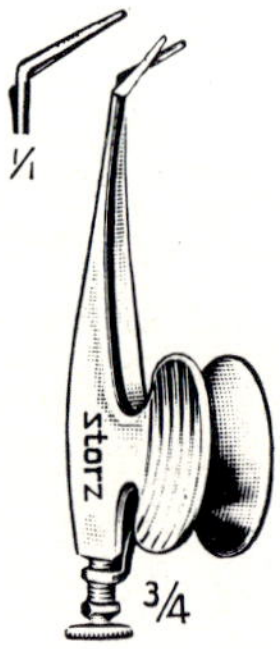

FIG. 54. Storz instrument No. E-3366.

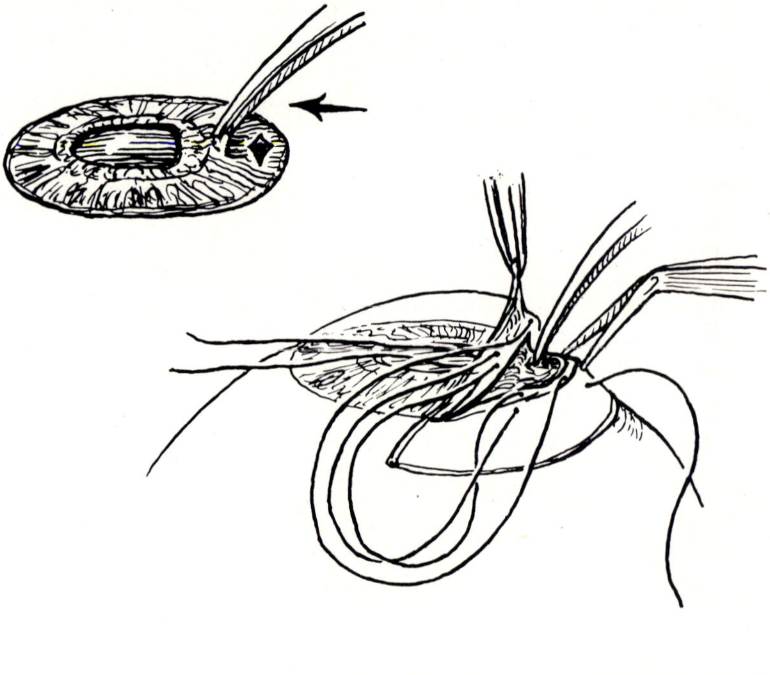

FIGURE 53

(Modified from Paton, Katzin, and Stilwell: Atlas of Eye Surgery, New York, Blakiston)

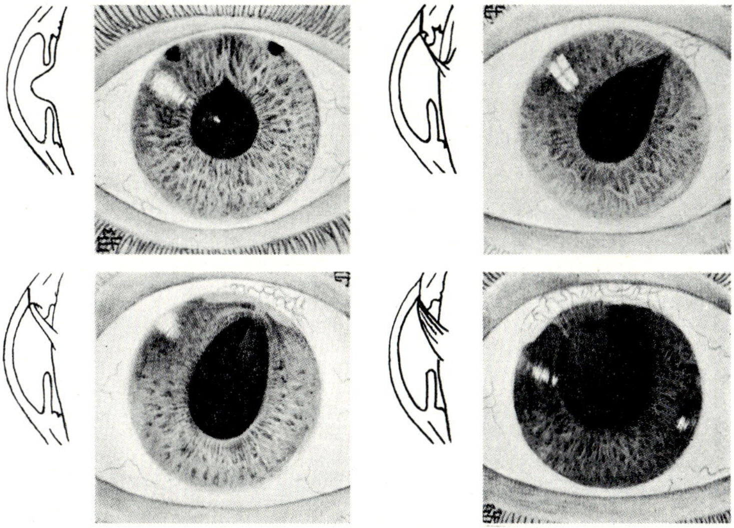

FIGURE 55

(Kirby, D. B.: Advanced Surgery of Cataract, Philadelphia, Lippincott)

be overcome by pressure and the other by a sphincterotomy.[26]

When this was discussed with Dr. Reese, it was mentioned that this diagnosis must be made at the time of surgery. The lens grasp must be released in the case due to sclerosis, and the sphincterotomy must be performed. Of course, this means that following the sphincterotomy the lens must be re-grasped.

If the pupil is too dilated to permit a peripheral iridectomy, stroking the iris with an iris spatula will partially constrict it and make the periphery accessible. Some surgeons will reach up with fine forceps to pull the iris down. Others advocate lifting the corneal or the scleral shelf in this area. The injection of pilocarpine directly into the anterior chamber will constrict the pupil and facilitate a peripheral iridectomy. However, the timing of the extraction of the lens must be such that the pupillary constriction will not impede removal of the lens.

Another approach to making a peripheral iridectomy in the presence of a widely dilated pupil is to perform the iridectomy after the extraction of the lens at which time the pupil is often narrower.

IRIDOTOMIES. Figure 53 shows the procedure used to do a small iridotomy. One method is the utilization of the Barraquer scissors (Fig. 54) without forceps to draw the pupil downward. This accomplishes the same end-result. I have used this technic on occasion and have found it to be excellent. (At present, I am doing peripheral iridectomies only in the young individual who wants to wear a contact lens.)

One of the most beautiful iridotomies or iridectomies that I have ever seen was that in a patient operated on in Holland by the late Dr. Weve. This was a very fine

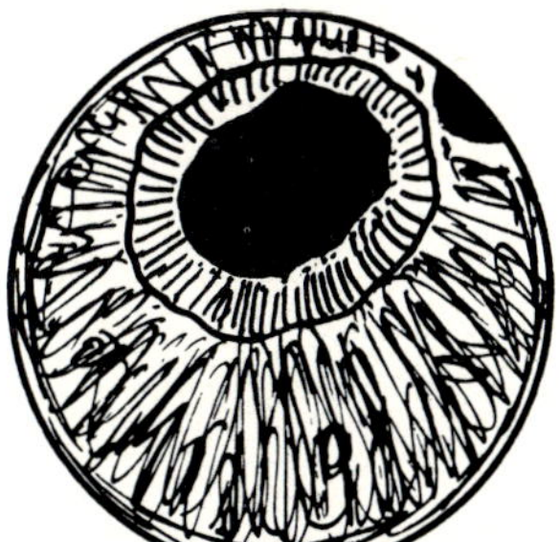

FIGURE 56

(Modified from Guillaumat, Louis, *et al.*: Traitement Chirurgical des Affections Oculaires, Paris, Doin)

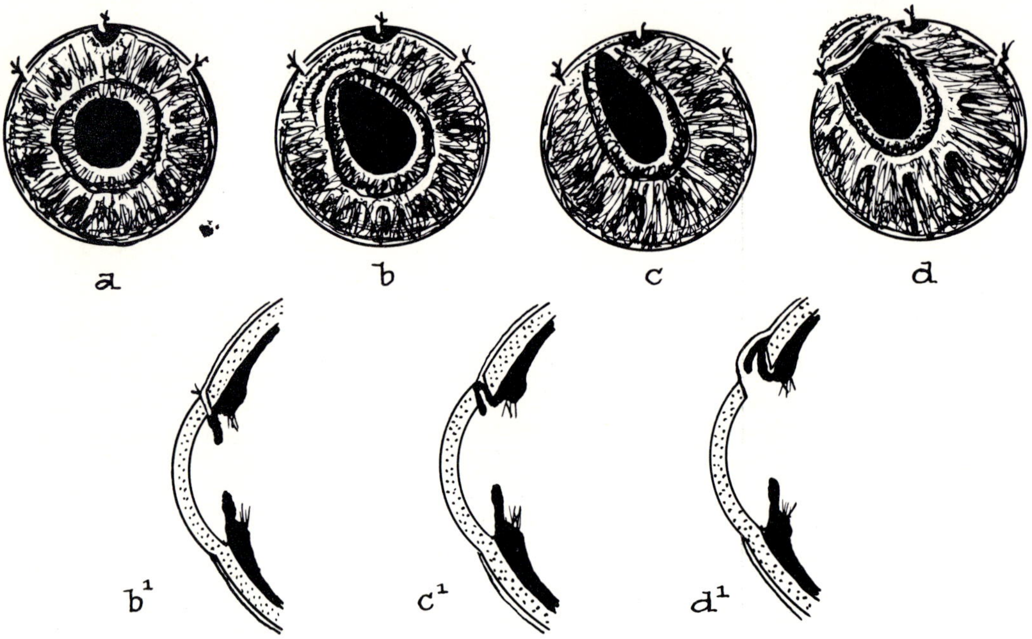

FIG. 57. Successive steps the pupil shows in a case of iris incarceration. (Modified from Guillaumat, Louis, *et al.*: Traitement Chirurgical des Affections Oculaires, Paris, Doin)

vertical iris slit at 12 o'clock. I never knew how Dr. Weve accomplished such a fine end-result, but I later accomplished the same thing by doing an iridectomy of the same nature with fine forceps *after* the lens had been removed and the sutures had been approximated and tied loosely with one knot. However, because of the danger of striking the vitreous, I do not recommend this as a routine procedure.

I am not one who favors a round pupil in every case. Figures 55 to 57 show the final result of some round pupils.

Figure 55 shows what can happen to a round pupil after vitreous is lost. Note that the pupil is no longer round.

In Figure 56 no vitreous has been lost. However, the iris has become adherent to the wound edge. This type of wound often can lead to a flat chamber.

Figure 57 is another view of a similar process in which no vitreous has been lost, but the iris has become adherent to the wound edge. The upper portion of this figure shows the iris in the anterior and the posterior positions and the lower portion shows the incarceration of the iris from a lateral position.

UPDRAWN OR "TEAR-DROP" SHAPED PUPIL can occur very early or not until 2 months or more following uneventful intracapsular extraction. Fortunately, it does not occur frequently.

The principal causes of this complication are thought to be: (1) an incomplete clearing of the wound before closing at the time of surgery; (2) faulty apposition of the wound lips; (3) gaping of the posterior wound lip caused by a tight suture; (4) squeezing after the akinesia of the orbicularis has worn off; and (5) trauma.

Atkinson reports three instances of updrawn or "tear-drop" shaped pupils occurring on the first postoperative day

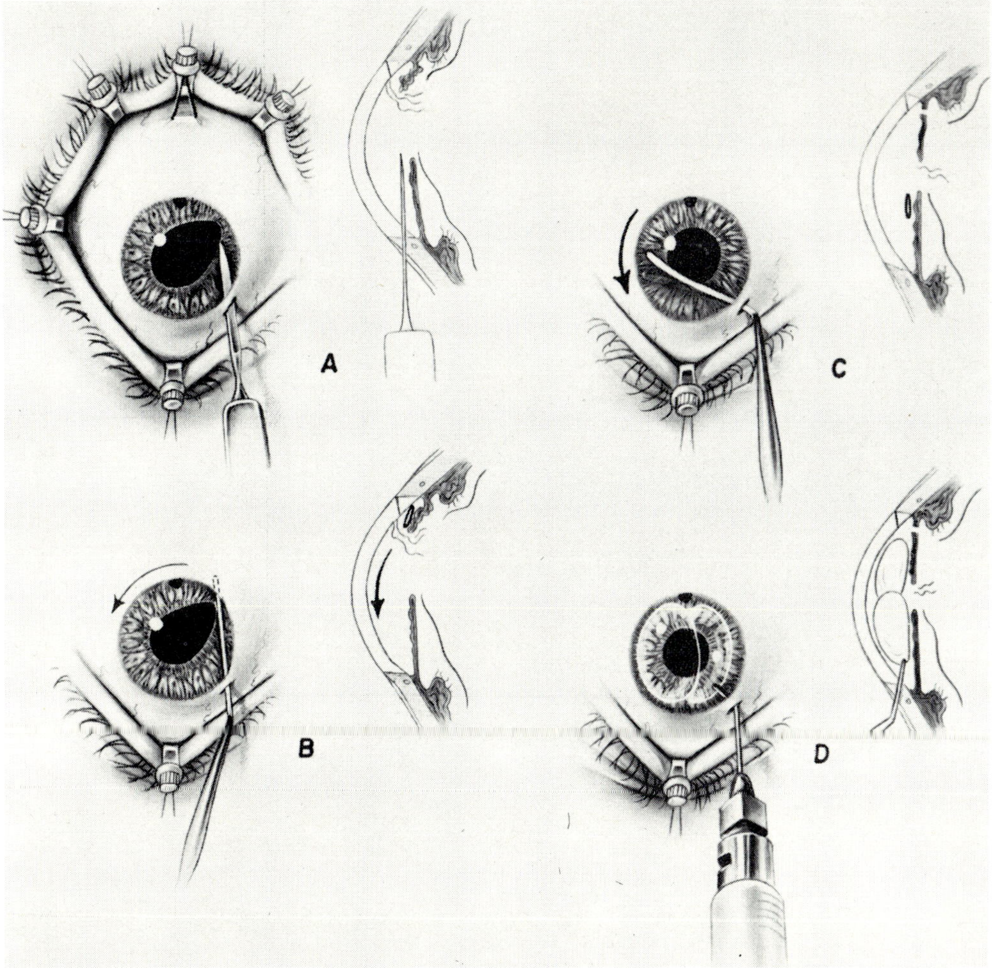

FIG. 58. (A) Slanting incision with Wheeler discission knife. (B) Introduction of a 15 mm. spatula 0.5 mm. wide into the anterior chamber between the vitreous fibers and the deflected iris. (C) Location of the spatula in the opposite direction of the deflected pupil to break the vitreous fibers. (D) Air injection into the anterior chamber. (Dr. Ramon Castroviejo)

following uncomplicated intracapsular extractions. The cause in these three cases was thought to be an adhesion of the iris to the wound or to a strand of the zonule, since slit-lamp examinations 3 weeks later showed the hyaloid to be intact.

In these three cases, Atkinson's operative procedure was as follows:

The same preanesthetic medication is used as for the cataract extraction: pentobarbital sodium (Nembutal) (0.1 gm.), meperidine hydrochloride (Demerol) (75 mg.), Phenergan hydrochloride (12.5 mg.). An hour and a half is allowed for the medication to take effect before the patient is taken to the operating room. Akinesia of the orbicularis is obtained by block of the facial nerve. Tetracaine (Pontocaine) hydrochloride (0.5 percent), epinephrine (1:1000), and pilocarpine (two percent) with hyaluronidase (Wydase) is given under the conjunctiva and Tenon's capsule in the sector corresponding

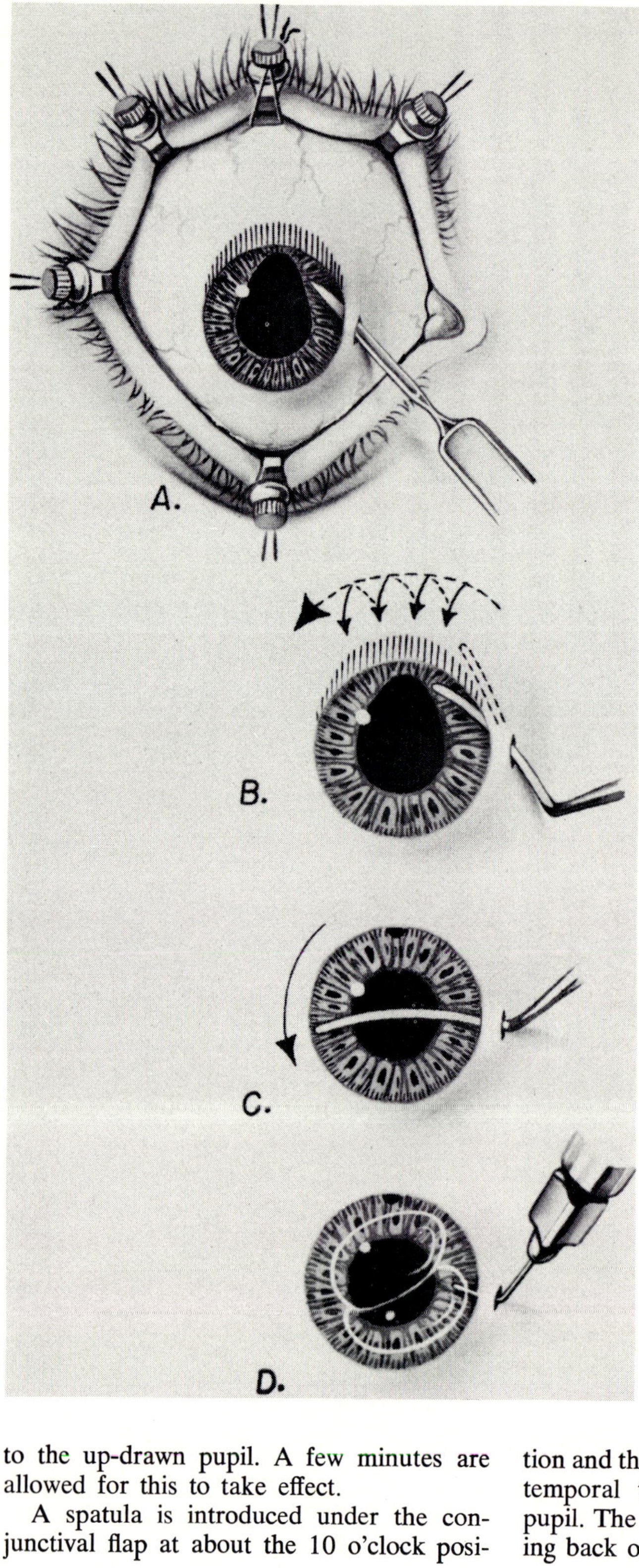

FIG. 59. (A) Slanting incision into the anterior chamber with Wheeler discission knife. (B & C) Cyclodialysis through the anterior chamber with a 15 mm. spatula 0.5 mm. wide. (D) Air injection into the anterior chamber. (Dr. Ramon Castroviejo)

to the up-drawn pupil. A few minutes are allowed for this to take effect.

A spatula is introduced under the conjunctival flap at about the 10 o'clock position and then into the anterior chamber angle, temporal to the point of the "tear-drop" pupil. The spatula is then swept down, pressing back on the iris as is sometimes done at

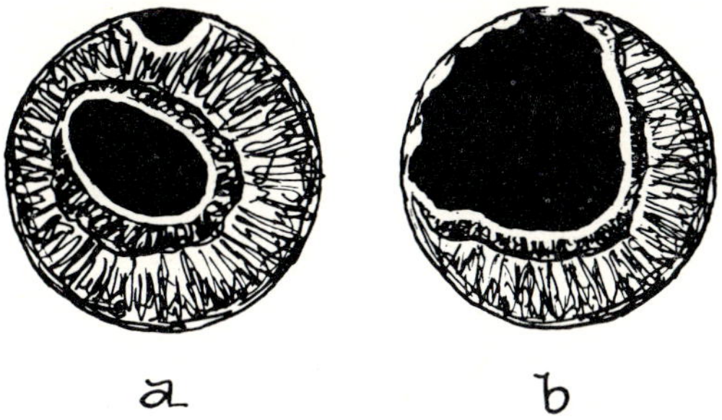

FIG. 60. Successive steps in pupillary deformity after vitreous loss (with peripheral iridectomy). (Modified from Guillaumat, Louis, *et al.*: Traitement Chirurgical des Affections Oculaires, Paris, Doin)

the time of operation to replace the iris. The pupil immediately becomes round and central and the spatula is withdrawn with very little loss of aqueous. Pilocarpine (two percent), eserine (0.25 percent) and Neosporin are then instilled and a monocular dressing applied.

Atkinson also reports two cases of "tear-drop" pupils occurring several months after cataract extraction. (In both these cases the pupils were round and central when examined 2 months postoperatively.) In one instance vision was reduced from 20/20 to 20/40 and in the other from 20/15 to 20/100. The eyes were quiet, and it was felt that

probably a "corepraxy" as advocated by Franceschetti or an iridectomy as reported by Chandler could be used to improve the vision in these eyes.[4]

The late occurrence of the updrawn pupil is an indication that the wound had been opened and is further evidence that the cataract incision requires 2 months or more for firm healing.

With this convincing evidence in regard to the length of time required for firm healing of the cataract incision it would seem advisable to caution our patients in regard to squeezing, rubbing the eye, and other trauma

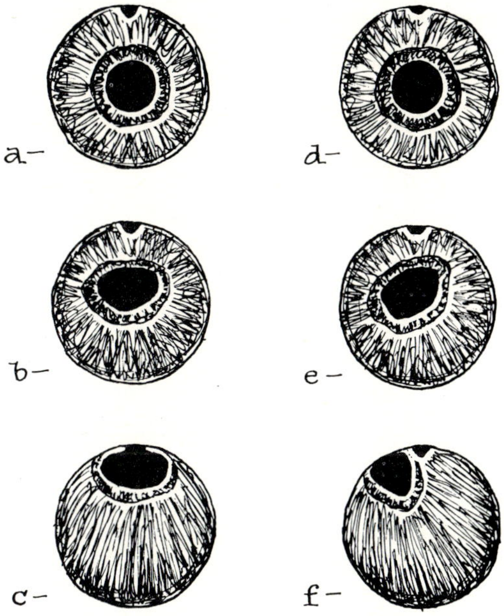

FIG. 61. Steps in the formation of a "hammock pupil" after vitreous loss when the iris had been reposited and the pupil had been centered immediately at the time of surgery. (Illustration shows two different eyes.) (Modified from Guillaumat, Louis, *et al.*: Traitement Chirurgical des Affections Oculaires, Paris, Doin)

for at least three or four months after the operation, possibly longer.[4]

If weeks or months after the cataract operation the pupil has remained deflected, either because of pulling of vitreous fibers attached to the incision or by peripheral adhesions to the incision, the two technics described by Dr. Castroviejo are recommended.[11]

Figure 58 shows the handling of the deflected pupil after cataract surgery in cases where there has been vitreous prolapse with small incarceration of the vitreous into the scar.

Figure 59 shows the maneuver to open the angle through the anterior chamber in cases of peripheral adhesions to the incision after cataract surgery.

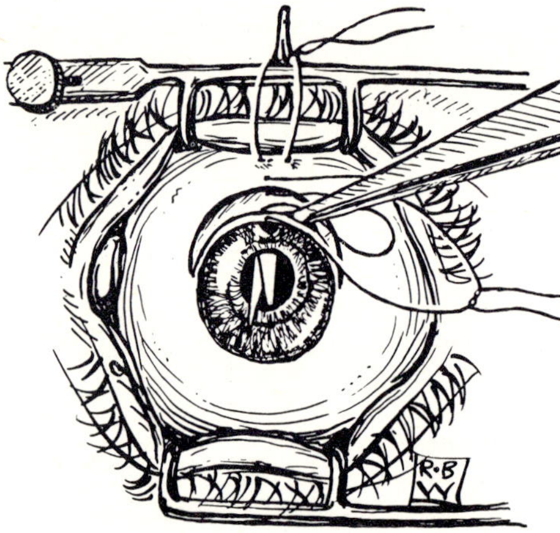

FIG. 62. Cutting of the sphincter of the iris in the lower part when the iris has a marked tendency to prolapse. (Modified from Arruga, H.: Ocular Surgery, Barcelona, Salvat Editores, S. A.)

At the end of the operation miotics are instilled to keep the pupil centrally located (see also Chap. 3 under "Vitreous Prolapse").

Figure 60 shows another round pupil with a peripheral iridectomy that has resulted in a pupil which is no longer round. In some cases the iris can prolapse backward, and glaucoma may follow. At present I know of no satisfactory method of repositing an iris that is prolapsed backward, either immediately or at a later date.

Figure 61 shows the successive stages of ascension of the pupil or a hammock pupil after a loss of vitreous even after the iris has been reduced and moved to the center of the pupil.

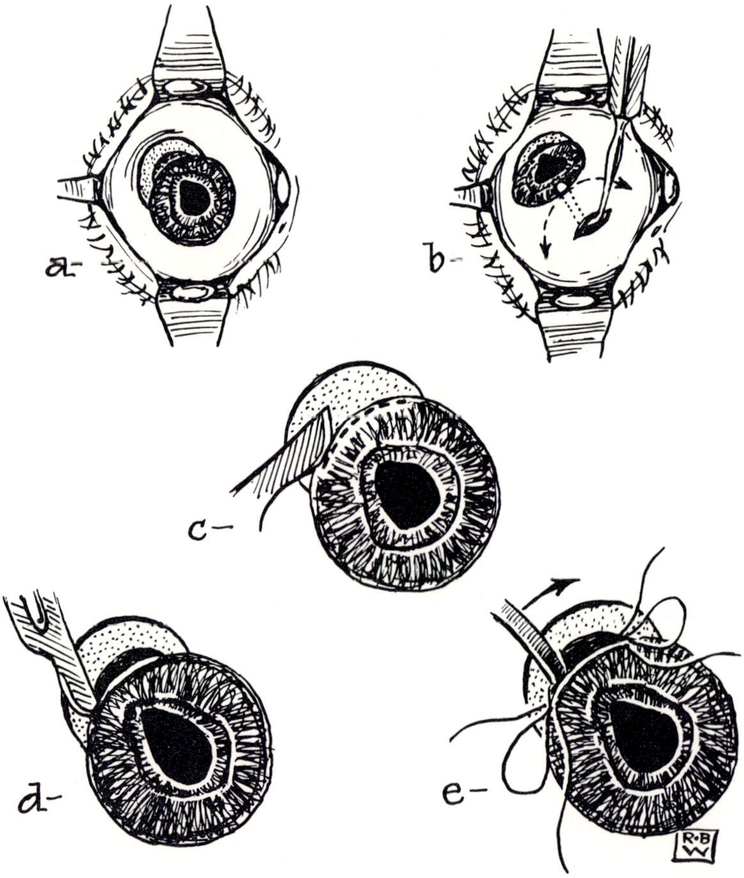

FIG. 63. Resection of a recent iris herniation. (Modified from Guillaumat, Louis, *et al.*: Traitement Chirurgical des Affections Oculaires, Paris, Doin)

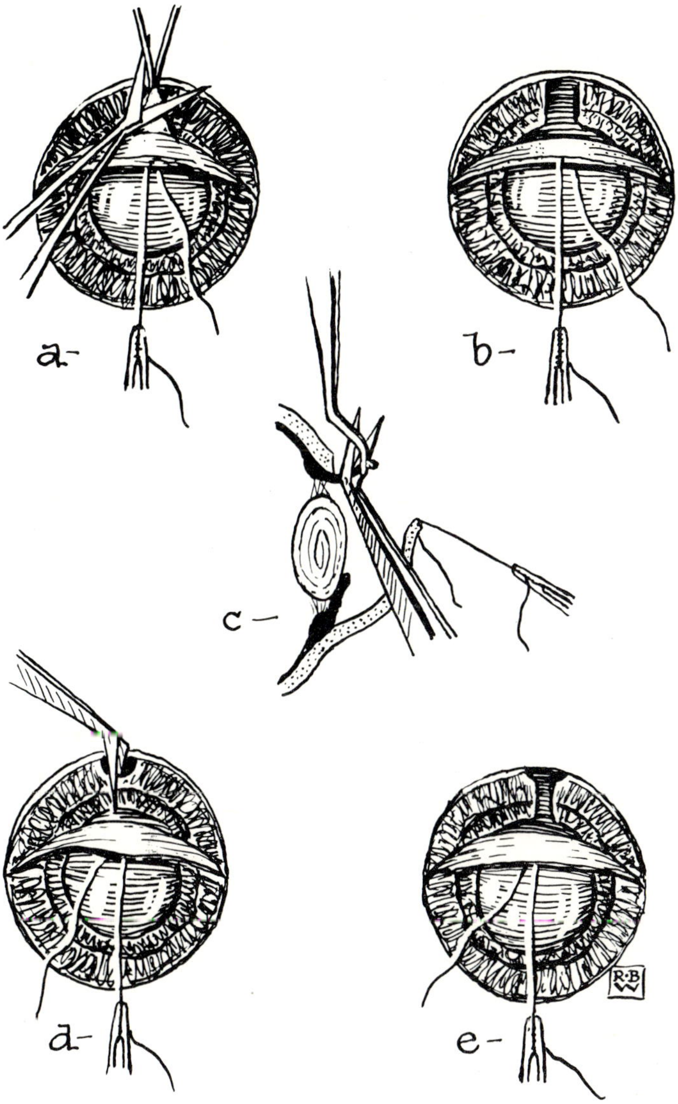

FIG. 64. Total iridectomy. (Modified from Guillaumat, Louis, *et al.*: Traitement Chirurgical des Affections Oculaires, Paris, Doin)

Figure 62 shows what to do if the iris has a tendency to prolapse when a round-pupil extraction is attempted. It might be wiser to convert a round pupil to one with a total iridectomy. Some will disagree with this.

Figure 63 shows other steps that may be taken if there is an iris prolapse after a round pupil. Section B in this figure shows a cyclodialysis done below in an effort to avoid subsequent glaucoma. Some would not use this approach.

Technic of Full Iridectomy. When asked about his technic of making a full iridectomy, a fine surgeon was quoted as saying, "I just grab the iris and cut away."

Figure 64 shows a way of creating a total or full iridectomy. A shows the usual technic, and B shows a beautiful keyhole type of full iridectomy which many surgeons do not accomplish. C shows a lateral view of the method of doing this type of iridectomy. A colleague of mine very often obtains this type of iridectomy. His

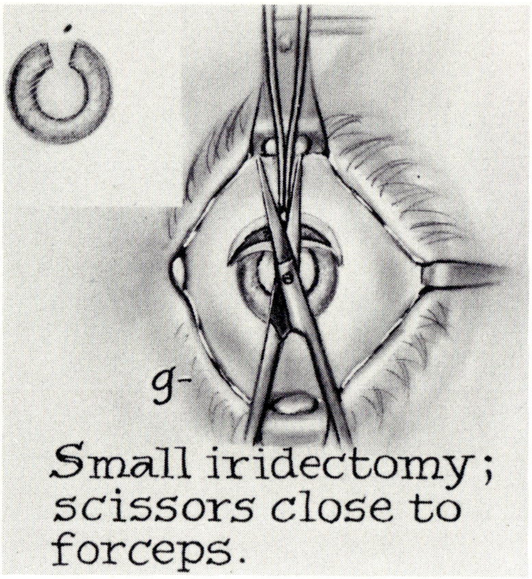

FIG. 65. Small iridectomy; scissors close to forceps. (Berens, C., and King, J. H.: An Atlas of Ophthalmic Surgery, Philadelphia, Lippincott)

trick for doing so is to make a small corneal incision, doing the iridectomy immediately afterward. However, this can be dangerous in that it is possible to cut the upper portion of the iris when inserting

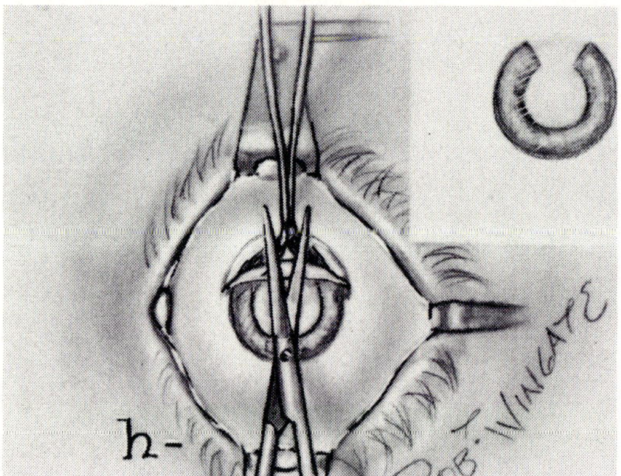

FIG. 66. Larger iridectomy; scissors away from forceps. (Berens, C., and King, J. H.: An Atlas of Ophthalmic Surgery, Philadelphia, Lippincott)

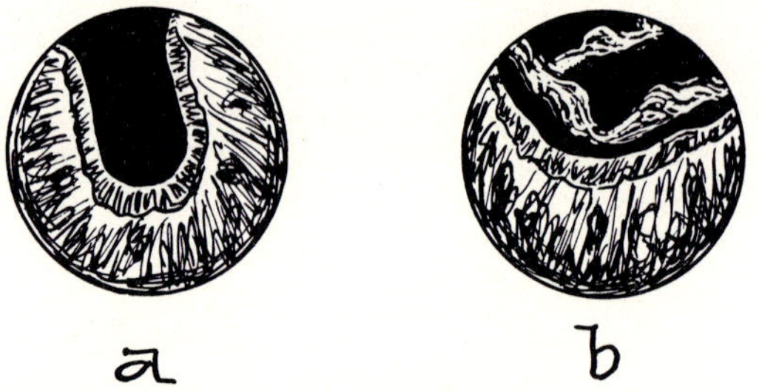

FIGURE 67

(Modified from Guillaumat, Louis, *et al.*: Traitement Chirurgical des Affections Oculaires, Paris, Doin)

the scissors for enlarging the corneal section. If one is not careful, vitreous will present at the same time. Another method of performing a small iridectomy is to grasp the iris in the middle position with fine forceps and then to cut with the scissors close to the forceps (Fig. 65). A larger iridectomy will result if the scissors are away from the forceps (Fig. 66).

If one wishes to create a total iridectomy and to have a fine looking pupil, an iridectomy above followed by the insertion of the scissors (as shown in Fig. 64, D) can result at times in an iridectomy like the one shown in Figure 64, E.

Two narrowly separated cuts of the iris

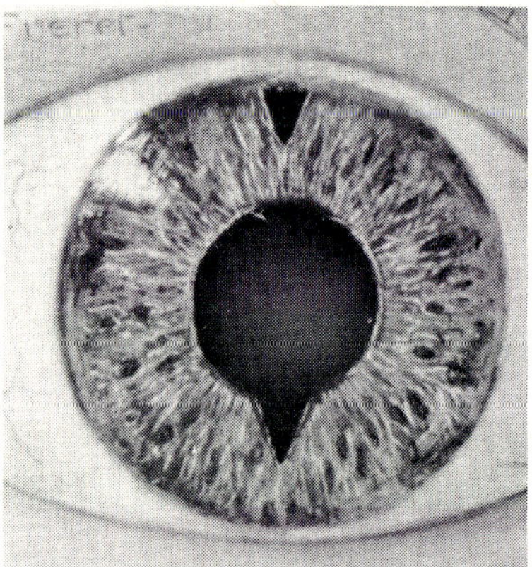

FIGURE 68

(Kirby, D. B.: Advanced Surgery of Cataract, Philadelphia, Lippincott)

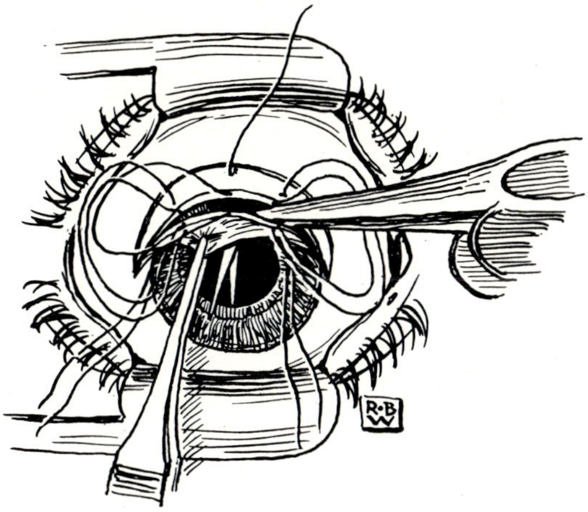

FIGURE 69

(Modified from Paton, Katzin & Stilwell: Atlas of Eye Surgery, New York, Blakiston)

followed by tearing the iris between these cuts is another method of making a fine keyhole slit. If there is a need for a full iridectomy in a case with glaucoma or suspected glaucoma, the tearing of the iris need not be "basal" to the extent that it will damage the ciliary body and start serious hemorrhage.

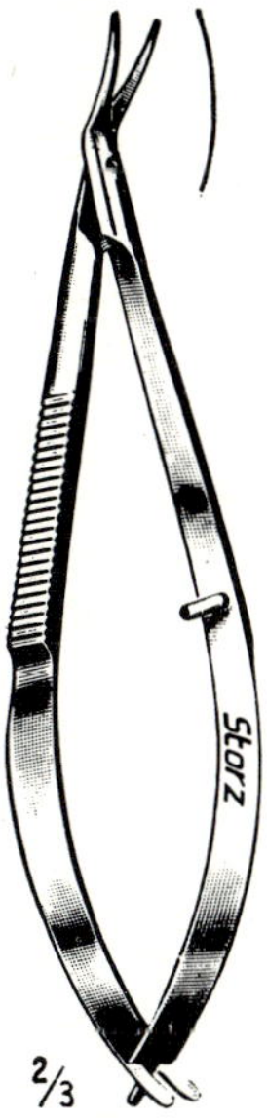

FIG. 70. Anterior synechia scissors, Castroviejo (Storz instrument No. E-3324).

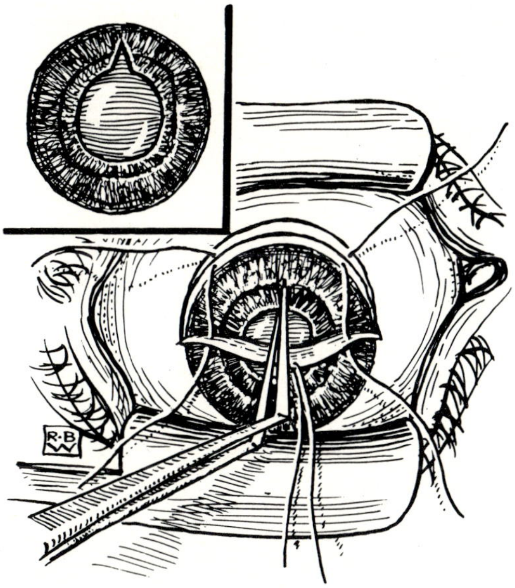

FIG. 71. In some cases, a central radial iridotomy above will suffice to provide access to the lens capsule above and adequate space for the delivery of the cataract. This may well be placed below if the surgeon plans to tumble the lens after a grasp of the capsule below. (Modified from Kirby, D. B.: Advanced Surgery of Cataract, Philadelphia, Lippincott)

Unfortunately, the end-result of a complete iridectomy can look like that shown in Figure 67, B. This is especially so if vitreous has been lost.

Figure 68 shows the appearance of an eye following the removal of a complicated cataract. Note the 12 o'clock peripheral iridectomy with a radial iridotomy at 6 o'clock.

Figure 69 shows the method used to perform the radial iridotomy at the 6 o'clock position. This combination would be indicated in order to avoid a subsequent hammock pupil. The anterior synechia scissors are excellent for the vertical iridotomy below (Fig. 70).

Previously, I performed approximately half of my cataract cases with round pupils and half with iridectomies or iridotomies. However, my feeling now is that both the surgeon and the patient will be happier in the long run with some form of full iridectomy or vertical iridotomy. The one real exception here is in the young person who wants to wear a contact lens.

Figure 71 shows a vertical or radial iridotomy at the 12 o'clock position. This is an ideal type of pupil, since, with the lid in position, it looks similar to a round pupil and does not have the cosmetically displeasing appearance of a badly performed total iridectomy. This has sometimes been described as the "pear type" of iridotomy of Verhoeff. This type of central, radial iridotomy will provide access to the lens capsule above if a capsule forceps is used and will create adequate space for the delivery of the cataract. This type of iridotomy may also be placed below.

RADIAL IRIDOTOMY. Both ends of my Barraquer scissors have been rounded for performing the radial iridotomy above. I use rounded scissors with a long corneal curve for the iridotomy below (see Fig. 70).

Dr. Michael John Roper-Hall has summarized beautifully the indications for radial iridotomy:

1. To prevent up-drawn pupil due to inflammation in extractions complicated by:
   a. Iritis and iridocyclitis.
   b. Following glaucoma operations.
   c. Where this has occurred in the other eye.
2. To prevent up-drawn pupil due to vitreous loss in extractions complicated by:
   a) Subluxation or dislocation of lens.
   b) Excessive myopia.
   c) Where this has occurred in the other eye.
3. To give access to the lens by widening the pupil when:
   a) It fails to dilate from any cause (senility, diabetes, iris atrophy, heavy pigmentation).
   b) An intumescent lens causes disproportion.
   (Performed at 6 o'clock or by completing an iridotomy at 12 o'clock.)
4. As a means of preventing pupillary block particularly in narrow angle glaucoma and where pupil block has occurred in the other eye.[28]

Summary and Conclusions. To summarize the preference for iridectomies or iridotomies over round pupils, the advent of alpha-chymotrypsin has made no essential changes in the surgery of the iris in cataract extraction. Derrick Vail says that he favors the ". . . complete iridectomy in all but selected cases . . . The fetish of the round pupil is one that needs, in my opinion, courageous scrutiny, reappraisal, honest criticism and evaluation."[38]

Townes showed that "eyes with complete iridectomies have fewer complications and heal more quietly than eyes with peripheral iridectomies." Also, surprisingly enough, he found no statistically significant difference in visual results.[31]

Those surgeons who favor the round pupil (and most do) repeatedly say that it is more normal and physiologic and acts as a natural barrier when there is vitreous loss. However, in terms of the patient's vision, especially when the pupil is decentered under the upper lid, in terms of glaucoma and permitting aqueous to flow readily between the anterior and the posterior chambers and in terms of the difficulty the surgeon experiences in finding holes in detachments following cataract surgery, the round pupil may likewise be considered a "natural" barrier.

However, it must be remembered that there are some very fine surgeons who use no iridectomy whatsoever—that is, a cataract extraction without an iridotomy or iridectomy. They feel that when the wound is adequately sutured there will be no iris prolapse and that the eye, except for the absence of the lens, is the most natural in appearance and in terms of function. In most cases my own personal preference is a compromise between a full iridectomy and a round pupil with peripheral iridectomies.

Tendency for Iris Prolapse

The question has often been asked, "What can the surgeon do when after opening the anterior chamber, he is confronted with the lens and the vitreous bulging forward and the iris threatening to prolapse?"

When I am presented with this situation, my first step is to determine whether the superior rectus muscle is playing a part in the problem; I do this by loosening the suture through this muscle. If the iris prolapse persists, I will check my lid clamps. (As a rule, I do not use a speculum for cataract surgery.)

If the local anesthesia is not adequate, I will consider supplementing it with intravenous Demerol or barbiturates. At this point one may (1) repeat it, or (2) do an iridectomy or its equivalent and proceed with the next steps if the situation seems to be under control. However, two other courses have been suggested. (1) If urea was not given preoperatively, the wound can be closed and urea can be given intravenously. (2) An iridectomy may be performed; the eye then is closed, and the cataract is extracted at a later time under more favorable conditions.[36]

If the iris continues to prolapse after the above steps and if I have planned a peripheral iridectomy, my own preference is a full or complete iridectomy. Under these circumstances, I will choose a sliding technic as opposed to a tumbling procedure in the extraction of the lens and will not use alpha-chymotrypsin.

If the situation is not well controlled after all of these steps have been taken, then I will go on to an extracapsular extraction with a complete anterior capsulectomy.

Iris Pigment Loss With the Use of Alpha-Chymotrypsin

When I first began to use alpha-chymotrypsin in the early stages of its use in this country, I noted an excess amount of pigmentation. This would occur after I irrigated the enzyme under the iris with a sweeping motion of the cannula to ensure even distribution throughout the zonular areas. The pigmentation resembled that which is seen in some diabetics at the time of cataract surgery when alpha-chymotrypsin is not used. I wrote to Dr. Barraquer asking whether he felt that this was due to a mechanical or a chemical defect. He replied that he thought it was largely due to mechanical processes but possibly was related to the particular batch of alpha-chymotrypsin I had been using. At that point I obtained a new supply of the enzyme and modified my technic so that the cannula, after being introduced at the 6 o'clock position, was no longer swept around the iris, and found that the enzyme would diffuse itself.

Dr. Barraquer's latest recommendations in minimizing this pigmentation include: (1) the use of a fine cannula with a blunt tip; (2) two-hand control of the injection (Dr. Barraquer steadies the cannula with a forceps in the other hand); and (3) slight pressure away from the iris pigment and toward the lens, followed by gentle irrigation of the enzyme.

Since modifying my technic with the cannula, I have not noticed this complication. However, it should be emphasized that the cannula must not be introduced so deeply that it may rupture the hyaloid membrane or injure the ciliary body.

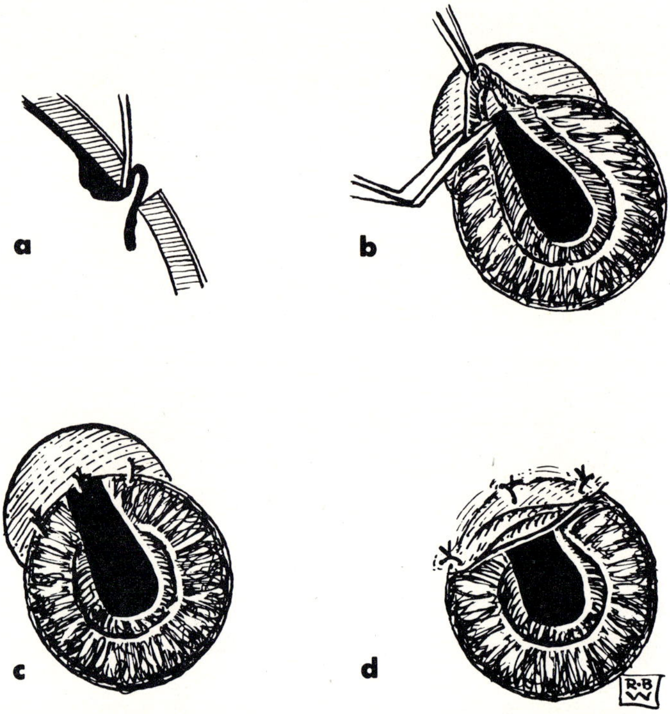

FIG. 72. Resection of a recent iris herniation. (Modified from Guillaumat, Louis, *et al.*: Traitement Chirurgical des Affections Oculaires, Paris, Doin)

IRIS PROLAPSE (RECENT)

If the iris prolapse is less than ½ mm. and is covered by conjunctiva, some feel that it might be best to leave it alone. However, if it is greater than ½ mm. and is increasing in size, it is a surgical and not a medical problem. A thick conjunctival flap should be created if possible, the iris excised, the wound edges curetted if necessary and the wound resutured with chromic sutures. Some feel that every iris prolapse is an emergency and, since both the patient and the surgeon are apprehensive, the repair should be done under general anesthesia. This is especially true following round pupil extractions. If one waits, the iridectomy necessarily will have to be larger.

Figure 72 illustrates a round pupil that has been converted to one with a total iridectomy following a recent iris prolapse. There are some who feel that strong miotics can reduce some of these recent prolapses. However, I have never seen a case in which this has actually been accomplished.

The instillation of pilocarpine into the anterior chamber immediately after the extraction of the lens may help to prevent some of these small iris prolapses. Some feel that when this occurs in the patient with an irregular pupil, he should be taken back to surgery on the first postoperative day. The few iris prolapses that I have encountered in surgery occurred when I first began to use alpha-chymotrypsin. In those cases, I brought the patient back to the operating room the following day and made a complete iridectomy in the area where the iris had prolapsed.

IRIS PROLAPSE (LATE)

Figure 73 shows one method of repairing an old iris prolapse which occurred following a round pupil. The upper por-

FIGURE 73

(Modified from Guillaumat, Louis, *et al.*: Traitement Chirurgical des Affections Oculaires, Paris, Doin)

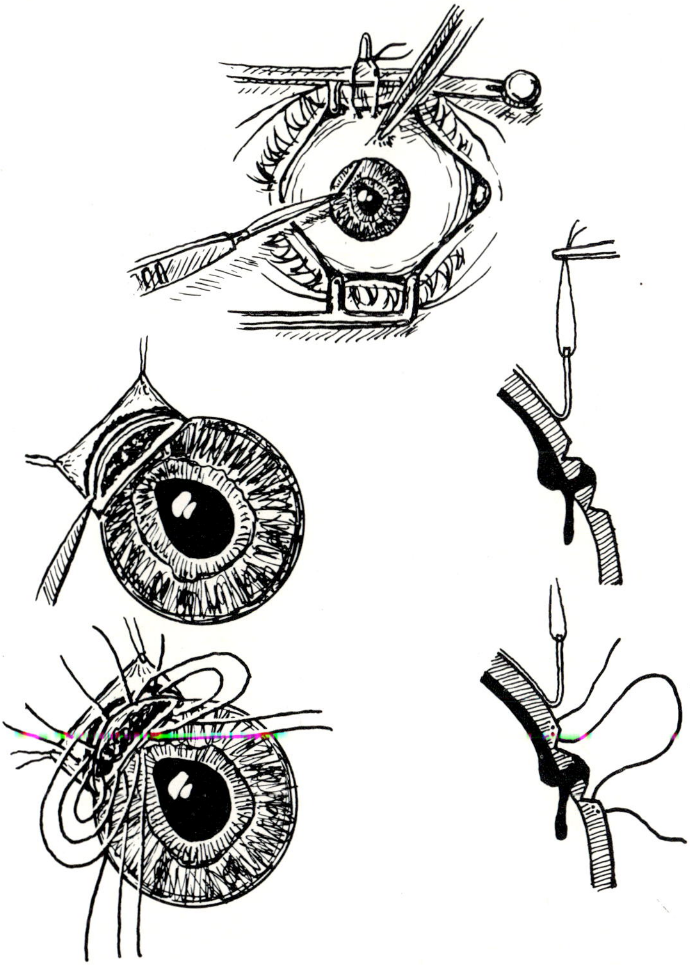

tion of this figure shows the dissection of the iris away from the wound edge. A needle-knife is most helpful here, especially if an extracapsular extraction has been performed. The capsule will help to hold back the vitreous while the wound edge is being repaired. Figure 73 also shows a lateral view of this procedure, and Figure 74 shows a more detailed picture of the final results.

HAMMOCK PUPIL

The operation that I favor for hammock pupil after the loss of vitreous is the creation of an opening through the iris with the keratome from below, followed by an optical iridectomy with the iris forceps. There are many modifications of this procedure.[12]

As is shown in Figure 75, the keratome enters the anterior chamber with a slanting incision. Figure 76 shows the iris grasped by smooth forceps passed through the slanting incision. It is a wise idea to have several pairs of forceps on hand. A Hess forceps is also very good for this maneuver if one must get over the shelf created by the slanting incision.

An iridectomy done close to the cornea and the forceps is illustrated in Figure 77.

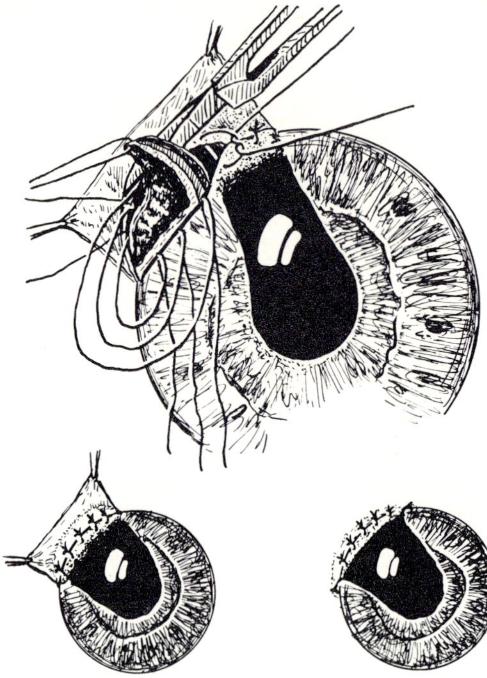

FIGURE 74

(Modified from Guillaumat, Louis, *et al.*: Traitement Chirurgical des Affections Oculaires, Paris, Doin)

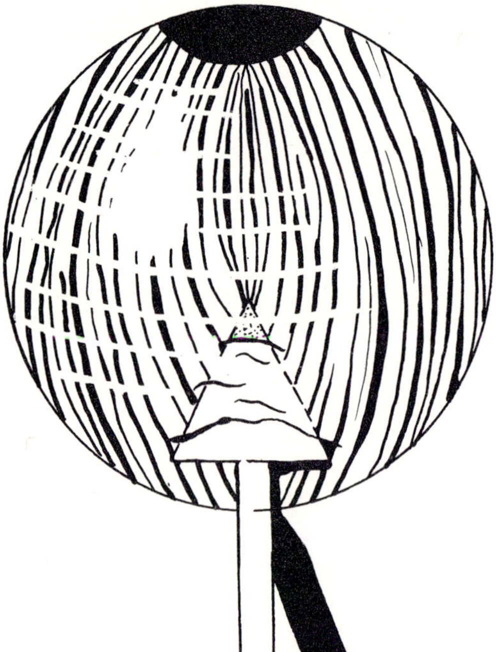

FIG. 75. Keratome entering the anterior chamber with a slanting incision. (Patterson *in* Fasanella: Management of Complications in Eye Surgery, Philadelphia, Saunders)

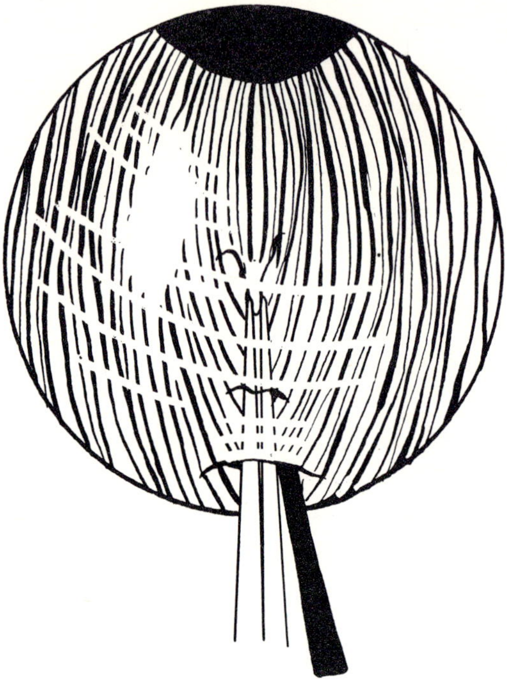

FIG. 76. The iris grasped by smooth forceps passed through the slanting incision. (Patterson *in* Fasanella: Management of Complications in Eye Surgery, Philadelphia, Saunders)

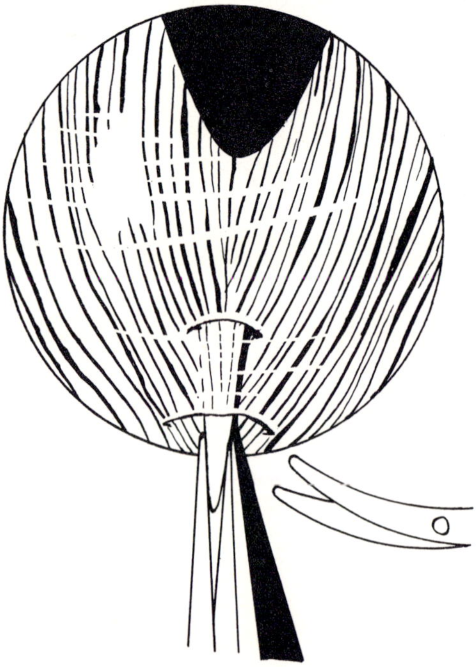

FIG. 77. Iridectomy done close to cornea and forceps. (Patterson *in* Fasanella: Management of Complications in Eye Surgery, Philadelphia, Saunders)

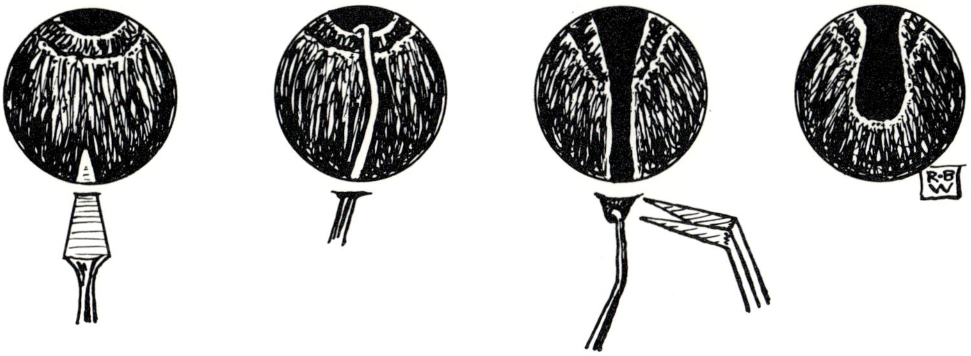

FIG. 78. Technic of Franceschetti for updrawn pupil. (Modified from Arruga, H.: Ocular Surgery, Barcelona, Salvat Editores, S. A.)

FIG. 79. (*Top*) Updrawn pupil with two keratome incisions at 5 and 7 o'clock at the limbus. (*Bottom*) Iris hook passed through incision parallel to the iris, grasping the iris at the pupil margin. (Patterson *in* Fasanella: Management of Complications in Eye Surgery, Philadelphia, Saunders)

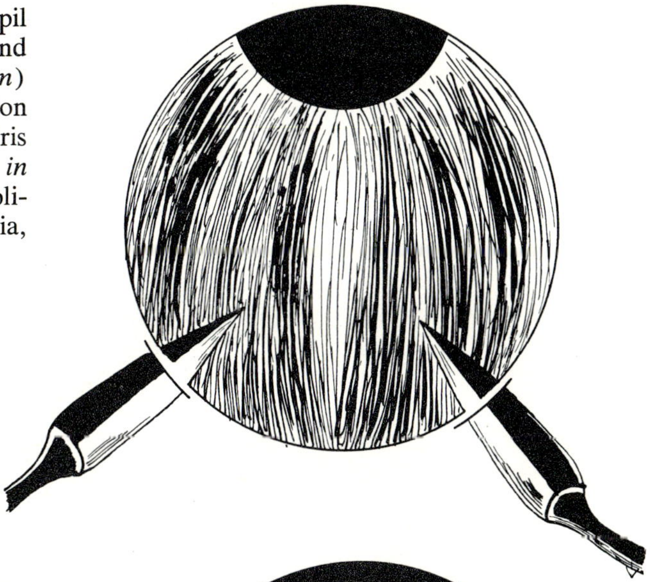

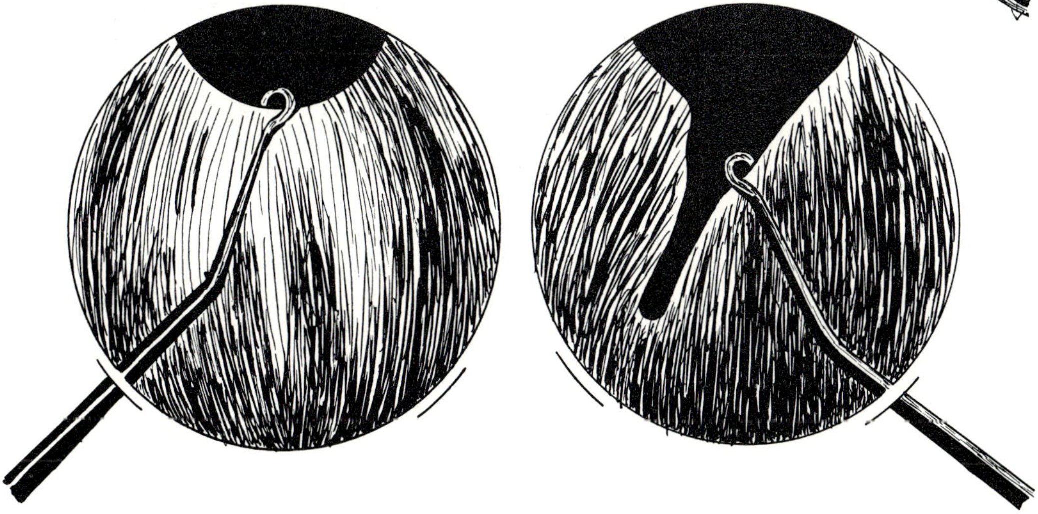

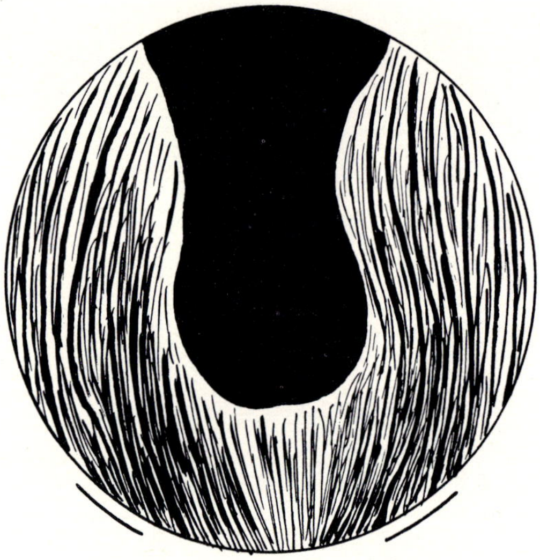

FIG. 80. Resultant pupil. (Patterson *in* Fasanella: Management of Complications in Eye Surgery, Philadelphia, Saunders)

One technic utilizing a hook and creating a typical iridectomy is shown in Figure 78. A typical iridectomy is also created with two keratome incisions as noted in Figures 79 and 80.

Figure 81 shows an updrawn pupil with two keratome incisions at 5 and 9 o'clock at the limbus. The central pupil and the capsule remain.

Today we are able to create a central opening like this with the light coagulator. My experience with this is the same as that noted by others—it is not always successful. First, there must be sufficient space between the cornea and the updrawn pupil or the iris to use the light coagulator. Otherwise, one can burn a hole through the cornea. The injection of saline into the anterior chamber can over-

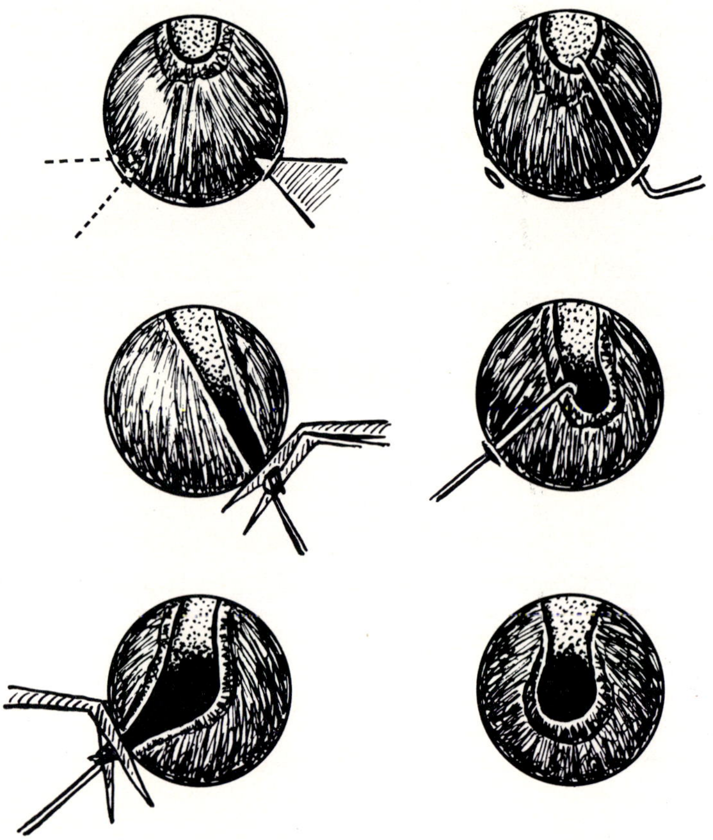

FIG. 81. Coropraxy, Franceschetti technic. (Modified from Guillaumat, Louis, *et al.*: Traitement Chirurgical des Affections Oculaires, Paris, Doin)

come this problem. Secondly, the cornea must be clear. Thirdly, secondary membranes and vitreous opacities behind the iris contraindicate the use of the light coagulator. By using the coagulator, there is less chance of causing hemorrhage in cases of rubeosis. With the coagulator there is no loss of vitreous or atrophy of the globe.

At the present time, there are two steps necessary to create the pupil with the use of the light coagulator. A high intensity of current must be used to make the first opening through the iris. If this penetrates both layers of the iris, it will often be accompanied by a popping noise as the opening is made. A barrage of four to five contacts around the central opening then should follow. The intensity of the light coagulator for these steps is much less than that for the initial opening. However, occasionally, an opening is made through only one layer of the iris. At times the vitreous face in this area is opaque and, in spite of an opening, no true vision can be obtained. Local cortisone, preferably in the form of drops, must be used every 2 hours. Mydriatics as well are helpful.

REFERENCES

1. Ackerman, A. L.: The action of urea in acute glaucoma, Am. J. Ophthal. *52*: 875, 1961.
2. Arruga, H.: La compresión pre-opertoria del ojo para obtener su hioptonia al extraerla catarata, Presented at the Sociedad Oftal., Hispano-Americana, Cordoba, 1959.
3. Atkinson, W. S.: Anesthetic complications *in* Fasanella, R. M. (ed.): Management of Complications in Eye Surgery, Philadelphia, Saunders, 1957.
4. ——: Correction of updrawn or "teardrop" pupil, Am. J. Ophthal. *47*:227, 1959.
5. ——: Symposium: Surgical management of cataracts, New York Eye and Ear Infirmary Alumni Meeting, April 10, 1962.
6. Barraquer Annals *3*:146, 1962.
7. Barraquer, Joaquin: Advances in surgery of the crystalline lens, Lecture Presented at the American Academy of Ophthalmology and Otolaryngology, Chicago, 1961.
8. ——: Iridectomias e iridotomias. Indicaciones y technica, An. Inst. Barraquer *3*:146, 1962.
9. Boyd, B. F.: Congenital cataracts—modern concepts, Highlights Ophthal. *4*:255, 1961.
10. Castroviejo, Ramon: Symposium: Complications of cataract surgery, New York Eye and Ear Infirmary Alumni Association, April 9-12, 1962.
11. ——: Personal communication.
12. Chandler, P. A.: Iridectomy for drawn-up pupil, Am. J. Ophthal. *36*:1253, 1953.
13. Dunnington, J. H.: Symposium: Complications of cataract surgery, New York Eye and Ear Infirmary Alumni Association, April 9-12, 1962.
14. Estrada, W. D.: Incisions and closures in cataract surgery, Ophthalmologia Ibero Americana *22*:24, 1961.
15. ——: Operative and postoperative complications related to the incision, An. Inst. Barraquer *3*:94, 1962.
16. Girard, L.: The problems of intracapsular cataract extraction in infants and children, III Curso Inter. Oftalmol., p. 145, May, 1961.
17. Jude, J. R., Kouwenhoven, W. B., Ing, and Knickerbocker, G. G.: Cardiac arrest, J.A.M.A. *178*:1063, 1961.
18. Kaplan, Morris: Personal communication.
19. Katzin, H. M., and Teng, C. C.: Personal communication.
20. Kirsch, R. E., and Steinman, W.: Digital pressure, an important safeguard in cataract surgery, A.M.A. Arch. Ophth. *54*:697, 1955.
21. McGarry, Isabelle: Annual review: glaucoma, A.M.A. Arch. Ophth. *66*: 871, 1961.

22. McLean, J. M.: Discussion: Incisions and sutures, An. Int. Barraquer *3*:122, 1962.
23. ——: Personal communication.
24. ——: A new corneoscleral suture, A.M.A. Arch. Ophth. *23*:554, 1940.
25. Martin, S. J.: Management of sudden cardiac collapse, Anesthesiology *27*: 738, 1961.
26. Reese, A. B.: An appraisal of the current trend in cataract surgery (Montgomery Lecture), Ireland, 1962.
27. Roper, K. L.: Preoperative care of the cataract patient, Inter. Ophth. Clinics *1*:563, 1961.
28. Roper-Hall, M. J.: An. Int. Barraquer *3*:153, 1962.
29. Scheie, H. G.: Incision and closure in cataract extraction, A.M.A. Arch. Ophth. *61*:431, 1959.
30. Schmidt, Kurt: Personal communication.
31. Shoch, David: A technique of cataract extraction, Inter. Ophth. Clinics *1*:585, 1961.
32. Sugar, H. S.: Extraction of cataract in glaucomatous eyes, III Curso Inter. Oftalmol., p. 261, May, 1961.
33. ——: Personal communication.
34. Swan, K. C.: Basal iridectomy for prevention and treatment of persistent shallow chamber after cataract extraction, Eye Digest, p. 5, Jan., 1958.
35. ——: *In* Clark, W. (ed.): Symposium on Glaucoma, St. Louis, Mosby, 1959.
36. Symposium: Complications of cataract surgery, New York Eye and Ear Infirmary Alumni Association, April 9-12, 1962.
37. Tarter, R. C., and Linn, J. G.: A clinical study of the use of intravenous urea in glaucoma, Am. J. Ophthal. *52*: 323, 1961.
38. Vail, Derrick: Inter. Ophth. Clinics, *1*:viii, No. 3, 1961.
39. Weinberger, H. A., van der Woude, R., and Maier, H. C.: Prognosis of cortical blindness following cardiac arrest in children. J.A.M.A. *179*:134, 1962.
39a. Weiss, *et al.*: A.M.A. Arch. Ophth. *68*: 341, 1962.
40. Yudkin, Arthur: Personal communication.

3

Problems Related to the Lens Extraction

VOMITING

It has already been mentioned that prior to the cataract extraction, nausea can be counteracted by the administration of oxygen and more sedation (barbiturates) or antiemetics. If vomiting occurs, the patient's head should be turned so that the operated eye is up and away from the vomitus. If vomitus should enter the eye before the lens has been removed, the eye should be irrigated, the wound should be closed, and further surgery should be postponed. If vomitus enters

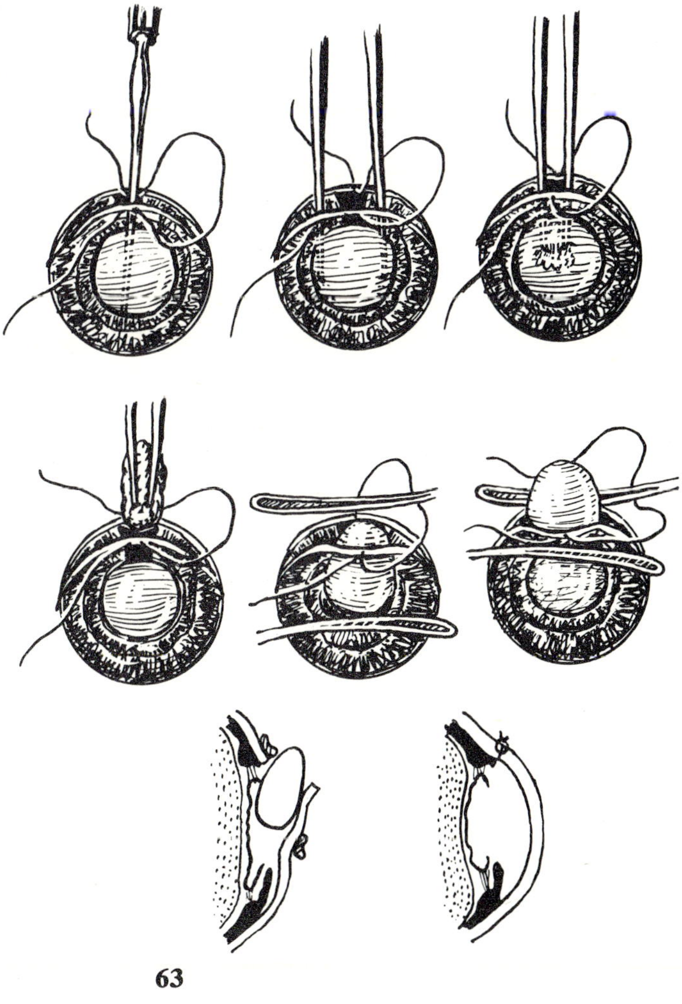

FIG. 82. Extracapsular extraction. (Modified from Guillaumat, Louis, *et al.*: Traitement Chirurgical des Affections Oculaires, Paris, Doin)

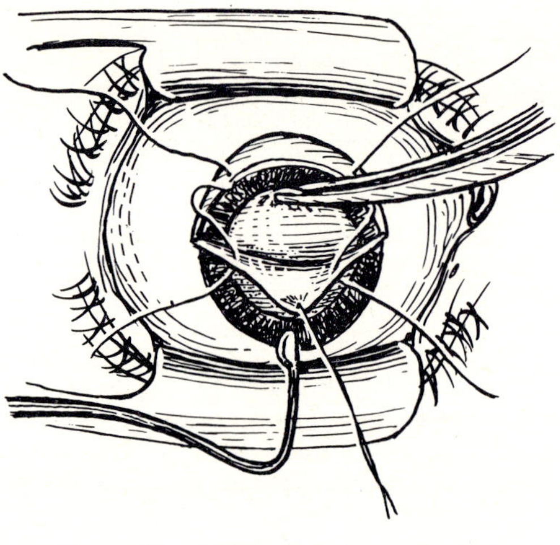

FIG. 83. Simultaneous contrapoint pressure is used to tilt the upper pole of the lens forward and to steady the lens for the upper pre-equatorial grasp of the capsule. The upper pole of the lens then is elevated and carried forward and downward by the forceps, as the point of the hook is insinuated into the limbus ring to hold the eye below or to make countertraction against the traction of the forceps. (Modified from Kirby, D.: Advanced Surgery of Cataract, Philadelphia, Lippincott)

the eye after removal of the lens, the eye should be irrigated and antibiotics should be started.[11]

EXTRACAPSULAR OR INTRACAPSULAR EXTRACTION

The main advantage of alpha-chymotrypsin is that it has increased the number of intracapsular extractions. However, if a surgeon is satisfied with extracapsulars or with his percentage of intracapsulars without the enzyme, he need not use alpha-chymotrypsin. Another conservative approach would be to use alpha-chymotrypsin in those selected cases where there are no contraindications and where the surgeon feels that he could not otherwise accomplish intracapsular extractions. Unfortunately, it is somewhat difficult to select these cases beforehand.

While visiting many of the eye clinics in Europe, I was surprised to find that many surgeons were doing the extracapsular type of extraction as a matter of routine. In Ireland, I asked a surgeon why he was doing extracapsulars, and he replied that he did them because he noted a great incidence of late herniation of vitreous following many of his intracapsulars with round pupils which he previously had done routinely. In some of these cases, he had done peripheral iridectomies and iridotomies. Unfortunately, a large number of these cases resulted in postoperative secondary glaucoma or late macular changes. He felt that the posterior capsule would protect against secondary glaucoma and macular changes due to late vitreous herniation following intracapsular extraction. Therefore, he reverted back to a well-planned extracapsular extraction (Fig. 82).

A very famous surgeon, who would prefer that I don't mention his name, told me that if he personally were to be operated on, he would want a well-planned extracapsular type of extraction. He has performed many of the most complicated intracapsular types of operation.

My former chief, who performed beautiful intracapsular extractions in almost every case, used to say to me, "I agree that if the sequence of events in the discovery of how to do a cataract extraction were such that the intracapsular had been discovered first, everyone, I feel, would be doing that 'wonderful,' safe, carefully performed extracapsular type of extraction."

One of the most recent arguments in favor of doing well-planned extracapsulars was presented at the Will's 1962 con-

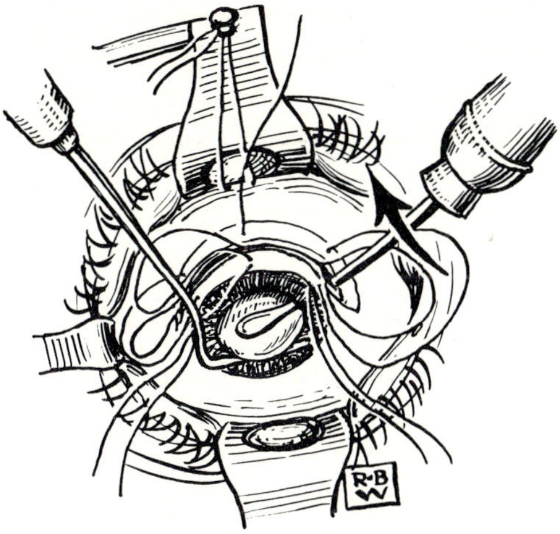

FIG. 84. More than half the zonule has been ruptured, and tumbling continues. (Modified from Paton, Katzin & Stilwell: Atlas of Eye Surgery, New York, Blakiston)

ference, where it was noted that there was a greater incidence of clear corneal grafts following this type of cataract extraction.

I myself prefer to do intracapsular extractions but will do a well-planned extracapsular in selected cases.

SLIDING VS. TUMBLING AND ALPHA-CHYMOTRYPSIN

Figure 83 shows the sliding technic. Figure 84 shows the tumbling technic. Sliding and tumbling continue to be another favorite source of argument among eye surgeons. There are still arguments in favor of both. In a recent letter Dr. Edmund Spaeth remarked:

> As to tumbling, I do not do it, it can be responsible for damage to the endothelium and *does* not facilitate extraction when using a forceps or erisophake—its real purpose, historically, is with the external pressure technique (*Smith Indian Principles*) to tuck the cornea in back of the lens, and it does predispose to vitreous prolapse and hyaloid damage. [See Figs. 85-87.]

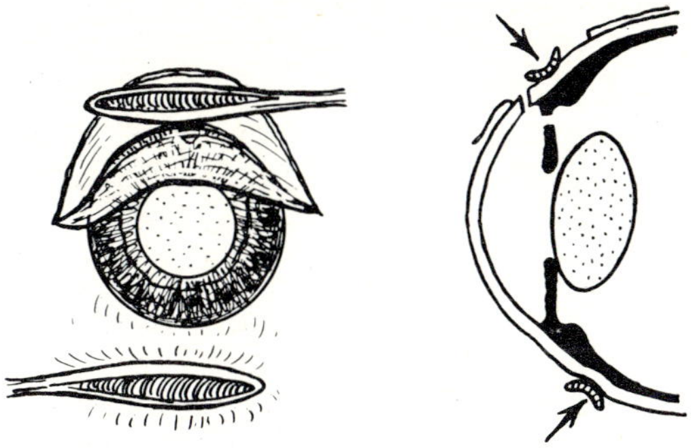

FIG. 85. A form of extraction of the lens by the Smith-Indian method. (Modified from Barraquer, Joaquin: An. Inst. Barraquer *2*:63, 1961)

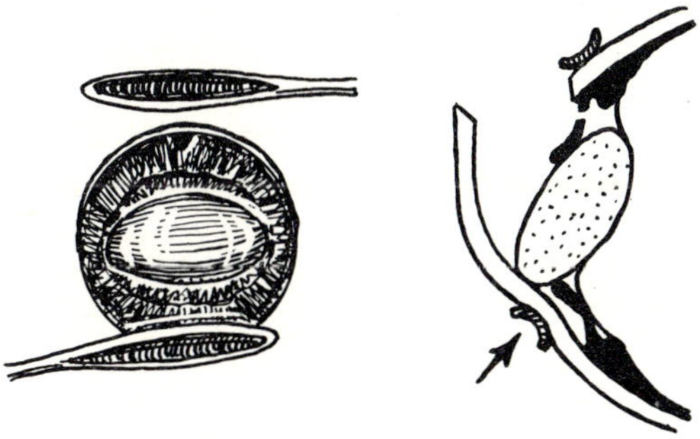

FIG. 86. Turning of the lens in the Smith-Indian method. (Modified from Barraquer, Joaquin: An. Inst. Barraquer *2*:63, 1961)

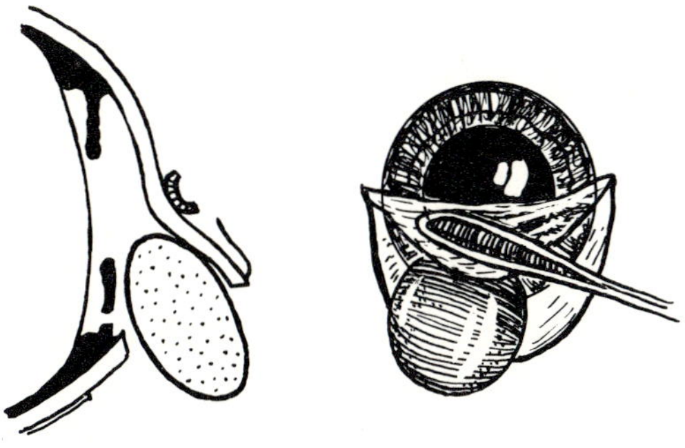

FIG. 87. Final step of the extraction. (Modified from Barraquer, Joaquin: An. Inst. Barraquer *2*:63, 1961)

Some of the best eye surgeons have changed from tumbling to a routine slide, while others have done just the opposite. In this country there has been a greater tendency to use the sliding technic since the advent of alpha-chymotrypsin. A fine German surgeon who performs very beautiful cataract extractions—intracapsulars with round pupils as a rule—remarked to me that he feels that there is always greater control in doing a sliding procedure; it is perhaps more difficult to perform, but if the surgeon gets into trouble, he can get out of these troubles more easily from a sliding position than he can from a tumble.

Dr. Salleras uses alpha-chymotrypsin in many cases. He slides or tumbles depending on the situation at the time of removal of the cataract. If the chamber is shallow, he prefers to slide rather than to tumble so that he will not damage the endothelium.[16]

In tumbling, there is a tendency (especially with the Bell erisophake) to break suction when the lens is pointing vertically or is just about to be delivered. Twisting the erisophake in one's fingers as shown in Figure 84 can help to prevent losing the contact of the erisophake at this point. Pressure through the cornea and pressure with the erisophake on the lens in a sense sandwiches the lens between the cornea and the erisophake. By removing the lens gradually one is able to avoid breaking the contact of the erisophake at this time.

In tumbling, one can be in very serious trouble when the zonules have broken below, the lens is pointing vertically upward, and vitreous is starting to present. The surgeon is in less trouble if the hook or the loop is still in contact with the cornea, as he can continue to tuck. A greater problem, whether or not alpha-chymotrypsin is used, is when the lens is hinged above and pointed vertically downward. In this particular situation, I know of no ideal solution. Some have suggested introducing a very small loop from the side and using this to steady the lens while it is regrasped with the erisophake or the capsule forceps. Fortunately, this situation is rare.

The lens may be completely dislocated with the use of alpha-chymotrypsin, but the mechanics of the delivery of the lens are thereby altered. However, by changing one's technic somewhat, these new mechanics can be managed adequately. Some surgeons feel that the use of the motor-driven erisophake is ideal with the use of alpha-chymotrypsin because no backward pressure need be exerted on the lens to initiate the grasp, especially if the lens is completely dislocated. In actual practice, the use of a small amount of the enzyme irrigated below with the head slightly elevated, thereby preventing the enzyme from reaching the upper zonules, will provide for a hinge above if one chooses to tumble.

In tumbling, especially with alpha-chymotrypsin, there is a greater danger of damaging the corneal endothelium, creating a striate keratitis and causing a dystrophy to progress. However, the greatest argument against this stand, which is taken by most American ophthalmologists, is that Dr. Joaquin Barraquer still will tumble routinely, unless he encounters a flat or a hard lens.

Dr. Barraquer feels there will be no more damage to the cornea than is usual if: (1) the corneal wound is large—180° to 200°, and (2) one avoids contact with the corneal endothelium and the excess alpha-chymotrypsin is washed out from the wound edge.[4]

I have noted no difference in the

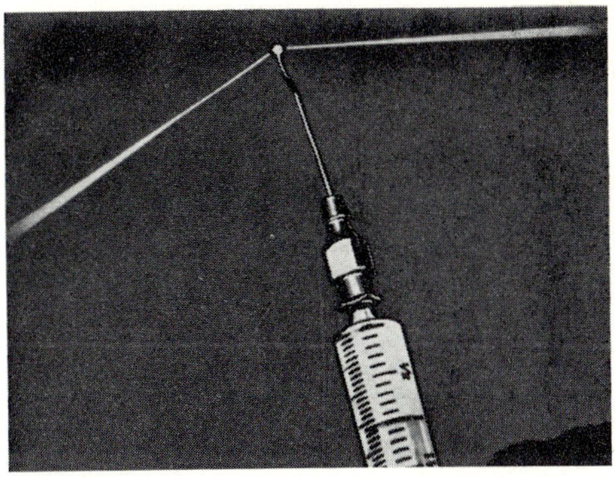

FIG. 89. Roper cannula. (Roper, K. L.: The Cataract Operation: A Study of Details, Am. Acad. Ophth. and Oto-laryng., 1961)

amount of damage to the corneal endothelium with the use of the Bell erisophake. To overcome this problem, the erisophake is applied to the lens surface at the end of approximately 1 minute and the forward displacement of the lens usually takes place at 2 minutes. The erisophake is held under the iris at the 6 o'clock position and after another minute the tumbling is started. Another method of avoiding endothelial damage is to inject a small amount of alpha-chymotrypsin (1 or 2 drops) in the position in which one desires to tumble. In most cases, the important step in removing a lens, whether it be a slide or a tumble, is the initial breaking of fibers. In a sense, this can be likened to tearing a thick paper-backed book. If one starts the tear through the middle of the book, it is relatively easy then to tear the book in two. With one or two drops of alpha-chymotrypsin in the area where one wants to start to tear the zonules, the excess will not damage the corneal endothelium. Likewise, it is relatively easy after this to extract the lens either by sliding or tumbling.

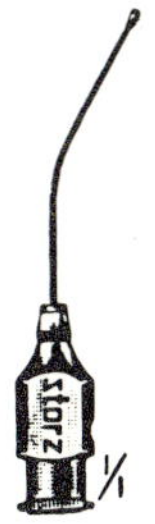

FIG. 88. Alpha-chymotrypsin cannula, Troutman (Storz instrument No. E-4414).

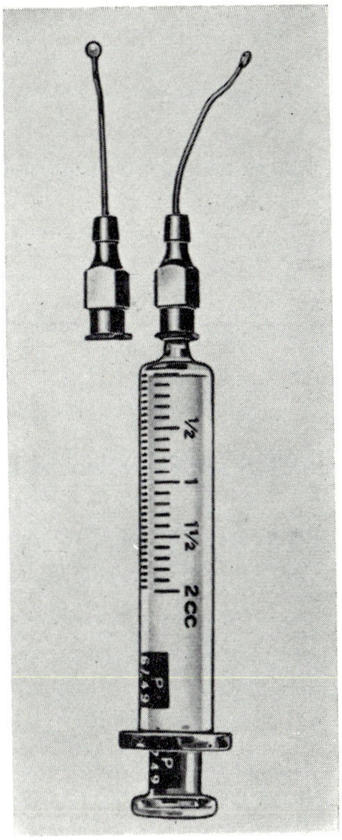

In mass cataract surgery in India, the routine use of a minimal amount of alpha-chymotrypsin (0.25 ml.) and the removal of the lens without washing out the excess solution was reported as not harmful to the eye and also as a great help in the surgery. There was a 2-minute waiting period during which an iridectomy was performed.[13]

ALPHA-CHYMOTRYPSIN IRRIGATING CANNULAS

A choice of cannulas for injecting alpha-chymotrypsin has been introduced.

My preference is a soft, rounded silver type which was purchased at the Barraquer Clinic. I feel that there is even less chance of rubbing off iris pigment with this than there is with the Troutman or the Roper cannulas. Troutman's cannula is very fine and is designed with an olive-like ending for introduction of the enzyme with minimal trauma to the intraocular structures (Fig. 88).

The Roper cannula (Fig. 89) has a flattened, round, symmetrical tip similar to the tip of Callahan's zonule stripper which eliminates an accidental tear of the anterior lens capsule or of the iris itself. The two openings at the sides of the flattened tip give a gentle diffusion of the solution both clockwise and counter-clockwise from the 2, the 6 and the 10 o'clock positions. Adequate irrigation of the superior zonules is obtained without having to introduce the tip through a peripheral iridotomy or iridectomy opening.

When using these cannulas it must be remembered that the tip should not be advanced so far that the hyaloid membrane may be ruptured or the vitreous is dislodged. However, the tip must be inserted far enough so that the enzyme solution will be sprayed across the fibers of the zonular ligament attached to the anterior capsule.

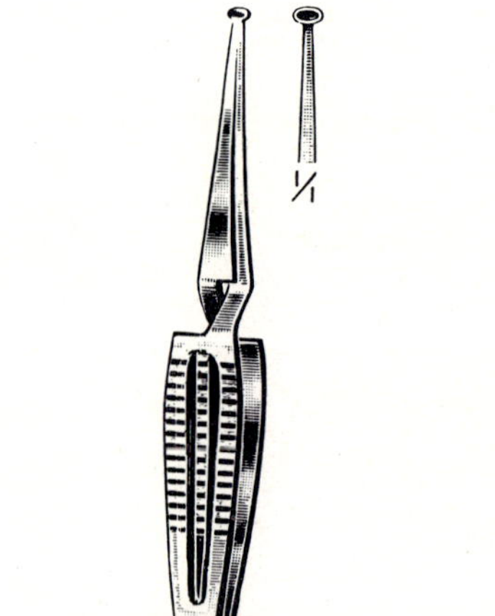

FIG. 90. (*Top*) McLean cross-action forceps (Storz instrument No. E-3304). (*Bottom*) Bell erisophake with rubber bulb (Storz instrument No. E-4840).

CAPSULE FORCEPS VS. ERISOPHAKE AND ALPHA-CHYMOTRYPSIN

The capsule forceps and the erisophake each have a definite place in cataract surgery, and one should become adept in using both. As Dr. Castroviejo pointed out, the mechanics of the forceps and the erisophake are essentially the same; the only difference is the bite on the capsule.[9]

Retrobulbar anesthesia, hyaluronidase and massage have made the eye softer. Because of this the lens is now somewhat more difficult to grasp than it was previously, but by exerting pressure on the external portion of the eye the lens will move forward, making it easier to grasp. When applying the erisophake on the lens one should allow a few seconds for it to "set." Both the erisophake and the capsule forceps should be carefully inspected before applying them.

Since the advent of alpha-chymotrypsin, most American ophthalmologists prefer the capsule forceps rather than the erisophake because they feel that there is less danger of creating endothelial damage. Forceps have been designed for use in sliding procedures, especially when alpha-chymotrypsin is used. These forceps have a cross-action principle to remove any tenseness from the fingers after the upper portion of the lens is grasped and, at the same time, grasp the upper portion of the capsule more adequately (Fig. 90, *left*). Dr. Arruga uses capsule forceps as a rule, and the Barraquers use the erisophake. The surgeon has his choice of a Bell type of erisophake (Fig. 90, *right*), modifications of this type, or one controlled electrically. I prefer the Bell erisophake and routinely use a balanced solution to fill it.

When using the Bell erisophake for a very mature lens, it is wise to expel only about one half of the air or the balanced solution in the erisophake. Suction in the Bell erisophake is generated by the amount of fluid or air in the rubber bulb. The elasticity of the bulb is important. If there is too little suction, the erisophake will come off; if there is too much suction, the capsule may rupture. One should err on the side of creating too little suction. It has been pointed out that filling the bulb of the Bell erisophake with solution rather than air for the autoclaving process will be a greater safeguard. Some feel that the erisophake is especially indicated for intumescent and morgagnian type cataracts, since there is less chance for the capsule to rupture. I sometimes prefer a modification of the Smith-Indian technic when removing a very mature lens with the use of alpha-chymotrypsin. This modification, I feel, lessens the danger of the loss of vitreous and at the same time is the best technic for removing the lens intracapsularly. If the capsule is strong and more complete suction is desired, the air or the balanced solution in the Bell erisophake must be expelled completely. Sometimes, unknown to the surgeon, particles of rub-

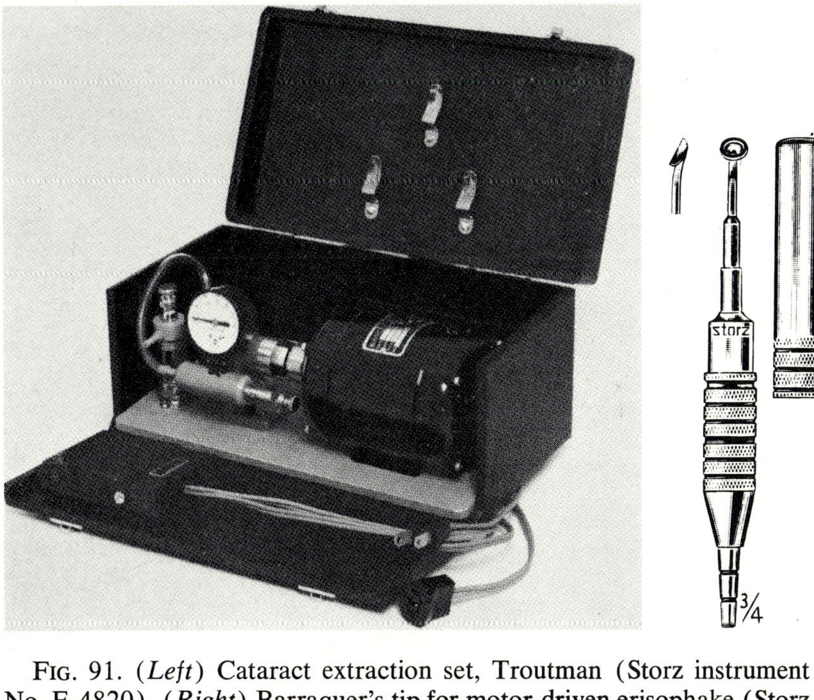

FIG. 91. (*Left*) Cataract extraction set, Troutman (Storz instrument No. E-4820). (*Right*) Barraquer's tip for motor-driven erisophake (Storz instrument No. E-4862).

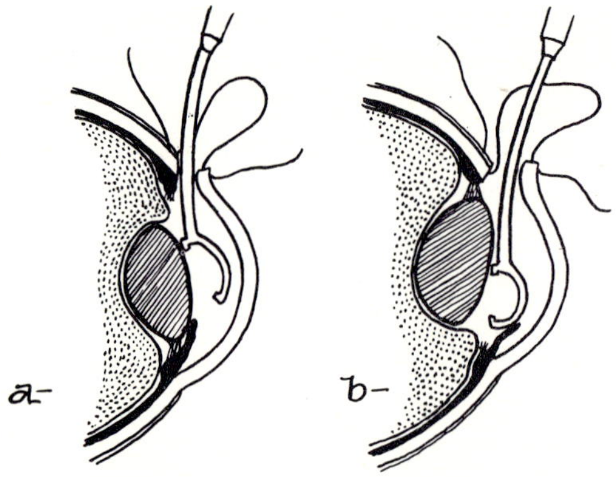

FIG. 92. Incorrect application of the erisophake. (Modified from Guillaumat, Louis, *et al.*: Traitement Chirurgical des Affections Oculaires, Paris, Doin)

ber can be extruded into the anterior chamber. For this reason, prior to actual use, the Bell erisophake should first be filled with a balanced solution, washed out and then refilled with a fresh balanced solution. The edges of the Bell erisophake must be examined carefully, for, if they are dented, suction can break easily. If suction is broken easily, a new rubber bulb might be tried. Another cause for breaking suction may be an accumulation of fine residues on the edges of the erisophake. Since soaking or brushing these surfaces is not always effective, fine emory has proved to be advantageous. One of the problems that I have noted with the Bell erisophake is that oil from the Post's solution used for sterilizing the instruments makes it difficult to catch the bulb and rotate it in one's fingers unless the excess is rubbed off.

I prefer not to have a curved handle on my Bell erisophake, as I tumble the lens entirely with motion in my fingers. As a rule, this is done from the 9 to the 12 o'clock position in the right eye and from the 12 to the 3 o'clock position in the left eye.

With the use of the motor-driven erisophake very little counterpressure is required; often no counterpressure is used at all. This is perhaps ideally used in conjunction with alpha-chymotrypsin because some downward pressure must be exerted when the Bell erisophake or one of its modifications is used. However, to overcome this complication when using alpha-chymotrypsin, I apply the erisophake before complete zonulolysis has taken place. In my first cataract extraction with alpha-chymotrypsin I feared that the lens might become dislocated posteriorly, and it oc-

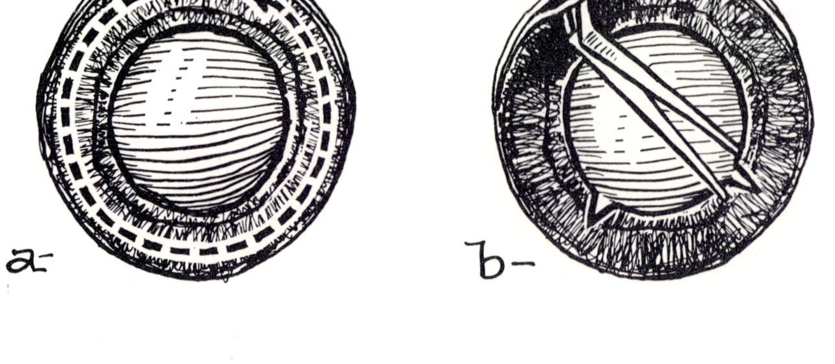

FIG. 93. Cataract extraction after an iridocyclitis, Barraquer's technic. (Modified from Guillaumat, Louis, *et al.*: Traitement Chirurgical des Affections Oculaires, Paris, Doin)

curred to my resident to put the alpha-chymotrypsin into the Bell erisophake. The erisophake was applied and squeezed the alpha-chymotrypsin under the iris while grasping the lens capsule at the same time. It occurred to me that the alpha-chymotrypsin might possibly damage the rubber bulb, but in examining some of these bulbs, no such damage was noted; however, I abandoned the idea of using alpha-chymotrypsin in the syringe of the Bell erisophake.

Recently the Barraquer motor-driven erisophake (Fig. 91) has been modified so that the noise from the motor is muffled with soundproof material and it will shut off automatically if vitreous is lost.

Figure 92 shows a pitfall—the incorrect application of the erisophake. It is obvious why the lens capsule is not grasped.

Figure 93 illustrates a complex situation in which a cataract is being extracted following an iridocyclitis. The synechiae are broken by the introduction of a spatula through the iridectomy, and a radial iridotomy is performed in the 5 and the 6 o'clock positions. In many cases the lens may then be extracted. Furthermore, in order to prevent the problems of a hammock pupil, I prefer a complete or a vertical iridotomy at the 12 o'clock position. In a case of this nature Dr. Sato[17] would have introduced his special knife at the 12 o'clock position, breaking the adhesion of the iris to the lens and then removing the lens in an extracapsular fashion. I do not favor such a method in that many of these lenses, in fact most in my experience, have been removed as intracapsular extractions. The alpha-chymotrypsin, if used, will have no effect whatsoever on the synechiae and therefore should not be applied until all the synechiae have been broken.

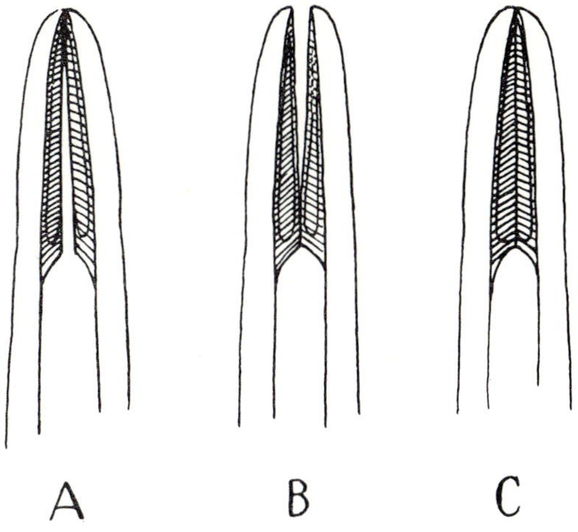

FIG. 94. Adjustment of blades of Arruga capsule forceps. (A) Blades touching first at point. (B) Blades touching first at heel. (C) Correct adjustment with blades meeting absolutely parallel. (Dr. A. B. Reese)

INABILITY TO GRIP THE CAPSULE

Inability to grip the capsule can be seen in intumescent lenses. If the surgeon finds that he cannot get a good grip on the capsule with the forceps or the erisophake, he should first make sure that his instruments are not at fault and that they are being used correctly. Figure 94 shows an Arruga forceps. These should be examined carefully with a loupe before they are used because some are manufactured with the toe or the heel of the blades touching first rather than with flat apposition. Unless there is simultaneous apposition of the blades, there is danger of pinching a hole in the capsule.[14]

In intumescent lenses, the erisophake is the instrument of choice. Obviously, the suction of the erisophake must be adequate for the type of cataract being extracted. The trick is to use a small amount of suction on the erisophake to prevent the capsule from breaking; often, even if it does break, most of the anterior portion of

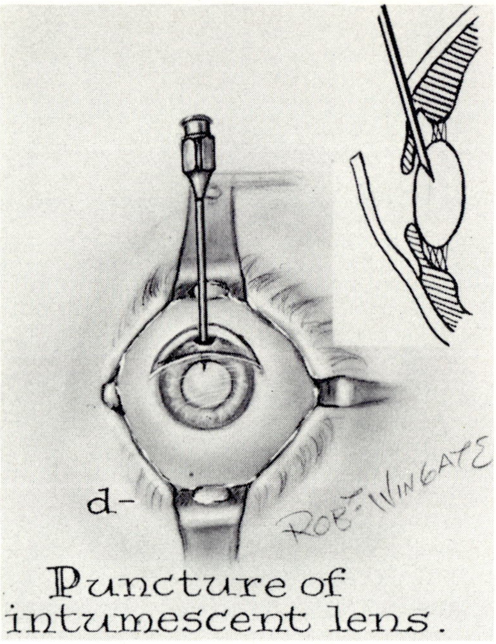

FIG. 95. Puncture of intumescent lens. (Berens, C., and King, J. H.: An Atlas of Ophthalmic Surgery, Philadelphia, Lippincott)

the capsule will come out with the erisophake. These intumescent lenses are large, and an especially large wound is required. An iridectomy is particularly important in this type of case because one has a greater chance to perform an intracapsular extraction.

Another approach is to prick the edge of the lens with a fine needle (Fig. 95); this will permit the surgeon to catch the capsule either with the erisophake over the hole or with the capsule forceps straddling the hole.

Because an intumescent cataract has very easily separated zonular fibers, a modified Smith operation should be considered. (For membranous cataracts, see Chap. 4.) Some feel that the chances of getting the lens out intracapsularly are greater if alpha-chymotrypsin is used. I think that the zonules are weaker in this type of case and that the extra manipulation needed to inject the alpha-chymotrypsin might cause rupture of the capsule.

LOSS OF GRIP ON THE CAPSULE

Prophylactically, one should have an adequate corneal incision and a well-dilated pupil. If the pupil cannot be well dilated, a total iridectomy superiorly and a vertical iridotomy inferiorly are necessary. Flat or hard lenses should be slid and not tumbled. During the tumbling procedure, contact with the erisophake is often broken if pressure through the cornea is not maintained. I like to prevent this by rolling the erisophake in my fingers and exerting a sandwichlike pressure on the lens through the cornea on one side with the erisophake on the other side. In this case, the lens acts as the "meat" in the sandwich.

In the case of losing one's grip on the capsule when using capsule forceps, a different type of capsule forceps should be tried (Fig. 96). In the case of the Bell erisophake, greater suction should be attempted. Or, if one is using the motor-driven erisophake, the amount of suction can be increased.

The loss of grip on the capsule may be due to the fact that the zonules are still intact. If one is using alpha-chymotrypsin, the possibility of adding more alpha-chymotrypsin should be considered.

Finally, one must remember that adhesions between the capsule and the hyaloid may be mistaken for tough zonules and that alpha-chymotrypsin does not overcome this problem (see p. 3).

RUPTURE OF THE CAPSULE DURING CATARACT EXTRACTION

There is no sure way of preventing rupture of the capsule. One seeks to deliver the lens in its capsule with the least amount of trauma to the surface of the vitreous and the smallest amount of traction on the zonular lamella transmitted to the retina and the vitreous.

Some of the reasons for a planned intracapsular extraction resulting in an extracapsular may be: (1) a short incision; (2) a lens which is larger than usual; (3) a corneal ledge; (4) tough zonules; (5) obstruction by sutures; and (6) faulty instruments.

When the lens is larger than usual, obviously the corneal or the corneoscleral incision must be made larger. For tough zonules, alpha-chymotrypsin is a most important aid. However, when the lens is mature, one must be especially cautious with the alpha-chymotrypsin cannula to prevent rupturing the capsule.

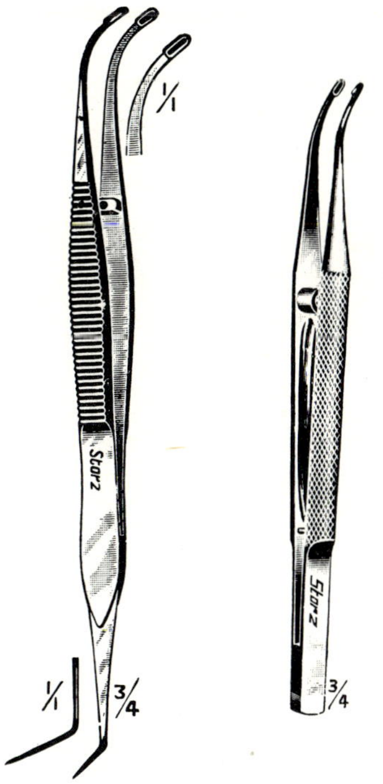

FIG. 96. (*Left*) Capsule forceps, Arruga-McCool (Storz instrument No. E-2070). (*Right*) Capsule forceps, Kirby (Storz instrument No. E-1320).

The capsule can also be ruptured with the toothed iris forceps in doing the iridectomy. I have found that fewer ruptures result with the use of the erisophake. Brown or hard nuclear cataracts often have very fragile capsules, and the erisophake is particularly suitable for such lenses.

If the capsule ruptures when one is attempting to slide and the rupture is at the site of application of the forceps, the lens can sometimes be tumbled or it may be delivered in its capsule by grasping it on the anterior surface with the forceps or the erisophake and continuing with a sliding procedure. As a rule, application of capsule forceps should be tangential to the capsule surface and a few millimeters to the side of the original grasp.

If the capsule ruptures during the cataract extraction and the zonules are intact, one should be guided by the behavior of the eye. If the situation is under control, one may proceed to an extracapsular type of extraction, making sure to remove most of the anterior portion of the capsule. As to the posterior capsule, even after the sutures are tight, I do not feel that it is wise to make an immediate opening into the posterior capsule. If the condition of the eye seems to be perilous and the wound tends to gape once the nucleus is

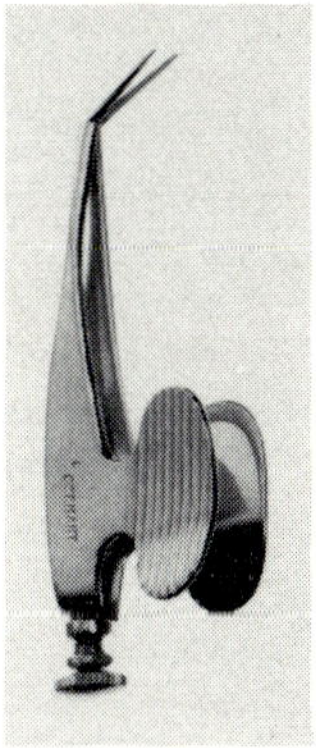

FIG. 97. New Barraquer fragment forceps (Storz instrument No. E-1878).

delivered, it is wise to close the wound without irrigation of the anterior chamber at this time.

On the other hand, when the zonules are broken and vitreous starts to present, the surgeon is confronted with a very troublesome combination. He must decide quickly whether the disadvantage of leaving some capsule and cortex is counterbalanced by the risk of vitreous loss. If the vitreous pressure is high, ideally the sutures must be pulled taut temporarily and steps must be taken to decrease the pressure if possible. If there seems to be no immediate or extreme risk and the eye is soft, one can be bolder and, under direct observation, actually lift the cornea with forceps or use irrigation. Portions of the capsule can then be carefully picked off with the use of the new Barraquer fragment forceps (Fig. 97) which are so narrow that they can be inserted even after the sutures have been pulled somewhat taut.

If no vitreous is presenting and especially if alpha-chymotrypsin has been used, I will attempt to remove the capsule entirely by pull. Undoubtedly, the alpha-chymotrypsin dissolves the zonules in these cases, and the capsule can come off as one piece.

When the capsule ruptures during the cataract extraction, I prefer to convert a round pupil to one with a total iridectomy. In addition, if there is danger of vitreous being lost or if a moderate to large amount has already been lost, I will do a vertical iridotomy at the 6 o'clock position.

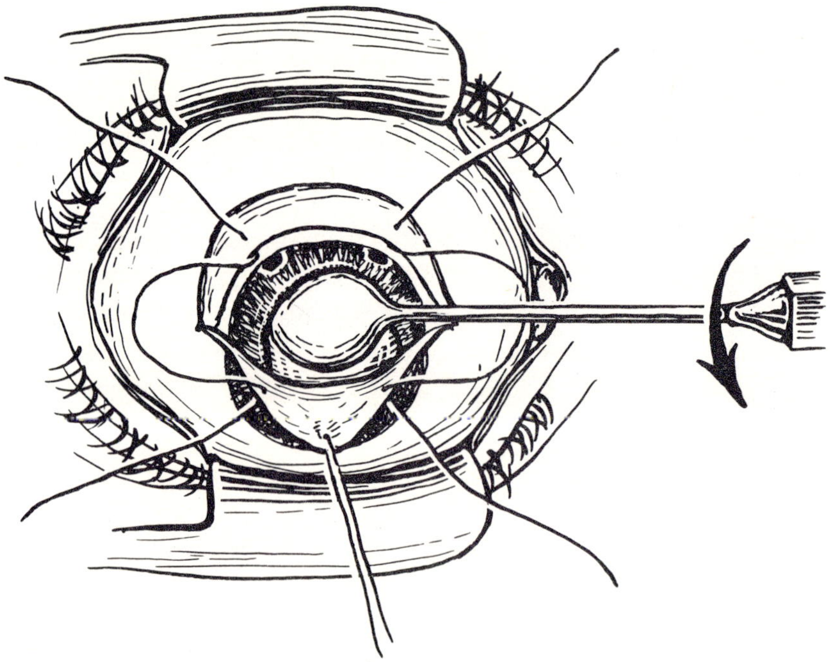

FIG. 98. In case the hole in the capsule is a little larger but is still discrete and has fairly regular edges, it may be covered with the grasp of the suction cup, and by inverse rotation, elevation and tilting, the effect of inverse tumbling may be produced. A cataract such as this as with a fragile zonule may be delivered in toto, even though the capsule has been torn. (Modified from Kirby, D. B.: Advanced Surgery of Cataract, Philadelphia, Lippincott)

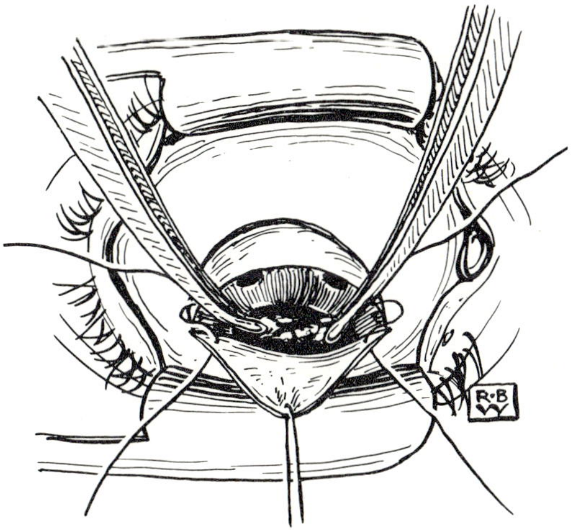

FIG. 99. Should any parts of the anterior capsule remain after the removal of the mass of the cortex and the nucleus, and if the edge or a piece of the capsule can be picked up as it floats in the stream of irrigating saline, it may be drawn out a little and lifted away from the posterior capsule with one pair of forceps, and then a second pair of forceps may be applied to another portion of the capsule elsewhere. Then, hand over hand, and advancing the grasp of the forceps as the capsule comes out of the recesses, the whole capsule may be delivered. (Modified from Kirby, D. B.: Advanced Surgery of Cataract, Philadelphia, Lippincott)

If a small hole is created in the capsule, an intracapsular extraction can still be performed as illustrated in Figure 98. If the hole has fairly regular edges, it may be covered with a grasp of the suction cup of the erisophake. Thus the chances of performing an intracapsular extraction are enhanced. Often, a small hole is purposely made in the capsule of a very mature cataract in order to release some of the fluid, and here, too, an intracapsular type of extraction may still be performed. If the hole is too large and the zonules are intact, as much as possible of the anterior capsule should be removed.

One method of removing the anterior capsule after the mass of the cortex and the nucleus have been removed is demonstrated in Figure 99. The edge or the pieces of the capsule can be picked up as the capsule remnants are floated in a

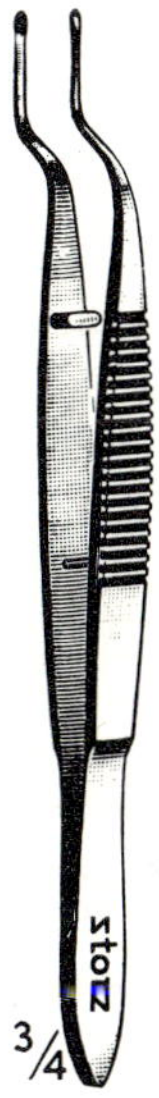

FIG. 100. Capsule fragment forceps, Guyton-Clark (Storz instrument No. E-2134).

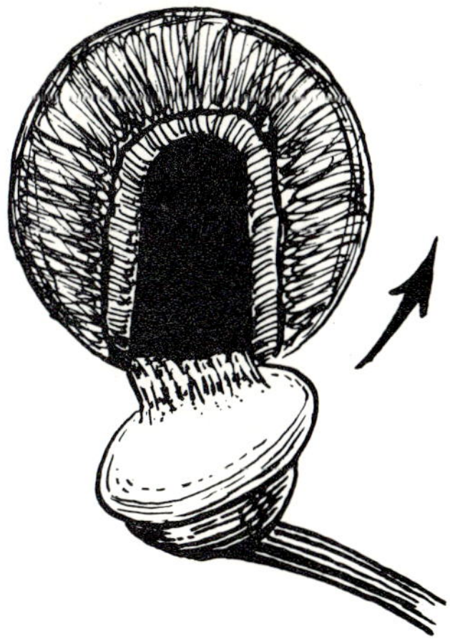

FIG. 101. Slipping out of the resistant upper zonular fibers by moving the lens toward the right. (Modified from Kirby, D. B.: Advanced Surgery of Cataract, Philadelphia, Lippincott)

stream of saline used for irrigation. Personally, I do not irrigate the anterior chamber while removing extra portions of the capsule. Furthermore, the capsule can be removed with the use of a pair of forceps by what is known as the "hand-over-hand" or "climbing-the-rope" maneuver (Fig. 100). Of course, the efficacy of this technic depends on a good assistant. Often, gently rocking the capsule from side to side will facilitate its removal—especially if alpha-chymotrypsin has been used. Finally, the use of some form of ultraviolet light for identifying portions of the lens is recommended by some.

Figure 101 shows resistant upper zonular fibers. The iris or the scleral edge of the wound will often shear these remaining zonules, thus preventing rupture of the capsule. (In addition, in the case of the round pupil, pausing a few minutes at the end of the procedure, lifting the flap and gently irrigating the zonules back into the anterior chamber often prevents an irregularity of the pupil.)

In summary, if one is attempting an intracapsular extraction and the capsule ruptures, it is better to do too little than too much.

POSTERIOR DISLOCATION OF THE LENS

If the lens is partially dislocated at the time of application of instruments, the use of a muscle hook or a small loop can sometimes steady the lens while the capsule forceps or the erisophake is applied. If the syringe-type erisophake is used, grasping the lens with the instrument should always be a two-hand job. This cannot be done with a Bell erisophake. In removing the lens, one must be careful not to traumatize the cornea. Occasionally a small and correctly shaped loop can be slid through the vitreous behind the lens. Some advocate spearing the lens with a sharp needle with or without cautery attached to the needle. This approach must not be used in a mature lens containing a morgagnian type of cataract because in this case the nucleus will drop to the bottom.

If the lens is luxated into the vitreous and the capsule is intact, some feel that it is best to remove the lens even with the loss of vitreous. It is difficult to visualize the lens even with a binocular headlamp or some form of ultraviolet light. If the vitreous is fluid, irrigation should be used as first pointed out by Verhoeff. Saline or, preferably, a balanced solution must be forced into the eye toward the ciliary body so that the lens will be forced out on the other side. If one irrigates directly back, this will not happen. If the capsule is intact and if irrigation of the eye fails to float the lens out, it is best to close the eye and make no further attempts at this time to remove the lens. If the capsule is intact, the lens usually will settle back in the eye where it may be tolerated for many years. If the eye is quiet, leave it alone. However, uveitis and secondary glaucoma are an indication for removing this type of lens.

If the capsule is ruptured and the nucleus is loose in the vitreous cavity, the surgeon is justified in attempting to remove the nucleus and as much of the lens matter as possible. The eye will be lost if the nucleus is not removed. Prolonged, vigorous irrigation is justified in an attempt to float the nucleus forward.

Hypermature Lens in the Vitreous

Later, if the tension rises, the surgeon may not know if this is lens-induced secondary to a hypermature lens or if it is due to other causes. The presenting findings are minimal. Occasionally a few cells may be found in the anterior chamber, even with an immature lens. Treatment consists of an iridectomy above combined with an iridotomy below. Then the lens is washed out with a forceful stream of balanced solution. Fortunately, at this time the vitreous is still fluid in most of these cases, and the lens now may be floated out. However, if the lens is attached to the retina, forceps extraction is necessary. Finally, multiple sutures and the injection of a balanced solution into the cavity should follow. Unfortunately, despite these measures a detached retina and phthisis bulbi may follow (see p. 135).

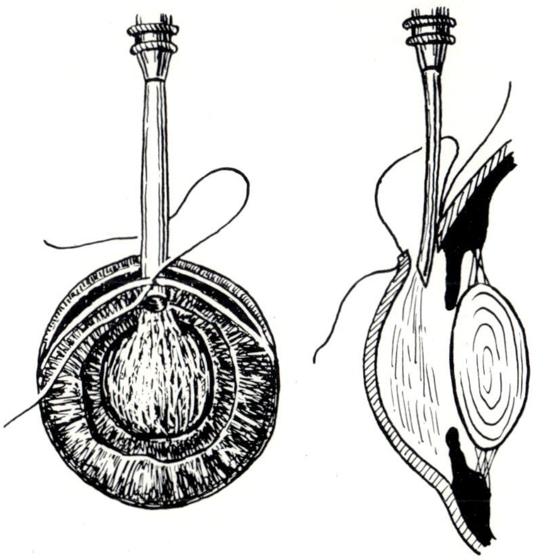

FIG. 102. Lavage of the anterior chamber. (Modified from Guillaumat, Louis, *et al.*: Traitement Chirurgical des Affections Oculaires, Paris, Doin)

LAVAGE OF THE ANTERIOR CHAMBER AND ALPHA-CHYMOTRYPSIN

If lavage of the anterior chamber is necessary, it must be done very cautiously. After the use of alpha-chymotrypsin, the needle used for lavaging the anterior chamber must not be put under the iris once the lens has been dislocated. At this stage it is very easy to cause vitreous to present. On one occasion (when alpha-chymotrypsin was not used) after I had completed an intracapsular extraction, the anterior vitreous face was broken by the stream of the lavage being driven too forcefully against it. Certainly in this case the alpha-chymotrypsin cannot be blamed for weakening the vitreous face. A safer procedure is to direct the stream on the sclera, the iris or the posterior surface of the cornea. Here one must be careful not to damage the endothelium.

Figure 102 shows lavage of the anterior chamber. Today, most surgeons feel that a balanced solution should be used. Many solutions contain calcium which prolongs the action of alpha-chymotrypsin; this must be considered when deciding which solution is to be used. Some balanced solutions which do not contain calcium are available.

Balanced Solutions

A warning has been sounded against using drugs containing methylcellulose during intraocular surgery. Studies on the irritating action of the methylcellulose seem to indicate that iridocyclitis is not due to this drug. It is probably the isotonic sodium chloride solution that causes the mild iritis and iridocyclitis. Popular balanced solutions today are Ringer's solution, Hank's balanced salt solution and Gey's balanced salt solution.

AIR IN THE ANTERIOR CHAMBER

I use air in the anterior chamber if vitreous has been lost. In a personal communication, Dr. Edmund Spaeth stated that now he *always* uses *air* in the anterior chamber. It is important in vitreous loss that this injection be made from below.[19] I will also use air in the anterior chamber when there is a question of dystrophy, when the chamber has not formed spontaneously, or when a flat chamber is noted at the end of the procedure. In using air in the anterior chamber, one must always avoid an excess because of the possibility of creating an air-block glaucoma. Balanced solutions are now being used more frequently in corneal transplants and following lens extractions because there is less danger of forming an air-block glaucoma (see p. 142).

VITREOUS PROLAPSE

Although flat chamber, hyphema and epithelial invasion are regarded as serious and distressing complications associated with cataract surgery, vitreous loss during or after cataract surgery has been and still is one of the major complications in eye surgery. Vitreous loss leads to a high incidence of retinal detachments, and to corneal and macular changes that are often irreversible. A very fine surgeon once remarked, "Vitreous loss is one situation over which I lose sleep." Since vitreous loss is related to the surgeon, the patient and the state of the eye and since the surgeon is responsible for his own actions and those of the patient, it can be readily understood why he may lose sleep over this situation.

Prophylaxis

1. Both the surgeon and the patient should be relaxed. A surgeon running to the operating room from a busy office can hardly be relaxed.

2. Succinylcholine should be avoided in general anesthesia, or the surgeon must wait long enough after the initial stages of induction with this anesthetic agent for the ocular pressure to return to normal.

3. Adequate akinesia including direct injection of the lids is important. Supplemental intravenous anesthesia such as a barbiturate and/or Demerol is helpful, especially for the tense, high-strung or heavy-set patient with a thick neck and shoulders. Some surgeons feel that no retrobulbar anesthesia is best; others advocate a blunt needle for the retrobulbar anesthesia to prevent retrobulbar hemorrhages and vitreous loss. Others substitute injections along the superior rectus muscle and into Tenon's capsule to avoid retrobulbar hemorrhages. I advocate a retrobulbar anesthesia incorporating hyaluronidase. One, 2 or even 3 ml. of the retrobulbar anesthetic plus hyaluronidase can be squeezed into the back of the eye. It doesn't matter how much is squeezed in; it can be squeezed out by digital massage. Massage must be continued until the eye is soft. Of course, one should not use massage where there are dislocated lenses.

4. Acetazolamide (Diamox) may be started 2 or 3 days prior to surgery, and intravenous urea[21] (or mannitol) may be given ½ hour before surgery.

5. I perform a canthotomy routinely as another precautionary measure against the loss of vitreous and also because I feel that it reduces postoperative hyphema. To minimize bleeding a Kelly clamp is applied for 1 minute. Studies with the tonometer show that even lid sutures can cause an increased intraocular pressure. This happens less often after a canthotomy. If the pressure is elevated, readjusting the pull on the lid sutures sometimes can lower the intraocular pressure.

6. After digital massage, easing of the speculum or the lid sutures and the use of the tonometer can assure the surgeon that

the intraocular pressure is normal prior to opening the eye.

7. One should loosen the superior rectus suture before the actual lens extraction.

8. If the Flieringa-Bonaccolto ring is used, it must be properly placed and checked with the tonometer while pressure is exerted on the sutures holding it prior to the incision (Fig. 103). A ring on the forward part of the eye often will cause the ocular pressure to be high if the sutures used to hold the ring are pulled. This can be proved by taking a pressure with the tonometer prior to opening the eye. If the ring is placed on, or more toward the equator, the intraocular pres-

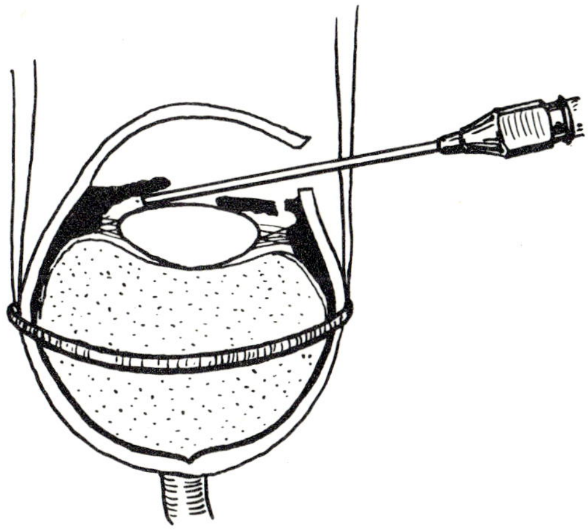

FIG. 103. The correct placement of the Flieringa-Bonaccolto ring. (Modified from Barraquer, Joaquin: An. Inst. Barraquer *2*:63, 1961)

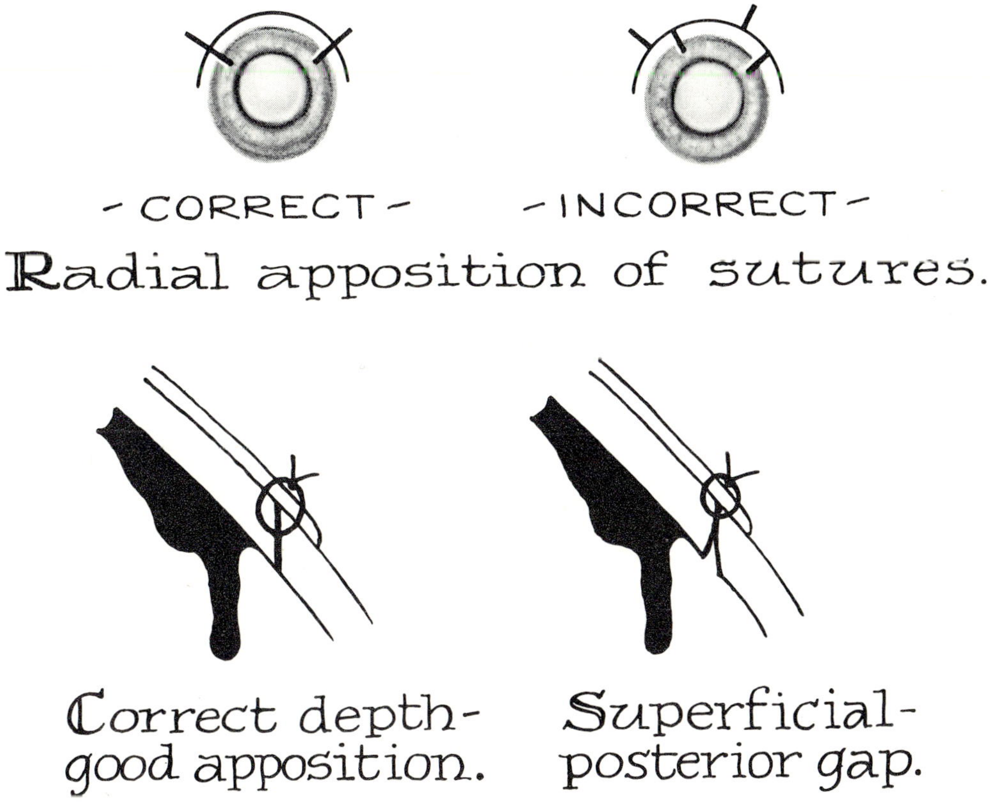

FIGURE 104.

(Berens, C., and King, J. H.: An Atlas of Ophthalmic Surgery, Philadelphia, Lippincott)

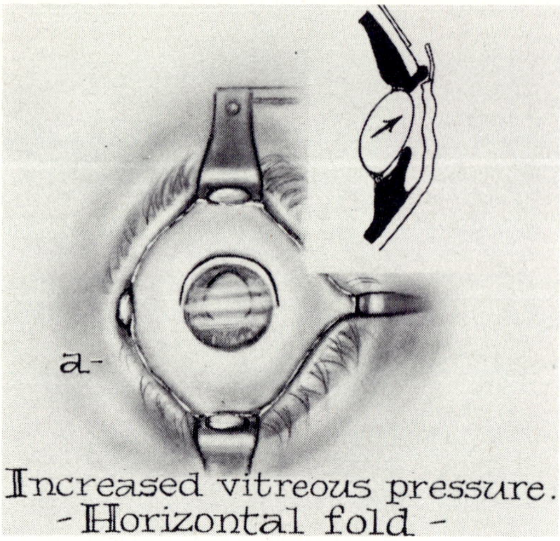

FIG. 105. A horizontal fold in the cornea after the section indicates increased vitreous pressure. (Berens, C., and King, J. H.: An Atlas of Ophthalmic Surgery, Philadelphia, Lippincott)

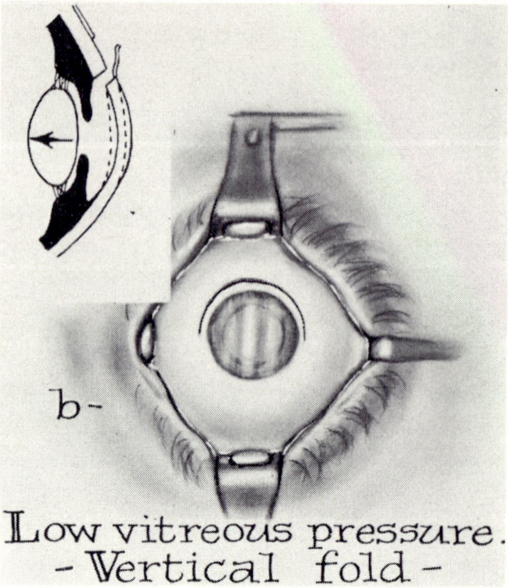

FIG. 106. A vertical corneal fold indicates a low vitreous pressure. (Berens, C., and King, J. H.: An Atlas of Ophthalmic Surgery, Philadelphia, Lippincott)

sure will be less. Girard feels that the ring should be at the equator and that there should be 1 mm. of clearance all around the ring. Therefore, it is wise to have a selection of rings.

9. "Hard sutures" are very important for preventing vitreous prolapse. These are defined as sutures that are placed in solid corneal and scleral tissue and not in loose, yielding conjunctiva or in insecure episcleral or limbal tissue. They pass through and not over the lips of the wound. When so placed and tied, they bring the tissues back to their exact preoperative position. "Hard sutures" must be placed properly in direction and depth. They must not be too deep. These sutures should be placed radially instead of vertically, since this leads to malposition and buckling of the cornea[15] (Fig. 104).

10. It is said that until the advent of the enzyme alpha-chymotrypsin the utmost surgical skill was required to remove the lens without rupturing the capsule. Now, surgical skill and a slight change in technic are required to prevent vitreous loss, since the enzyme makes this a more likely operative complication than rupture of the capsule.[15] The enzyme should not be used in cases with fluid vitreous, where there are subluxated lenses, or where the hyaloid is not intact as in most traumatic cases.

When one intends to use alpha-chymotrypsin, one must be certain that the lens has not risen forward against the cornea, indicating the threat of vitreous loss. If this occurs, it is much better to omit the use of the enzyme and to rupture the zonular ligaments with the zonule stripper at the lower equator. Then the lens can be tumbled out with an erisophake or a forceps, holding back the vitreous inside the eye with the upper pole of the lens which is the last part to leave the eye if tumbling is used.

If the iris prolapses, one may: (1) re-

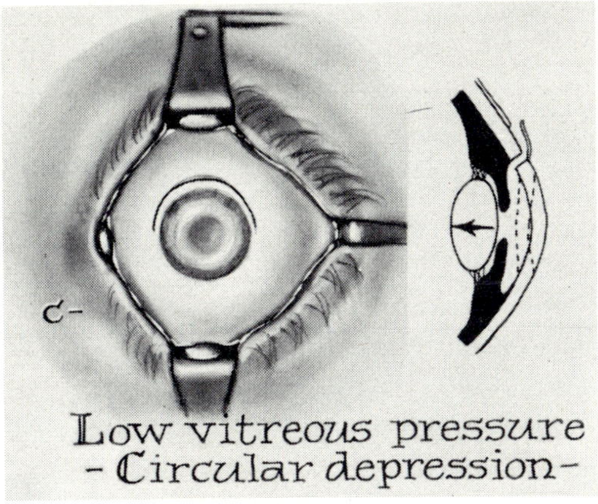

FIG. 107. A circular corneal fold indicates a low vitreous pressure. (Berens, C., and King, J. H.: An Atlas of Ophthalmic Surgery, Philadelphia, Lippincott)

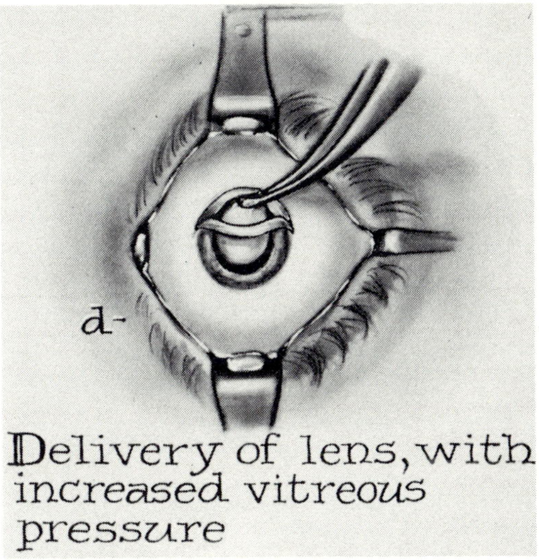

FIG. 108. In the presence of increased vitreous pressure it is safer to deliver the lens in a sliding fashion. (Berens, C., and King, J. H.: An Atlas of Ophthalmic Surgery, Philadelphia, Lippincott)

posit it, or (2) do an iridectomy or the equivalent and proceed with the next steps if the situation seems to be controlled. However, two other courses have been suggested: (1) the use of urea (if urea had not been given preoperatively, the wound can be closed and intravenous urea can be given); and (2) an iridectomy may be performed, the eye then being closed. In this case the cataract is extracted at a later time under more favorable conditions.[18]

After the section, increased vitreous pressure can be detected by a horizontal fold in the center of the cornea between the extremities of the incision (Fig. 105). Low vitreous pressure is indicated by a vertical fold (Fig. 106) or by a circular depression of the cornea (Fig. 107).

If the lens and the iris present on opening the wound, I definitely will not use the enzyme and, in these cases, will do a complete iridectomy and remove the lens in a sliding fashion, exerting a pull chiefly from *above* with minimal to no push from below (Fig. 108). My second choice in this situation is to do a complete iridectomy and a planned extracapsular extraction.

It is important that the surgeon employ a method of injecting alpha-chymotrypsin into the posterior chamber that will not allow it to penetrate the vitreous body. When using alpha-chymotrypsin a blunt cannula should be used with two-hand control. The cannula must not be pushed into the vitreous, and the enzyme must be injected slowly. I prefer 1 or 2 drops of alpha-chymotrypsin. It must be remembered that the *zonules need only be weakened, not dissolved.*

11. The section must be adequate, 180° to 200°. This is helpful for an intracapsular or an extracapsular extraction. In the latter case it permits removal of the nucleus and most of the cortex.

12. In applying forceps or erisophake or in delivery of the lens, the keywords are *gently* and *slowly*.

13. If tumbling is used, a tucking of the cornea behind the lens can help to prevent vitreous loss.

14. The sutures must be drawn up gently. If the sclera is thin or elastic, it is possible to break the vitreous face if the sutures are pulled up too quickly.

15. One must not manipulate iris repositors or irrigate directly on an intact hyaloid.

Actual Management of Vitreous Prolapse: Further Generalizations

If one anticipates the loss of vitreous, one should lose it under controlled conditions and through a posterior sclerotomy. This should be done at the ora serrata which should be ringed with diathermy. In some cases, acetazolamide (Diamox), given 2 to 3 days preoperatively, and, at the time of surgery, intravenous urea or mannitol, retro-orbital injections (including hyaluronidase), massage and the Flieringa-Bonaccolto ring properly placed are auxiliary measures that may prove to be important.

At the time of vitreous loss the doctor or his assistant must not try to explain this loss to anyone. Silence is the best rule when any complication arises, since the patient is often awake and may be keenly aware of such comments.

If the vitreous protrusion is small and the hyaloid membrane is intact, an attempt should be made to release all tension on the globe to allow the vitreous to retract into the globe. Occasionally the hyaloid may retract if one gently lifts the corneoscleral sutures. During this maneuver the vitreous may fall back into place. Franceschetti is credited with suggesting the application of sterile distilled water to cause shrinkage of the vitreous.[3] Ideally, the distilled water should be cool—and so should the surgeon!

Since vitreous and retained lens matter is a bad combination, one should try, even at the risk of losing more vitreous, to obtain an intracapsular extraction.

As a rule, the loss of fluid vitreous causes fewer problems than the loss of solid vitreous. It has been said that the surgeon should consider the loss of fluid vitreous to be no more serious than the loss of aqueous. However, it is important that one try to anticipate the type of vitreous one might encounter. In the presence of a dense cataract the presence of fluid vitreous can be suspected if there is a

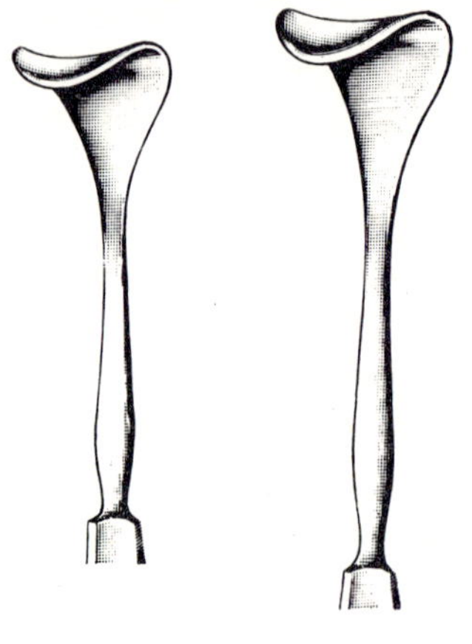

FIG. 109. (*Left*) Lid retractor, Desmarres: size 2, 15 mm. wide (Storz instrument No. E-982). (*Right*) Lid retractor, Desmarres: size 3, 17 mm. wide (Storz instrument No. E-983).

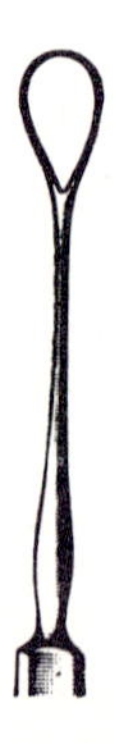

FIG. 110. Loop (Storz instrument No. E-664).

history of high myopia, uveitis, detachment or retinal disease.

Clinically, the appearance of the opposite eye may give a clue. In the involved eye a tremulous lens, a deep chamber or exfoliation of the lens capsule should make one suspicious of fluid vitreous.

Complications following loss of fluid vitreous can include choroidal, macular or even expulsive hemorrhage. There may be increased vitreous opacities, a soft eye and a detached choroid. Although postoperative pupillary block can occur with fluid vitreous, it is rare. In the few cases in which this does occur, it is due to a thickening of intervening peripheral solid vitreous which can block the pupil. Since fluid vitreous is seen in high myopia, uveitis and retinal disease, detachments can and do occur.

In general, following the loss of fluid vitreous the surgeon should follow his usual technic. However, with the use of additional sutures and the injection of a balanced solution into the eye which has lost fluid vitreous at surgery, the end-result is often a pleasant surprise.

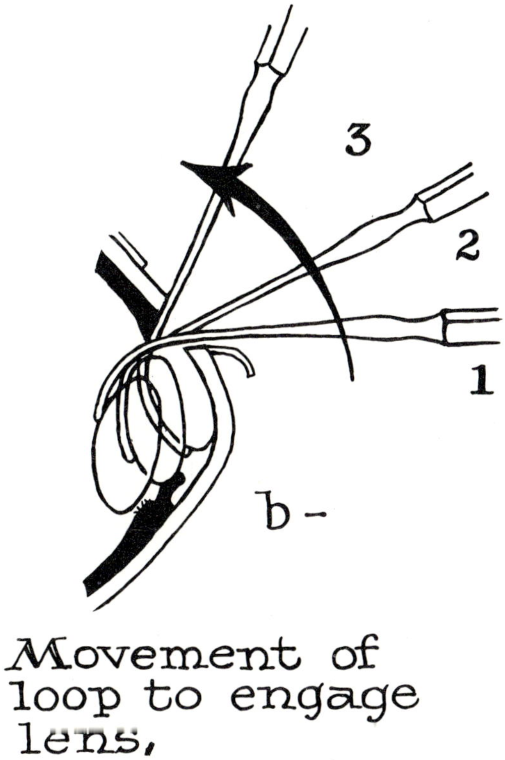

FIG. 111. Illustrates the movement of the loop to scoop the lens out. (Berens, C., and King, J. H.: An Atlas of Ophthalmic Surgery, Philadelphia, Lippincott)

LOSS OF FORMED VITREOUS

"Solid vitreous belongs inside the eye."[10] If formed vitreous is lost before the lens is extracted and one has a firm hold on the lens capsule, it is best to remove the lens by traction alone. If the lens is not firmly held, then it should be removed by the loop. The loop sometimes can be used to support the lens until another grasp is made. Ideally, a variety of loops should be available at all times, but this is especially true when a difficult cataract extraction is anticipated. I have suggested that a "vitreous emergency kit" should be available just as an emergency kit for cardiac arrest or for tracheotomies is kept ready. Lid retractors should be available (Fig. 109). The variety of loops should include "soft" ones (Fig. 110) so that they can be bent easily and the normal curve exaggerated to really scoop the lens out (Fig. 111). Ideally, right and left

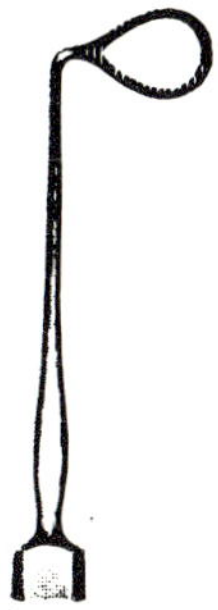

FIG. 112. Loop, Weber-Elschnig (Storz instrument No. E-668)

angled loops (Fig. 112), small loops (Fig. 113) and loops with an added guard in the center (Fig. 114) to prevent small lenses from falling through would be included in this set. A McGannon forceps for hard lenses and a solid spoon (Fig. 115) for sliding the lens out (Fig. 116) and dehydrated synthetic* or bank vitreous and urea might be considered in completing the "vitreous emergency kit." Since synthetic vitreous will probably represent the approach to the management of retinal detachment in the future, it is my feeling that some form of vitreous would be justified in massive loss of vitreous. I feel that some form of preserved human vitreous would be better than balanced solutions such as Gey's or Ringer's solutions or is even better than a synthetized vitreous which might cause endothelial damage if it comes in contact with the cornea. Ideally, preserved human vitreous or new synthetic forms of vitreous should be soluble, biologically active, noninflammatory and easy to remove if necessary. Following massive vitreous loss the substitutes would be best placed directly into the corneal opening used for the cataract extraction at the time of surgery rather than through a new perforation of the globe because these openings, even though small, are partially responsible for new formed tissue in the vitreous cavity at a later date. These new formed tissues may

* Vitreous infusion hyaluronic acid.

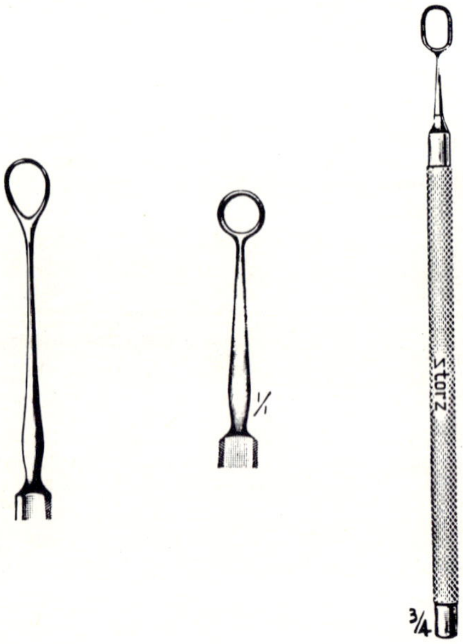

FIG. 113. (*Left*) Loop, Lewis (Storz instrument No. E-648). (*Center*) Expressor ring, Verhoff, (Storz instrument No. E-608). (*Right*) Loop, Amenabar (Storz instrument No. E-660).

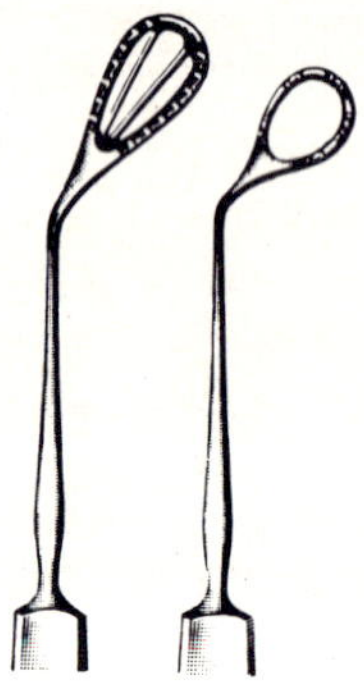

FIG. 114. (*Left*) Loop, Berens (Storz instrument No. E-652). (*Right*) Loop, Berens (Storz instrument No. E-654).

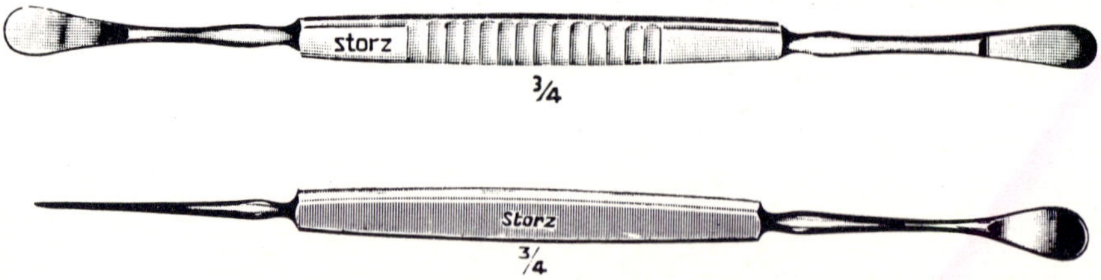

FIG. 115. (A) Spatula, Green (Storz instrument No. E-744). (B) Spoon and needle, Fisher (Storz instrument No. E-748).

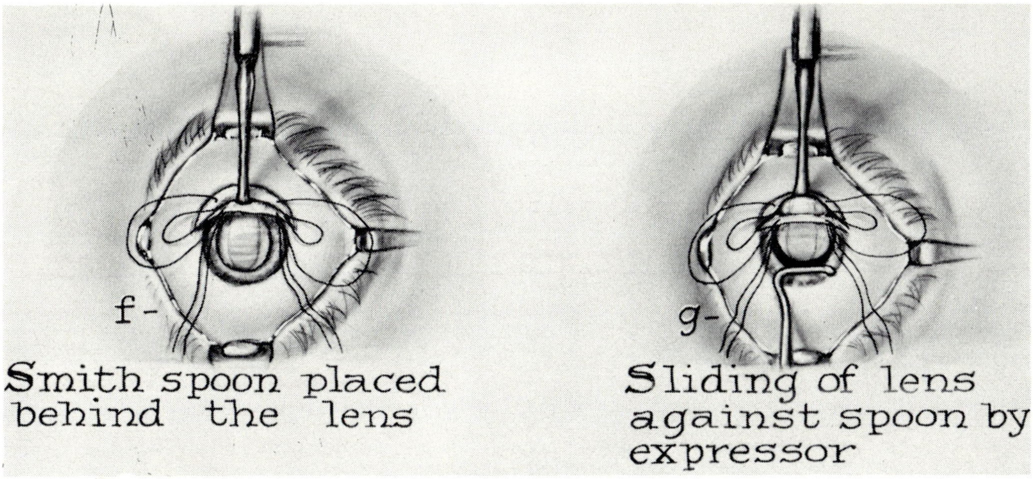

FIG. 116. (*Left*) Method of sliding lens out using the Smith spoon placed behind the lens. (*Right*) Sliding of lens against spoon by expressor. (Berens, C., and King, J. H.: An Atlas of Ophthalmic Surgery, Philadelphia, Lippincott)

be explained by the size of the hole, mild infection or reaction to the injected material. In turn these tissues may cause fixed retinal folds and retinal detachment.[12]

As noted previously, additional "hard sutures" are important. The following steps are most important:

1. Management of the iris (see "When Not Preserving the Round Pupil," p. 86, and "If the Round Pupil Is To Be Preserved," p. 88). I personally will do a complete iridectomy above and one or two radial iridotomies below.

2. Management of vitreous (see "When Not Preserving the Round Pupil," p. 86).

3. Air injection (early). A layer of balanced solution or air should be used. This is one of the greatest indications for air. It is important that this be given early, i.e., at the time of surgery. The air bubble should be small and introduced from *below* with a small, blunt needle (Fig. 117, *left*). Introducing the air from above the area of the vitreous loss is an ineffective procedure and sometimes can be dangerous.[19] (See "Air-Block Glaucoma," p. 142.) The air bubbles are sometimes helpful in showing where there are vitreous strands. Although its use has been suggested, I do not use the dissecting microscope to visualize these strands. Traction bands from the wound edge to the retina are responsible for causing detachments.

4. Mechanical separation. A narrow cyclodialysis spatula (Fig. 117, *center*)

FIG. 117. (*Left*) Cannula, air injection (Storz instrument No. E-499). (*Center*) Cyclodialysis spatula, Castroviejo (Storz instrument No. E-495). (*Right*) Iris hook (Storz instrument No. E-546).

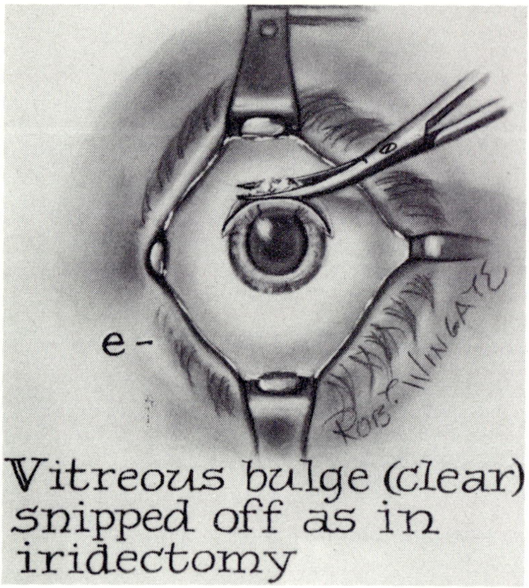

FIG. 118. Illustrates (clear) vitreous bulge cut off as in iridectomy. (Berens, C., and King, J. H.: An Atlas of Ophthalmic Surgery, Philadelphia, Lippincott)

from both sides should be used to push the vitreous strands back from the edge of the wound.

5. Urea. Intravenous urea may be used as indicated at the time of surgery.

6. Postoperative care. In these cases, acetazolamide (Diamox), binocular dressings and bed rest for 48 hours with the bed flat will help to preserve the air bubble and keep the vitreous from touching the corneal endothelium. Since these are steps that one would use to overcome the irreversible changes of corneal scarring following a late vitreous touch, they are steps that should be applied early. Prophylactically, it is wise to give a 4-day course of a systemic antibiotic to avoid infection (my present choice is 2 Gm. of chloromycetin stat and 1 Gm. daily for 3 days) and a systemic steroid (for 1 week or longer) to keep down the inflammatory reaction. If the vitreous is clear of the wound edge, keeping down inflammation may help to reduce the number of detachments and may keep macular changes to a minimum.

When Not Preserving the Round Pupil

I favor a *complete iridectomy above*, using a hook (Fig. 117, *right*) if necessary to catch the iris, and the addition of *one or two vertical iridotomies below* to avoid an updrawn pupil. With the injection of air the vitreous face will be away from the corneal endothelium. The radial iridotomy below will help to prevent updrawn pupils and will aid the vitreous in gravitating downward and away from the wound edge.[6] Dr. Edmund Spaeth feels that with vitreous presentation and prolapse one must emphasize the necessity for a sphincterolysis. It pleases me that at a recent meeting Dr. Dunnington said,

> In reference to maintenance of the round pupil following vitreous loss, I have not been so fortunate in maintaining the central round pupil. True, the eyes look fine for two weeks or even two months but then the pupil becomes up-drawn and an iridectomy is needed later. Therefore, I prefer the classical approach when vitreous is lost.[10]

If there is a vitreous bulge and the hyaloid membrane is not intact, usually I will cut the vitreous off as in an iridectomy (Fig. 118).

Dr. Castroviejo states,

> Regarding cutting massive vitreous prolapse with scissors, making it concave and adding a layer of saline, this is a procedure which I use in the very unfavorable cases of total penetrating keratoplasty when cornea, iris and lens remnants have to be removed and from the moment the eye has been entered, vitreous prolapses freely. Then, rather than to leave the vitreous in contact with the total penetrating transplant, I prefer to cut enough vitreous to create a concavity which will be filled with saline and the cornea then re-

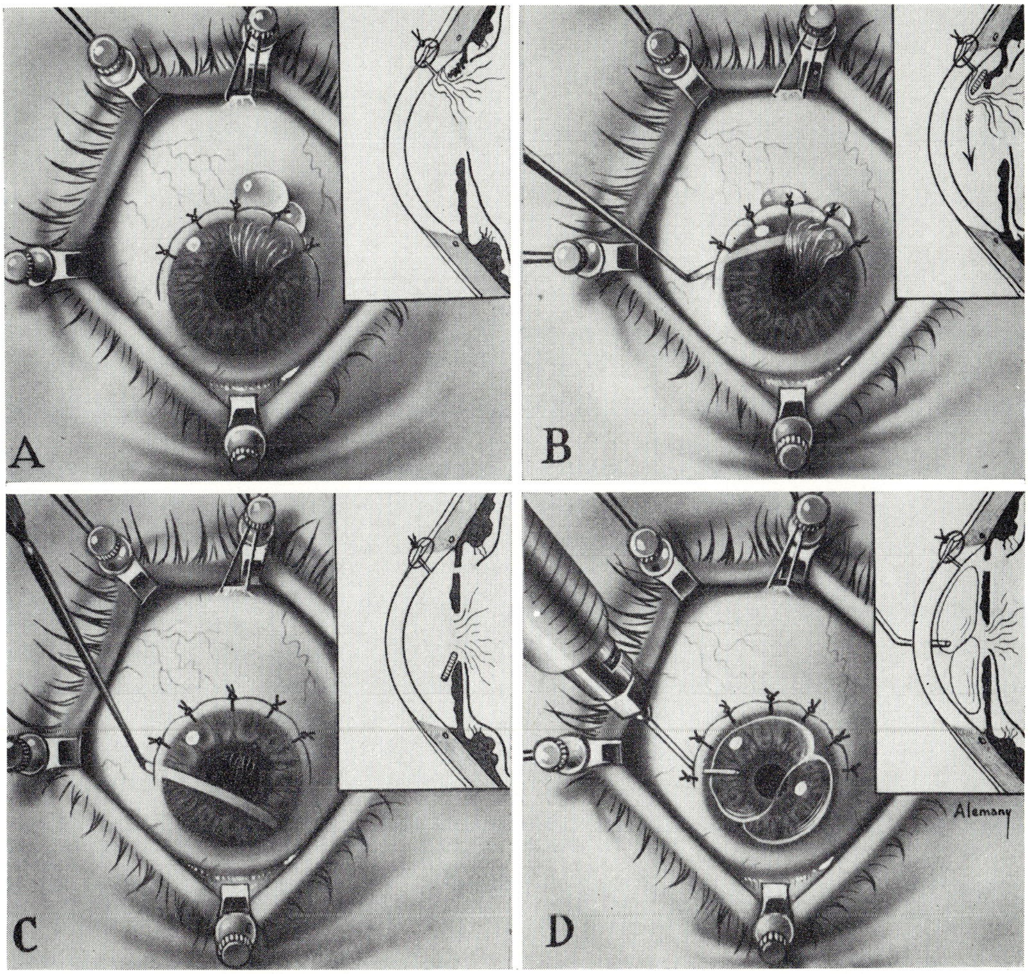

FIG. 119. Illustrating the maneuver to separate the vitreous from the incision in vitreous prolapse during cataract extraction. (Castroviejo, Ramon: Am. J. Ophthal. *48*:397)

mains in contact with saline rather than with vitreous with less chance of developing endothelial disease.[8]

Dr. Castroviejo's first choice is that described under "If the Round Pupil Is To Be Preserved." I myself wonder if the method of cutting massive vitreous prolapse with scissors until it is concave might not be advisable for cases of moderate vitreous loss. This, I feel, would be less traumatic to the eye than trying to search for pockets of fluid vitreous.

For reasons that I have outlined previously, if the amount of vitreous loss were total or almost total, I would not hesitate to inject "bank vitreous" followed by a layer of a balanced solution at the time of the loss. Of course, there are those who disagree with this approach. We have made a practice of having stored vitreous in the refrigerator in the operating room. I have used this successfully with excellent results in total loss of vitreous following injuries. Since I have used this type of human vitreous and know its characteristics, I, like Donald Shafer, prefer it to dehydrated vitreous, which I keep in reserve. I have not as yet used the newest synthetic vitreous for these cases.

Treatment should include local and systemic antibiotics and steroids as outlined previously.

If the Round Pupil Is To Be Preserved

In recent years most ophthalmologists who perform cataract surgery and prefer preserving the round pupil seem also to prefer the maintenance of the round pupil even after vitreous loss. They point out that the round pupil is a natural barrier to the prevention of vitreous prolapse during cataract extraction. I feel that the iris also can act as a natural barrier when one attempts to push vitreous back through the pupil. They add that the standard 12 o'clock full iridectomy and 6 o'clock iridotomy result in an open gate for vitreous to move forward and become attached to the cornea, thus causing edema and keratopathy. Furthermore, they feel that if vitreous is carefully reposited, the round pupil will be maintained, the vision will be better and there will be no greater incidence of uveitis, glaucoma, retinal detachment or corneal edema and bullous keratopathy.[5]

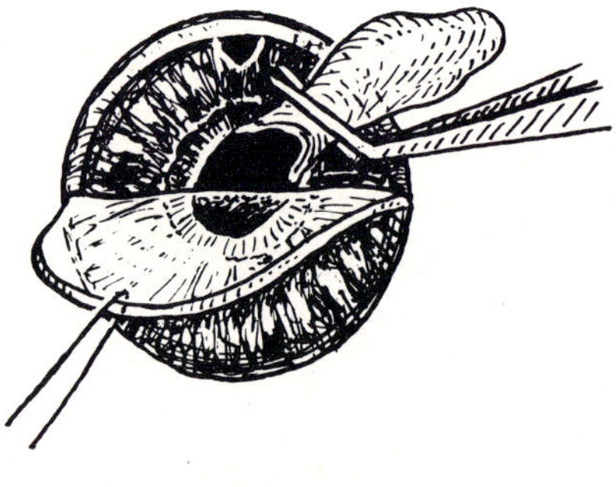

Fig. 120. Method of cutting the vitreous if the round pupil is to be preserved. (Modified from Barraquer, Joaquin: Trans. Am. Acad. Ophthal. Oto-laryng. *66*:46)

Castroviejo's technic is as follows:

When vitreous prolapses during a cataract operation, the incision is closed by five corneosclero-conjunctival sutures [Fig. 119, A]. A cyclodialysis spatula 15 mm. long and 0.50 mm. wide is introduced into the anterior chamber through the incision. The spatula is then moved across the surface of the iris, following the angle of the anterior chamber until the tip is at a point opposite to that at which it was introduced and lies between the iris and the vitreous strands incarcerated in the incision [Fig. 119, B]. The point of the spatula is then brought down over the pupillary area to break the vitreous strands from their points of attachment. If the maneuver is successful, the pupil is freed and assumes its normal central position [Fig. 119, C].

Air is then injected into the anterior chamber by means of a syringe with a 27-gauge needle, the tip of which has been bent and the point cut off to avoid damage to the internal structures of the eye. By holding the syringe with one hand and rotating the piston with the other, the surgeon can prevent the injection of too much air, injecting exactly the right amount needed to separate the iris and the vitreous [Fig. 119, D]. Eserine ointment is applied to contract the pupil so that its central position will be preserved.[7]

Dr. Salleras feels that in using the cyclodialysis spatula as described by Dr. Castroviejo, one must be sure in sweeping in the angle that he does not cause a cyclodialysis and hemorrhage.

Joaquin Barraquer follows essentially the same technic described by Castroviejo. Minor variations are made by Barraquer who cuts the strands of vitreous with deWecker-Barraquer scissors at the pupil and at the inferior scleral edge of the incision (Fig. 120). Then the vitreous is swept off the iris into the pupillary space with a fine marten-hair brush. After the incision has been closed carefully, air is injected into the anterior chamber. Any vitreous strands still incarcerated are swept away from the incision with a fine spatula modified by Barraquer from the vitreous spatula of Castroviejo. Barraquer points out that his entire maneuver can be facilitated if the vitreous volume is reduced by aspirating some fluid vitreous by passing a multiperforated cannula through the pupil[2] (Fig. 121).

Maumenee, McLean and Boyd pointed out that particularly in elderly individuals there is a certain amount of fluid vitreous present in a pocket located in the superior portion of the vitreous chamber because, as a rule, solid vitreous gravitates inferiorly.

When removing vitreous, it is advisable to preserve a round pupil. The needle must be a blunt No. 18 needle, and it must be placed well back into the eye. Since the vitreous is attached to the ora serrata, one must go through formed vitreous with the blunt needle. Since there is a tendency to put the needle only a little way into the eye, it should be emphasized that the needle must be placed far enough back. It should be put up above and posteriorly. The suction should be applied only when the needle is in the back of the eye. If the needle seems to be plugged, it should be unplugged by pushing the plunger forward. Removal of fluid vitreous is said not to be harmful to the eye.[20]

Discussion

In the face of vitreous loss, one must not yield to panic and must move slowly and deliberately. Hasty retreat causes more complications. I still favor doing a complete iridectomy at the 12 o'clock position and one or two radial iridotomies on the lower portion of the iris. If at the time of the prolapse it is difficult to grasp the iris to perform an iridectomy at the 12 o'clock position, a blunt hook is useful.

The use of a blunt needle or even one with multiple perforations does not seem practical to me, since it is difficult to tell in this type of emergency which is solid and which is liquid vitreous. I feel that solid vitreous can be changed to liquid vitreous even through a large-gauged needle. This may possibly explain the beneficial effects of such a procedure. I question, too, whether looking for the pocket of fluid vitreous is not as traumatic as through-and-through discissions of congenital cataracts. Of course, here one might say that this is a calculated risk and the lesser of two evils.

It was Thorpe who pointed out that the injection of air should be made from below and not from above. Those who have injected air from above know how many difficulties are encountered.

Again, it bears repetition that too large a bubble of air can cause an air-induced

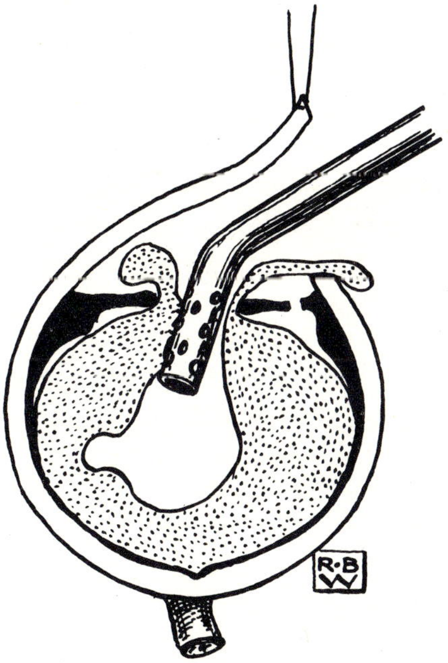

FIG. 121. Joaquin Barraquer's multi-perforating cannula for aspirating liquid vitreous from the back of the eye. (Modified from Barraquer, Joaquin: Trans. Am. Acad. Ophthal. Oto-laryng. *66*:46)

glaucoma. The injection of a balanced solution plus a small amount of air would seem to be the better choice. The injection of air after the use of multiple sutures is helpful in rechecking the sites of any vitreous strands. The use of the operating microscope has been suggested for further checking these strands of vitreous and might help, too, in directing the position of a long Castroviejo cyclodialysis spatula to break these strands.

Among my reasons for not trying to preserve the round pupil, especially after the loss of vitreous, are that not all of these pupils will stay round. In addition, many will become eccentrically placed, often with the center hidden under the lid. It is difficult for even the best optician to place the optical center over a pupil that moves upward or is hidden under a lid. An eccentric or updrawn round pupil would create a need to make a more central opening in the iris for visual purposes. In addition, vitreous is not accommodating and does not respect iridotomies and iridectomies which can more easily be plugged, leading to a secondary glaucoma. The natural course of many round pupils—even in unoperated eyes—is to become more rigid with the passage of time. Likewise, the incidence of detached retinas increases with time and particularly with vitreous loss.

Since the standard and accepted treatment for an updrawn pupil or vitreous adhesion to the cornea that occurs weeks or months after cataract surgery is to enter the anterior chamber and perform iridectomies and separate the vitreous from the cornea, I am one who still favors doing this at the time of vitreous loss. Delayed separation of the vitreous can be followed by irreversible corneal edema, bullous keratopathy and permanent corneal scars. The best treatment of the pupillary-block component of aphakic glaucoma is an iridectomy. This is another reason for my wanting to do this at the time of surgery of the cataract with vitreous prolapse. The surgeon and the patient are so much ahead if an iridectomy has been done at this time.

As to the argument that the full iridectomy at the 12 o'clock position and iridectomies below open the gate for vitreous to move forward and attach to the corneal endothelium resulting in corneal edema and bullous keratopathy, I like to point out that delayed vitreous prolapse can occur in round pupils or for that matter those with full iridectomies, even without immediate vitreous loss. The crucial factor causing corneal edema and bullous keratopathy is damage to the corneal endothelium. This damage can and should be prevented at all times.

A more radical idea on prevention of vitreous prolapse was suggested to me by Dr. Enrique Ariza H. who works with Dr. José Barraquer. To anticipate loss of vitreous, especially in children where multiple other problems such as an elastic sclera, adherent hyaloid, anesthetic problems, etc., play such a large part, the aspiration of vitreous at the pars plana prior to the actual removal of the cataract was suggested. The reinjection of this vitreous after the lens was removed and the sutures were in place was proposed. However, the approach was not helpful in children because the vitreous was so solid that it was difficult to remove, and, once removed, other factors such as lens-vitreous adhesions, elasticity of the sclera, etc., prevented good results. Vitreous loss in children carries a very great penalty. However, the possibility of an Ariza-Barraquer procedure in adults where fluid vitreous is present is food for thought.[1] I have not as yet used this approach.

SUMMARY

In vitreous loss, to prevent an updrawn pupil, to avoid glaucoma and to study possible postoperative detachments, I strongly favor a complete iridectomy at 12 o'clock and one or two vertical iridotomies below. Injection of air or a balanced solution from below and freeing the wound of strands with a repositor should follow. The essential mechanism of detachments is traction on the retina by vitreous bands in the wound. Therefore, these should be prevented by the steps outlined.

EXPULSIVE CHOROIDAL HEMORRHAGE

While there is no real way of anticipating or preventing expulsive choroidal hemorrhage, fortunately, this dreaded complication is rarely seen. One can sometimes be forewarned by the patient's complaint of sudden, severe pain. Immediately after this pain the wound begins to gape. If the wound can be closed satisfactorily, nothing more need be done at the moment. Several days later subchoroidal blood can be evacuated. However, if the wound gapes and the lens is spontaneously extruded and followed by vitreous and iris, the treatment of choice still is rapid drainage of the subchoroidal space by a posterior sclerotomy using a cataract knife. The posterior sclerotomy is performed over the area of hemorrhage or in the lower quadrant of the eye by inserting the cataract knife perpendicular to the limbus and then turning it on its side. Some eyes may be saved by this procedure.

Since this book was submitted for publication, Kamel (Am. J. Ophthal. 55:451, 1963) has reported that in eyes that have shown expulsive hemorrhage on the first operation, a prophylactic scleral trephination about 8 mm. from the limbus on the temporal side is made with a 2 mm. trephine hole. The trephining operation is extended through the sclera and is not a vitreous fistula. This can act as an exit for blood in case of expulsive hemorrhage.

REFERENCES

1. Ariza H., Enrique: Personal communication.
2. Barraquer, Joaquin: Advances in the surgery of the crystalline lens, Lecture Presented at the American Academy of Ophthalmology and Otolaryngology, Chicago, 1961.
3. ——: Complications operatorias en relacion con la extraction, III Curso Inter. Oftal., p. 181, May, 1961.
4. ——: Personal communication.
5. Boyd, B. F., Maumenee, A. E., and McLean, J. M.: Advances in cataract surgery, Highlights Ophthal. *3*:246, 1959.
6. Buxton, J. N.: Symposium: Surgical management of cataracts, New York Eye and Ear Infirmary Alumni Association, April 9-12, 1962.
7. Castroviejo, Ramon: Handling of eyes with vitreous prolapse, Am. J. Ophthal. *48*:397, 1959.
8. ——: Personal communication.
9. ——: Symposium: Complications of cataract surgery, New York Eye and Ear Infirmary Alumni Association, April 9-12, 1962.
10. Dunnington, J. H.: Symposium: Complications of cataract surgery, New York Eye and Ear Infirmary Alumni Association, April 9-12, 1962.
11. Dunphy, E. B.: Society Proceedings, New England Ophthalmological Society, Am. J. Ophthal. *52*:990, 1961.
12. Ferguson, E. C.: Drainage of subretinal fluid in scleral bucklings, Inter. Ophth. Clinics *2*:181, 1962.
13. Pritikin, R. I.: Zonulysin and instrumentation in mass eye surgery, Guildcraft, p. 30, Nov., 1961.
14. Reese, A. B.: An appraisal of the cur-

rent trend in cataract surgery, Montgomery Lecture, Ireland, 1962.

15. Roper, K. L.: The Cataract Operation; A Study of Details (Manual), Am. Acad. Ophthal. Otolaryng., 1961.
16. Salleras, A.: Practical advices on corneal surgery. Interum Congress of the Pan American Association of Ophthalmology, Lima, Peru, 1/25/62-2/3/62.
17. Sato, T.: *In* Holmes, W. (ed.): Geographic Ophthalmology, Springfield, Ill., Thomas, 1959.
18. Symposium: Complications of cataract surgery, New York Eye and Ear Infirmary Alumni Association, April 9-12, 1962.
19. Thorpe, H. E.: Panel discussion: Complications of intra-ocular surgery, New York Society for Clinical Ophthalmology, January 16, 1961.
20. ——: Panel Discussion: Complications of intra-ocular surgery, New York Society for Clinical Ophthalmology, January 16, 1961.
21. Urrets-Zavalia, Alberto: *From* Boyd, B. F.: Congenital cataracts—modern concepts, Highlights Ophthal. *4*:255, 1961.

4

Cataract Extraction in Special Cases

CONGENITAL CATARACTS

INTRODUCTION

Today there is still a great difference of opinion as to the best surgical approach for congenital cataracts. While perhaps the most widely accepted method is the linear extraction,* there are many who favor discission† or multiple discissions because they are easier to perform and, especially, because complications are minimal and the results are good. Aspiration (or suction) methods and combinations of linear extraction, discission and aspiration are becoming increasingly popular. The aforementioned operations are sometimes listed under modified extracapsular extractions as distinguished from intracapsular extractions—a form of surgery which most surgeons agree should not be used in children.

Although there are those who feel that early surgery may overcome some forms of nystagmus and amblyopia, at present most surgeons favor delaying surgery in total or severe involvement of bilateral congenital cataracts until the patient reaches 1 year of age. At this time, if the cataract is mature or almost mature, an operation is indicated on that eye. I am totally in accord with this approach as at this age the child can better tolerate general anesthesia and the eye itself responds more favorably to surgery. I will operate on the second eye when the child is 2 or 3 years of age.

In regard to zonular (lamellar), partial or monocular cataracts, a conservative course with an attempt to overcome amblyopia by the use of cycloplegics or partial occlusion is still considered to be the treatment of choice. However, for complete monocular cataracts, some advocate early surgery and the early use of a contact lens.[7] Usually the best time for surgery is when the patient is 6 or 7 years of age and the eye is more fully developed and a more definite acuity can be determined. In the monocular incomplete cataract when vision is noted to be 20/60 or better, it is better to avoid surgery. This decision is partly related to the fact that

* In this text, simple linear extraction signifies a technic for extracting a cataract by utilizing a keratome for the section and expressing opaque lens matter into a curette or a long shallow spoon; following this the residue in the anterior chamber is washed out with an irrigator.

Another description of simple linear extraction is given as follows: "The incision is made one mm. inside the limbus and five mm. wide; the capsule is lacerated with a cystotome and the lens material is expressed."[15]

In this text we will use the term simple linear extraction interchangeably with the Barkan type of linear extraction with a round pupil.

(Cordes comments that "It is the feeling today that a full iridectomy should be done in at least fifty percent and perhaps even more of the cases. This of course means a limbal incision."[16])

† Discission or "needling": Unfortunately, these terms have been used loosely and include cutting the anterior capsule and/or some cortex, and, on some occasions, for cutting all layers of the lens. Discission also has been used to mean incising or dividing a secondary cataract. The description of the operations listed in Chapter 5 under "Capsulotomies and Capsulectomies" will define this term more clearly in each individual case.

besides the complications of early surgery, there are other ocular defects in addition to the cataracts in many of these cases. Since one cannot determine an acuity in infants, the degree to which one can see the fundus gives a fairly good indication of what the child can see. If one can see well enough to get an outline of the disk, the vessels and the other structures, the child is probably going to be able to see fairly well, contraindicating surgery.[14]

Most congenital cataracts are stationary; however, in some cases—such as the zonular—the opacity may increase in *density* and will eventually require surgery. In microphthalmic eyes or in the presence of persistent hyperplastic primary vitreous or retinal dysplasia the prognosis is too poor to justify surgery. The presence of nystagmus indicates that the best possible vision will be no better than 20/50.

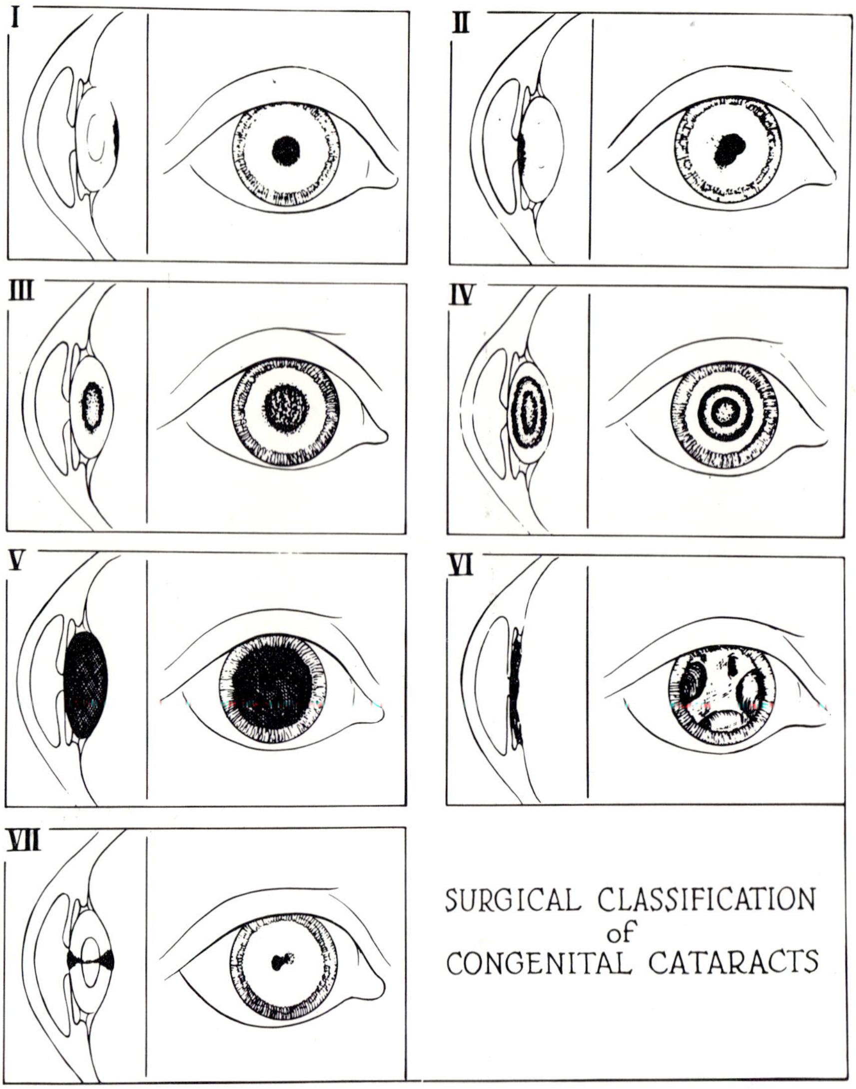

FIG. 122. The cross section and the front view of the 7 types of congenital cataracts. Note that only a representative group of type VII is illustrated. (Carbajal, U. M.: Am. J. Ophthal. *52*:361)

TABLE 1. SURGERY OF CONGENITAL CATARACTS

CLASSIFICATION	SUGGESTED SURGERY (IF INDICATED)	COMMENTS
I Posterior capsular and/or subcapsular	Discission and/or linear* followed by discission or cutting scissors	Difficult to handle by any method. Visual prognosis is poor because of hyaloid remnants and other anomalies.
II Anterior capsular and/or subcapsular	Discission and/or linear	This type is somewhat less difficult than Type I.
III Nuclear	Discission and/or linear	Good type for Moncreiff operation.
IV Zonular (lamellar)	Discission and/or linear	Results are good with discission and/or linear and suction (aspiration) preceded by a discission.
V Total	Discission and/or linear	An ideal type for discission and/or linear or for suction (aspiration)
VI Membranous	Discission, "hooks" or cutting scissors. (See Chap. 5 under "Capsulotomies and Capsulectomies.")	Linear and suction (aspiration) are definitely contra-indicated.
VII Mixed	Discission and/or linear	Results are difficult to predict by any method.

* See definition on page 93.

Although recent experimental work by Newell[31] and clinical work by others[44] might indicate a need for surgery as early as 3 months of age, I am still in favor of the approach outlined.

SURGICAL CLASSIFICATION OF CONGENITAL CATARACTS

Carbajal has grouped the forms of congenital cataracts. Figure 122 shows diagrammatically some of the major types of congenital cataracts.[10]

The surgeon has a wide choice of surgical procedures for the management of congenital cataracts. These include: (1) iridectomy for optical purposes; (2) discission; (3) linear extraction; (4) aspiration (or suction); (5) a combination of discission, linear extraction and aspiration (or suction); and (6) intracapsular extraction.

These different technics all will be described, but greater emphasis will be given to the more popular and some of the more modern ones. So that the reader may better visualize the type of cataract and the wide choice of surgery proposed, I have modified Carbajal's chart and listed some suggested surgery in Table 1. At present, my own preference is a combination of discission followed by a linear type of extraction in most cases. This is listed in the first column, but this does not mean that it is necessarily the best approach. It cannot be stressed too strongly that each type of surgery must be tailored to the problem at hand and that the chart stresses suggested surgery only *if indicated*. In many instances, some surgeons would prefer discissions alone and others a linear extraction alone.

Some surgeons may prefer a combination of discission and aspiration (suction). In some instances such as in the total type (V) some might use suction alone. Others (Carbajal) suggest aspiration (suction) followed by discission in many of these cases.

Iridectomy for Optical Purposes

Today iridectomy for optical purposes is not often used. It has been used particularly in the dense central type of cataract; the opening in the iris is usually made down and in. Newton has reported some fine results in selected cases with nuclear cataracts.[32] Optical iridectomy is of special value in retarded children where fine vision is not essential. The method is safe and relatively simple to perform.[38] Iridectomy in the inner, lower quadrant gives the best result.

Technic. Since the periphery of the iris must be preserved for optical reasons, the smallest fold of iris which can be grasped at the pupillary margin is drawn out and cut off at the tip. In this manner, a coloboma, limited to the pupillary border of the iris, is produced (Fig. 123).

The incision inside the cornea is made with a keratome with the wound of entrance a little inside the limbus.

Dr. Cordes suggests that

> . . . if an optical iridectomy is to be done, it would best be done above. Most of them are not too successful and, thus, if it has been done above, one doesn't have a distorted pupil if another procedure is done.[16]

Extracapsular Extractions (Modifications)

Discission. Single or repeated, discission is probably the oldest of all opera-

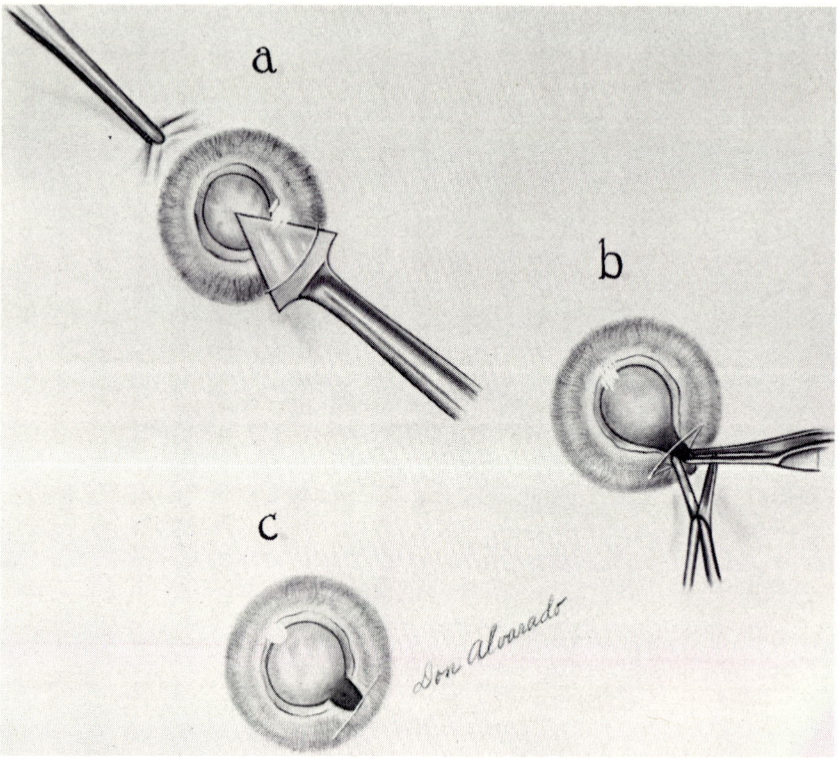

Fig. 123. (A) A keratome incision is made a little inside the limbus in the lower nasal quadrant. (B) The iris is grasped at the pupillary margin, drawn out and cut off at the tip. The blades of the iris scissors are held perpendicular to the corneal incision. (C) Postoperative appearance of the coloboma produced. (Cordes, F. C. *in* Haik, G. (ed.): Symposium on Diseases and Surgery of the Lens, St. Louis, Mosby)

tions for congenital cataracts. Today it is still used by many surgeons. It is considered a safe, effective and easy surgical procedure which some consider suitable for most congenital cataracts. The need for co-operation on the part of the patient is minimal. It may be of the Ziegler through-and-through type. Trauma to the vitreous and predisposition to retinal detachment are the main objections to this operation. However, it is pointed out that if the cases are selected carefully and the procedure is done correctly, multiple discissions will be unnecessary. The correct management includes cutting the anterior capsule and the nucleus without cutting the posterior capsule. However, if a membrane remains, no further discission should be done, but resort should be made to a capsulotomy or a capsulectomy (see p. 161) so that traction may be minimal. It has been pointed out also that the majority of operations for congenital cataract require a posterior capsulotomy or capsulectomy as a final step anyhow, and this must cause some trauma to the vitreous.

DISCISSION WITH ZIEGLER-LIKE KNIFE.* Dr. Ira S. Jones, who favors discission, describes his technic as follows:

> A Ziegler or Knapp knife-needle is entered under the conjunctiva at the limbus into the anterior chamber [Fig. 124, A]. The anterior capsule is opened by two or more cuts [Fig. 124, B]. These are no longer than half the diameter of the lens face and are placed so that lens matter swells into the pupil and not behind the iris. The number of cuts and the amount of stirring up of the cortical material can be varied. Care is taken that the posterior capsule is not opened. After withdrawal of the knife, atropine is instilled. So long as unabsorbed cortex is present additional needlings may be done at intervals of no closer than twelve weeks apart. When the cortex is gone, then if a secondary membrane remains, it may be divided with a sharp Wheeler discission knife in either the Wheeler or the Ziegler manner, preferably the former.[21]

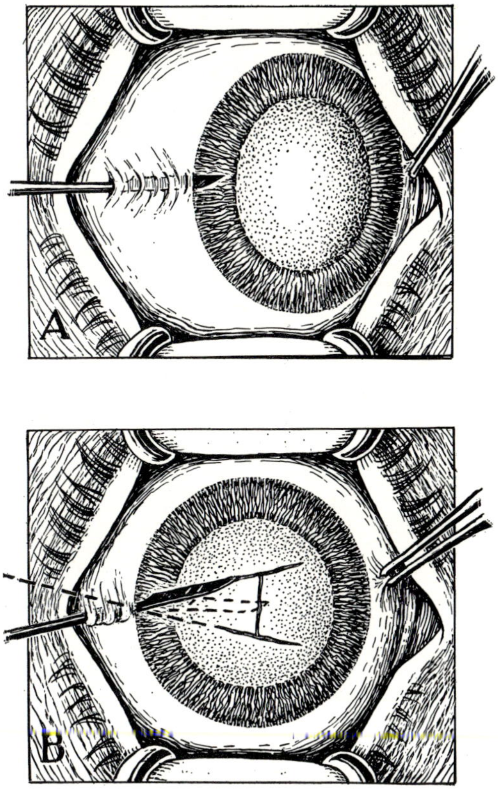

FIG. 124. (A) The technic of the needling operation. The incision under conjunctiva at the limbus. (B) Incisions in the lens capsule. (Jones, I. S.: Am. J. Ophthal. *52*:347)

Just before withdrawing the needle-knife from the eye after performing a discission for congenital cataracts, Dr. Saul Sugar always does an iridotomy. He feels that this helps to prevent a block of the pupil which causes a secondary glaucoma after the swelling material or even the dislocated nucleus bulges out.[42]

A membranous cataract can be thick or thin depending on whether the anterior, the posterior or both portions of the cap-

* The reader must differentiate the Ziegler through-and-through surgery in which the discission goes through the lens into the vitreous. This has been almost universally discarded. However, the Ziegler knife is still used.

sule remain after absorption of the lens proper. With thin membranes a sharp needle-knife may be used. However, if there is any resistance to getting the knife through the membrane, the knife should be removed, and, following a keratome incision and iridectomy, the membrane should be treated so as to avoid excessive traction (see p. 161). Discission of the central membranous opacity can be extremely difficult and, in some cases, impossible.

MONCREIFF'S OPERATION is a form of discission. In this procedure an incision is made through the anterior capsule into the cortex with a knife-needle. Multiple

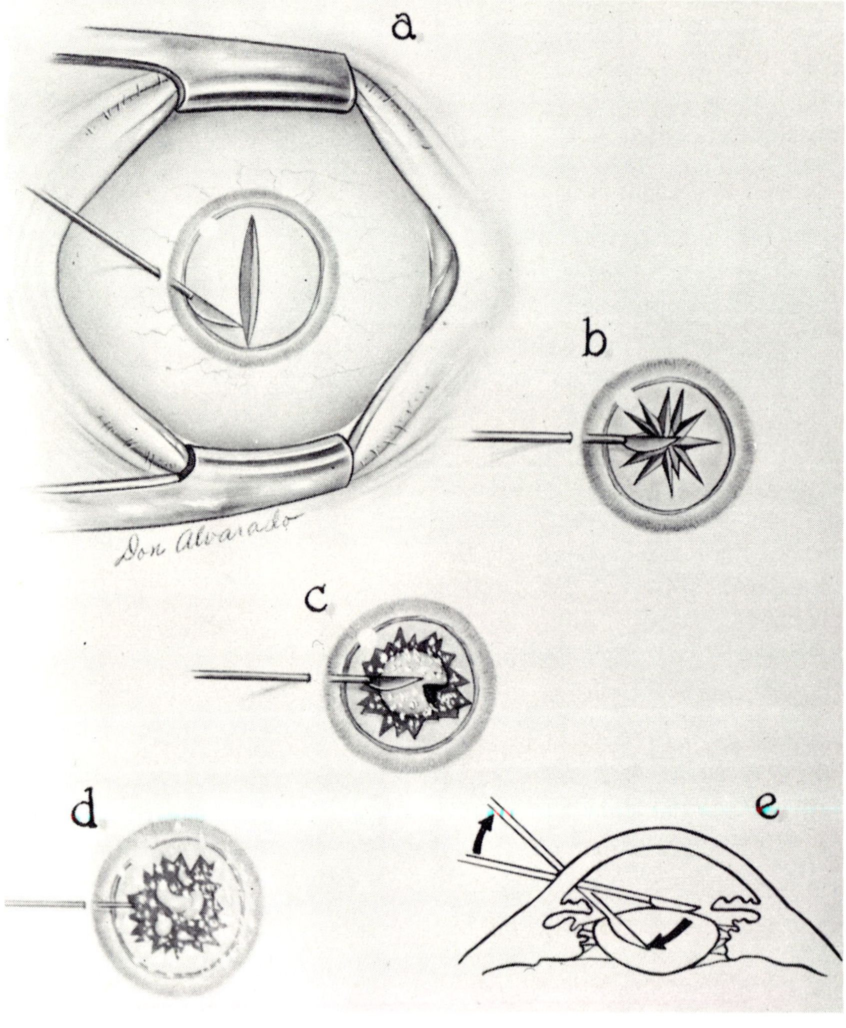

FIG. 125. Moncreiff operation. (A) An initial incision is made through the anterior capsule into the anterior cortex with a knife-needle. (B) Multiple incisions are similarly made in all directions down to the nucleus. (C) The nucleus is cut into fragments. (D) Cortical material remaining in the capsular sac is washed into the anterior chamber with an anterior-chamber irrigator. (E) Diagrammatic representation of the incision down to the nucleus. (Cordes, F. C. *in* Haik, G. (ed.): Symposium on Diseases and Surgery of the Lens, St. Louis, Mosby)

incisions then are made in all directions down to the nucleus. The nucleus is cut into fragments by repeating this procedure until the anterior cortex and the capsule are reduced to shreds. When the knife is withdrawn, a little aqueous is allowed to escape. Cortical material remaining in the capsular sac is washed into the anterior chamber with an anterior chamber irrigator[14] (Fig. 125).

WHEELER DISCISSION, some surgeons feel, is indicated in cases of shrunken membranes or after cataract. A Wheeler discission knife is introduced through the cornea 2 mm. within the limbus, superiorly (usually at the 12 o'clock meridian). The point of the knife is carefully advanced toward the pupillary margin at the 6 o'clock meridian. It is then thrust through the membrane and the handle is carried forward, the blade moving in an arc about the point of insertion through the cornea which serves as a fulcrum. It is important to withdraw the knife gradually as the incision is made. A diagrammatic representation of the procedure (side view) is shown in Figure 126. It is important that the knife be very sharp. The objective is to do the least possible damage to the vitreous in order to avoid late detachment of the retina. Complications in the Wheeler discission include cutting of the ciliary body. This can be avoided by not inserting the knife too far back. Another complication is pushing the membrane before the knife. If the membrane bends in front of the knife, the knife should be held still for a second, at which time the membrane may break because of the stretching effect. If it does not, a short cutting movement should be made. If the procedure is not carried out carefully, the corneal wound may enlarge and vitreous may follow. Such an opening should be cauterized and, if necessary, sutured to prevent fistula formation. (If the membrane is very tough, so that the needle-knife does not cut it, some feel that the deWecker scissors should be used.) (See Fig. 127.) In a recent letter, Dr. Edmund Spaeth stated that

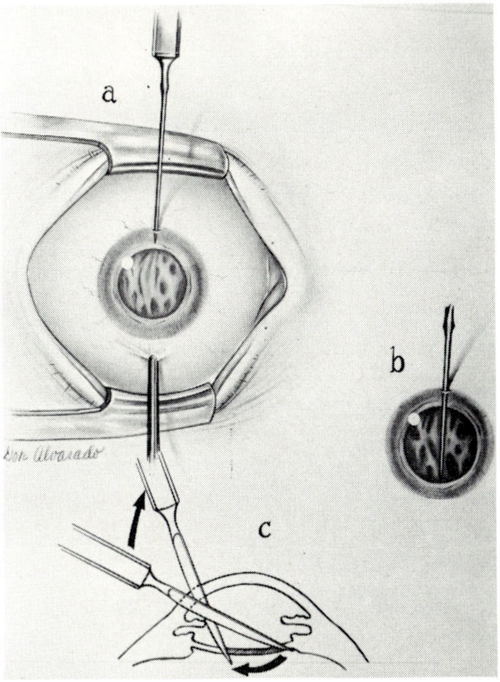

FIG. 126. Wheeler discission. (A) A Wheeler discission knife is introduced through the cornea 2 mm. within the limbus, superiorly (usually at the 12 o'clock meridian). (B) The point of the knife is carefully advanced toward the pupillary margin at the 6 o'clock meridian. It is then thrust through the membrane and is carried forward with a sawing motion, the point of insertion through the cornea serving as a fulcrum. It is important to withdraw the knife gradually as the incision is made. (C) Diagrammatic representation of the procedure (side view). (Cordes, F. C. *in* Haik, G. (ed.): Symposium on Diseases and Surgery of the Lens, St. Louis, Mosby)

With membranous cataract I feel that the operation of choice is a keratome incision and deWecker scissors incision of the membranous cataract—not a knife needle because of the damage to vitreous with knife needle.

(See author's choice, p. 161.)

Linear extraction is said to be the safest operation for the majority of forms of congenital cataracts as far as both the immediate results and the avoidance of late complications are concerned. The visual results are felt to be the best following this technic. Linear extraction greatly reduces the anesthetic and the operative risks of removing congenital cataracts and cuts down the total number of days in the hospital. In the average soft cataract, linear extraction done in one sitting is said by many to be the operation of choice.

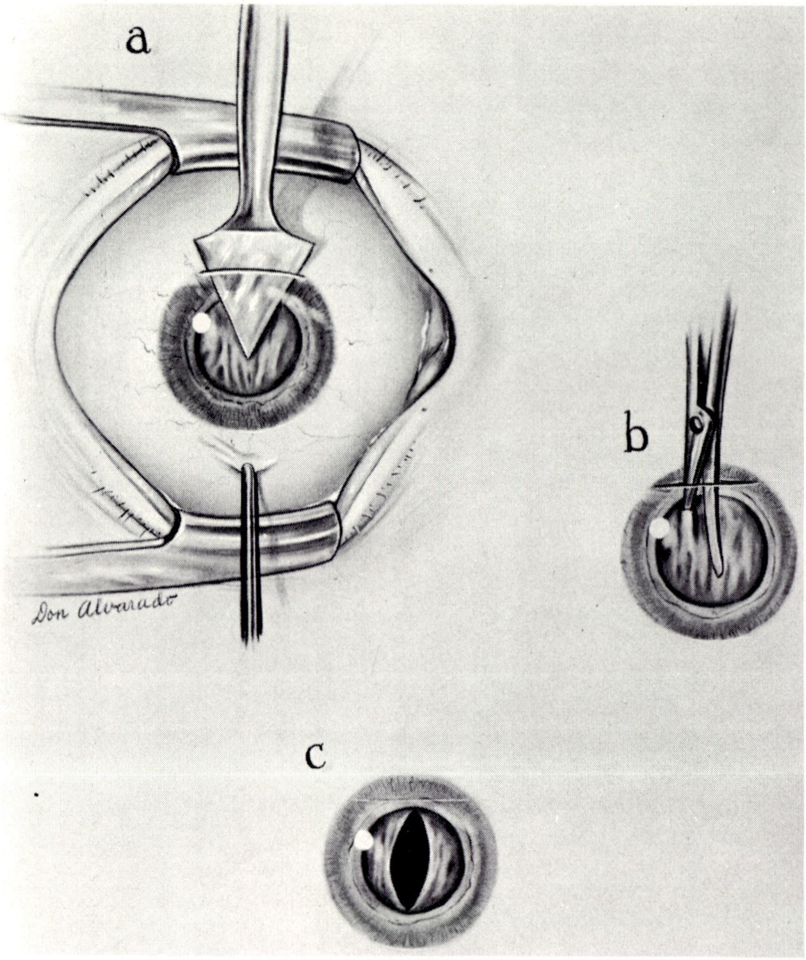

FIG. 127. Capsulotomy with occlusion of the pupil. (A) A keratome incision about 5 mm. long is made just within the limbus. (B) The scissors (Berens or deWecker) are introduced with their blades closed. When they have entered the anterior chamber, the blades are slightly opened and the sharp tip of the posterior blade is pushed gently through the membrane. The blades are then carried downward, one behind and the other in front of the membrane, until a cut of the desired length has been secured. (C) Postoperative appearance of the opening. (Cordes, F. C. *in* Haik, G. (ed.): Symposium on Diseases and Surgery of the Lens, St. Louis, Mosby)

Linear extraction is good for rubella cataracts.* In these cases it is wise to combine an iridectomy with a linear extraction. In posterior polar cataracts in which the major opacity is confined to the posterior capsule, a linear extraction followed later

* This same type of cataract follows other viral diseases.

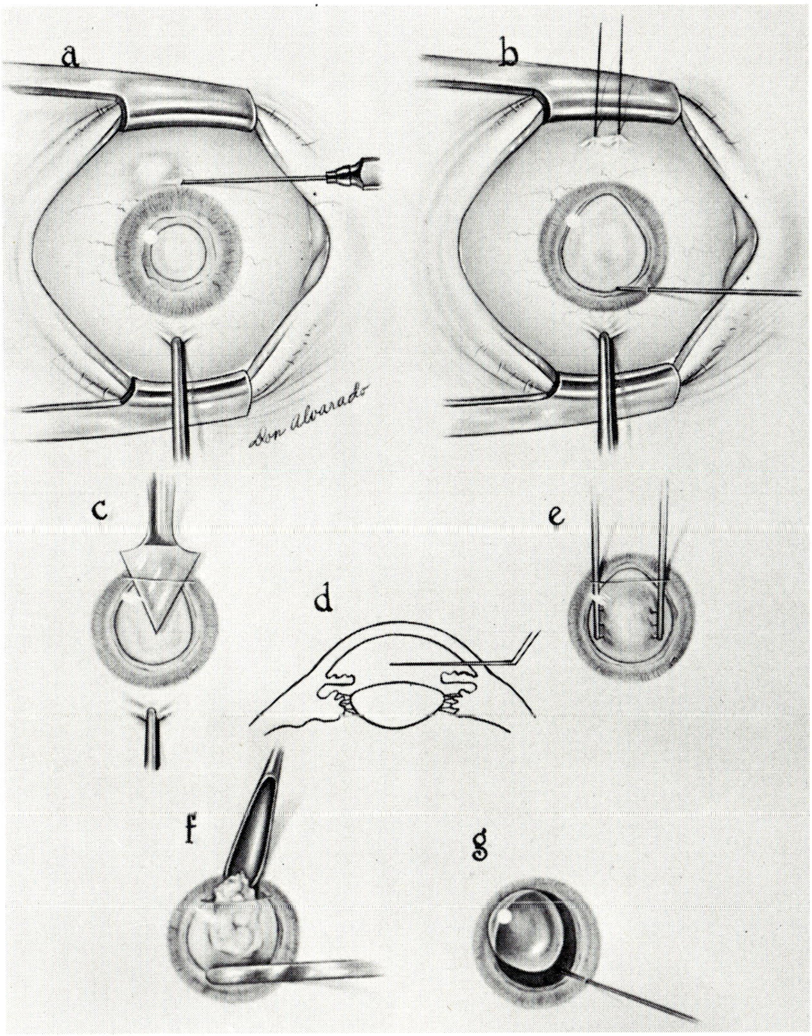

FIG. 128. Linear extraction. (A) Adrenalin (1:1,000) is injected subconjunctivally at the limbus at the 12 o'clock meridian to promote wide dilatation of the pupil. (B) A stab wound is made within the limbus in the lower temporal quadrant to facilitate injection of air after completion of the operation. (C) A keratome incision is made 1.5 to 2 mm. inside the limbus, superiorly, parallel to the iris surface. (D) Diagrammatic representation to show angle of keratome incision (side view). Note the valvelike opening. (E) A large capsulotomy is done with a Fuchs capsule forceps. (F) The lens substance is expressed out of the anterior chamber. (G) Air is injected into the anterior chamber through the stab wound created previously. (Cordes, F. C. *in* Haik, G. (ed.): Symposium on Diseases and Surgery of the Lens, St. Louis, Mosby)

by a Wheeler discission is the choice of some surgeons. The prognosis must be guarded in these cases because of the possible anomalies in the posterior segment. If there is a membranous type of cataract, linear extraction is not indicated.

TECHNIC. Dr. Frederick Cordes' technic is modified from that of Otto Barkan. Dr. Cordes feels that with careful attention to detail there is a greater chance of avoiding some of the complications such as delayed restoration of the chamber, updrawn pupil, occlusion of the pupil, membrane formation, vitreous loss, glaucoma and retinal detachment (Fig. 128).

After the routine preoperative preparation and anesthesia, two drops of epinephrine hydrochloride (1:1,000) are injected at the limbus above, the open part of the needle being directed toward the limbus. After five or ten minutes, the pupil is widely dilated, especially at the site of the impending incision and a suture is placed in the superior rectus. The dilation of the pupil resulting, as it does, from the contraction of the sympathetic fibers, persists when the anterior chamber is opened, and this keeps the iris out of the wound. Prior to the incision a stab wound is made into the anterior chamber below and temporally to facilitate the injection of air after the completion of the operation. As an aid in locating the opening, the knife needle is wiped on a piece of wet filter paper that has previously been impregnated with fluorescein, and the fluorescein is allowed to dry on the knife before the stab wound is made. This leaves a green stain along the course of the stab wound, which persists during the entire operation.

A keratome incision is made 1.5 to 2.0 mm. inside the limbus and parallel to the iris surface, to produce a valve-like opening. A large capsulotomy is now performed with Fuchs capsule forceps. It is important to remember that the capsule forceps should be used only once, because of the danger of biting through the posterior capsule into the vitreous. The lens substance is now expressed and the anterior chamber washed out with isotonic sodium chloride solution. [Dr. Cordes makes the suggestion that air be injected first through the keratome incision. If this is not possible, then air is injected through the previously made puncture wound.]

With a small Luer syringe and a 28-gauge needle, air is injected through the previously made puncture wound. If the tip of the needle is dulled a little, it has less tendency to catch in the course of the puncture wound. The air remains in the anterior chamber for several days and prevents the iris from coming into contact with the keratome wound in the cornea, and thus prevents the formation of anterior synechias. The long-continued use of atropine after the operation is important.[15]

LINEAR EXTRACTION WITH POOR PUPILLARY DILATATION. Dr. Cordes continues,

In those cases where the pupil will not dilate easily and widely preoperatively or in which surgery on the other eye has shown that it is impossible to keep the pupil well dilated postoperatively, a full iridectomy should be done. Where there is no dilation, in addition to the iridectomy, an iridotomy of the sphincter should be done below. This will prevent the pupil from drawing up as it may do if only an iridectomy is performed. The recent tendency has been to do a full iridectomy in all cases of congenital cataract surgery. Rubella cataract certainly falls into this category.

The procedure is as follows:

A five-mm. keratome incision is made at the limbus. The iris is then grasped about midway between its root and the pupil, in as small a bite as possible. The iris is pulled out, and the iridectomy is done with the scissors at right angles to the incision [Fig. 129]. The capsulotomy is now performed and the extraction completed in the usual manner. Atropine is administered after operation.

The importance of the use of atropine or scopolamine after any type of congenital cataract surgery for as long as two months after the eye seems to have cleared entirely cannot be overemphasized. If mydriatics are discontinued before all the cortex is absorbed, there is usually an occlusion of the pupil or posterior synechia formation.[15]

In doing an extraction with iridectomy, Dr. Cordes now makes a conjunctival flap and closes with two 6.0 catgut corneoscleral sutures and one conjunctival suture.

Aspiration or Suction Technics. Under aspiration or suction, I have included only Fuchs', Scheie's and Kara's technics. Lyle and Troutman have modified Fuchs' method. The Troutman modification, the Rodriquez Barrios modification, the Vargas, the Maumenee and the Carbajal types might be described under aspiration (or suction) or discission but have been included in this text under "Combined Procedures" (see p. 107).

The aspiration methods are based on similar principles with variations in the type of needle or syringes used or in the type of incision. The Troutman type is essentially a 4-layer incision (sometimes called 3-layer incision, if conjunctiva is not included, or mitred, step, half-lap or shelving) with the utilization of the Fuchs large size cannula.[7]

Aspiration (or suction) makes earlier surgery possible and is said to produce less trauma and inflammation; in many cases fewer procedures are necessary.

The indications and the contraindications for all the aspiration types are essentially the same as those indicated under Fuchs' aspiration technic.

The advantages of aspiration are that since a large amount of the lens material is aspirated there is very little postoperative reaction and less need for performing multiple operations. Usually one operation and one short period of anesthesia is all that is necessary. The anesthesia does not have to be as deep as that for those procedures requiring larger openings of the eye and can be interrupted if necessary. Since by the aspiration technic, solutions are aspirated and irrigated at the same time, the anterior chamber depth can be maintained or restored and there is less chance of complications associated with rupture of the posterior capsule. Since the opening through the cornea is small, few if any sutures are needed and the postoperative dangers associated with wound disruptions are minimal.

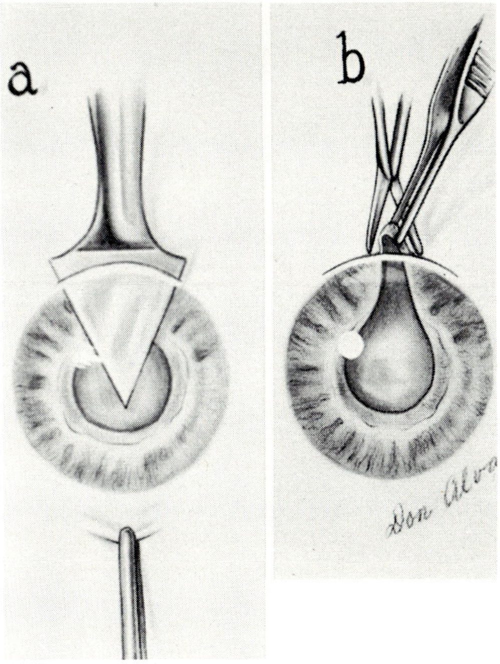

FIG. 129. Iridectomy. (A) A limbal keratomic incision is made superiorly. (B) A complete iridectomy is done. (Cordes, F. C. *in* Haik, G. (ed.): Symposium on Diseases and Surgery of the Lens, St. Louis, Mosby)

FUCHS' TECHNIC: In a personal communication, Dr. Cordes commented, "It is interesting to me that the Fuchs Aspiration technique, used some 40 years ago is again being revived with various modifications." The Fuchs two-way syringe with two side opening cannulas is

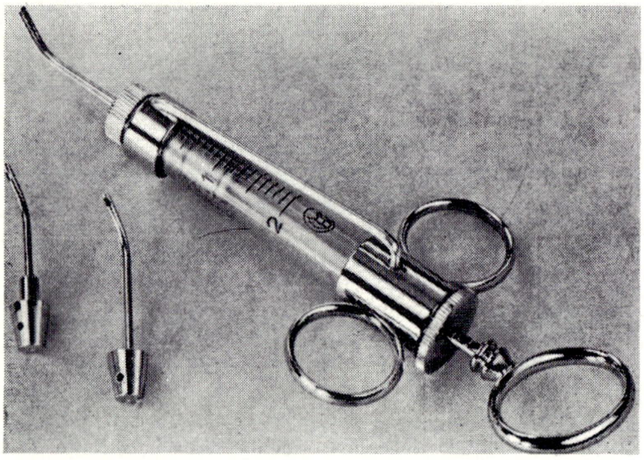

FIG. 130. Fuchs' two-way syringe (Storz instrument No. E-4882).

not new, but it is increasing in popularity, especially in congenital cataracts. The syringe is intended for use in the removal of lens residue and substance, irrigation following hemorrhage, and in conjunction with the removal of soft traumatic, congenital or juvenile cataracts of the zonular (lamellar) and total or hypermature types. It is not meant for membranous, hard cataracts or mixed types such as anterior and posterior polar, which cannot pass through the cannula easily.[7] Some congenital cataracts can be needled (avoiding the through-and-through type), and several days later this syringe can be used for lens residue. Dr. Fuchs of Stuttgart, Germany, designed the syringe and introduced it in the United States at the International Congress of Ophthalmology in New York in 1954. It was also presented at the 1958 meeting of the American Academy of Ophthalmology and Otolaryngology by Dr. Louis Daily. The two-way syringe with double cannulas supplies simultaneous irrigation and aspiration. The fluid in the anterior chamber can be changed several times with one motion and without varying the volume of the anterior chamber. This fluid introduction and simultaneous removal causes a swirling action within the anterior chamber. As the piston moves downward within the barrel of the syringe, the fluid is forced from one of the double cannulas. At the same time, the upper part of the barrel, being vacated by the downward moving piston, creates a vacuum which causes the fluid within the anterior chamber to be drawn into the second of the cannulas which is connected by a tube to the upper chamber of the syringe (Fig. 130). Drs. Joaquin Barraquer and Richard Troutman feel that the Fuchs two-way syringe is very useful in cataract extraction in children.[3] (See "Troutman's Technic," p. 110.)

SCHEIE'S TECHNIC. The following is Dr. Harold Scheie's new technic for aspiration of congenital cataracts or soft cataracts when the cataract is (a) complete; (b) incomplete; or (c) accompanied by incomplete pupillary dilatation. This aspiration technic is valuable for the removal of cataracts of any etiology occurring before the nucleus is firmly formed, i.e., in individuals up to 30 years of age. It is indicated for juvenile cataracts and is very helpful in the management of traumatic cataracts in young people.

A. Complete Cataract

When the cataract is complete, a small conjunctival flap is reflected toward the limbus. An eye speculum is inserted and a superior rectus suture is placed. A small conjunctival flap is dissected toward the limbus superiorly. The eye is fixed with a fixation forceps at the 6 o'clock position and a Ziegler type knife-needle is inserted in a plane parallel to the iris 1.5 to 2.0 mm. behind the limbus. A wide cruciate incision is made through the lens capsule and the knife-needle withdrawn, enlarging the scleral opening very slightly as it is removed to create a puncture just large enough to admit the needle and for suction.

The needle is a specially made thin-wall No.-19 needle with an oval tip of the type described by Atkinson for retrobulbar anesthesia. It is inserted, bevel down, through the knife-needle incision at the 12 o'clock position [Fig. 131, a]. Because the needle is made with a thin wall, the aperture is equivalent to that of a No.-18 needle. It is attached to a two-cc. syringe containing approximately 0.25 cc. of saline solution.

When the tip of the needle is at the lower pupillary border, the needle is rotated so that the bevel is turned forward with the aperture facing the cornea [Fig. 131, b]. This point in technique was first made by Dean. I have never seen damage to the corneal endothelium occur from the force of the suction or needle tip.

With the needle in place, suction is created by withdrawing the plunger of the syringe. If the lens does not aspirate readily, fluid can be forced into the anterior chamber and sucked out several times which helps to break up and remove the lens material. When the cataract is complete, however, there is

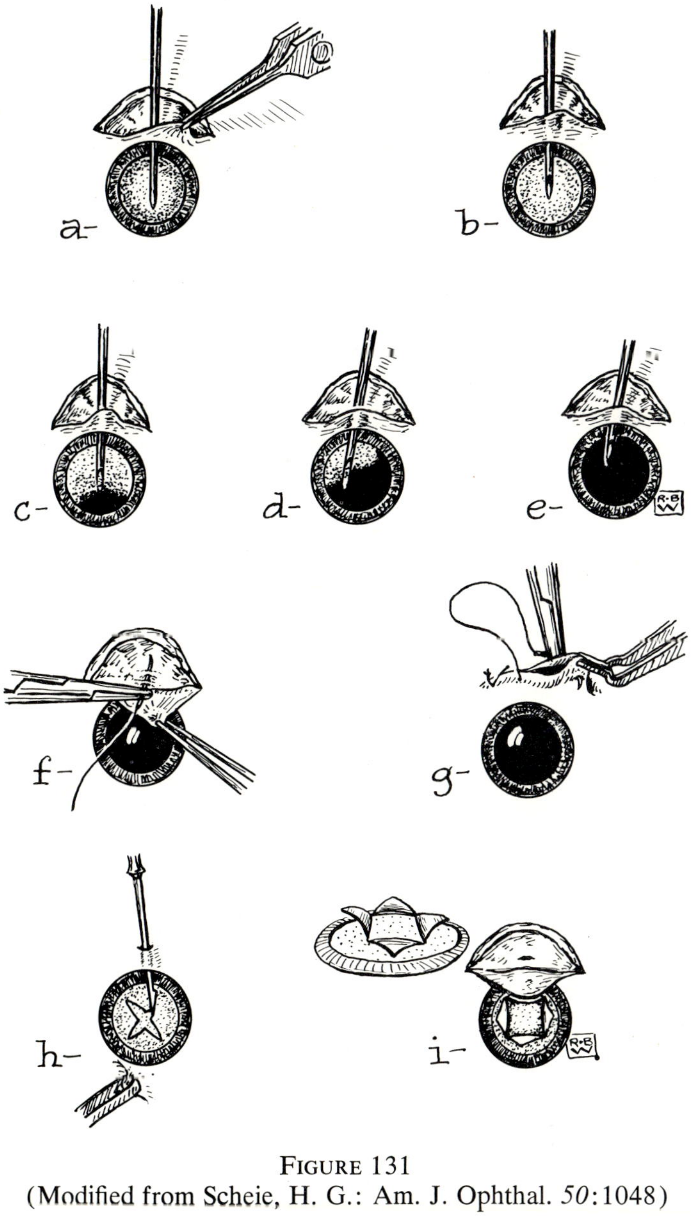

FIGURE 131
(Modified from Scheie, H. G.: Am. J. Ophthal. *50*:1048)

usually no difficulty in removing the lens material. As the lens material is aspirated, the tip of the needle can be directed to various positions in the anterior chamber to gather up any material that remains. It is of interest that even dense central nuclear plaques or membrane can be sucked into the lumen of the needle and removed. When the chamber is clear, the needle is removed [Fig. 131, c, d & e]. If lens material remains, the needle can be inserted into the chamber more than once by injecting saline to deepen the chamber as the needle is inserted. This protects the face of the vitreous.

Occasionally the pupillary border is displaced as the needle is withdrawn, indicating that the iris is caught in the scleral puncture. It can be freed by directing a current of saline into the opening by an anterior chamber irrigator held against the incision. To insure prompt reformation of the chamber, even though the incision is small, a 6-0 mild chromic catgut appositional suture with an atraumatic needle is placed across the knife-needle incision [Fig. 131, f & g]. Finally, the conjunctiva is closed. Pupillary dilation is maintained postoperatively with the continued use of atropine and if necessary phenylephrine (10 per cent).

B. Incomplete Cataract

If the cataract is incomplete, a preliminary needling should be done. A knife-needle is inserted into the anterior chamber through the conjunctiva and sclera about 1.5 to 2.0 mm. back of the limbus [Fig. 131, h]. A large cruciate incision is made in the anterior lens capsule. No attempt is made to stir up the cortex because of danger of injury to the posterior capsule. The eye is observed carefully for the next few days and when the lens is completely opaque and softened, as a result of action of the aqueous, aspiration is done. The interval is usually two or three days to a week. At that time, the operation as described for complete cataract is carried out. A conjunctival flap is turned, but another knife-needle incision usually is not necessary because the No.-19 needle can be inserted through the original puncture made for the discission [Fig. 131, i]. Aspiration of the lens material is done as previously described and the wound closure is identical. Pupillary dilatation, again, must be maintained postoperatively.

C. Aspiration With Incomplete Pupillary Dilatation

If the pupil does not dilate well preoperatively, the above operations must be combined with complete iridectomy. The technic is modified somewhat. A conjunctival flap is reflected toward the limbus. The knife-needle incision is made as already described and, except that following the discission, the wound is enlarged slightly but to no more than three mm. Slight pressure on the globe with the lips of the knife-needle incision separated permits the root of the iris to present into the opening. The iris is teased out by hand-over-hand action with iris forceps and a complete iridectomy done. Care is taken to replace the iris pillars. If the cataract is complete the No.-19 needle is then inserted as described and the lens removed.If the cataract is incomplete, the conjunctival incision is closed and removal of the lens material is done several days later as already described under Section B.[38]

It must be emphasized that in this last instance where the pupil will not dilate, it is important that there be a full iridectomy.

One of my residents created some of these needles for me by grinding the points of No. 19 needles. He has included bends in some of these needles for work at different angles. These bends help in inserting the needles into the eye but impede rotation at the aperture. I have performed almost the same suction-irrigation procedure with a long glass irrigating tip on a rubber bulb which I like because the control of the irrigation and the suction is entirely in the fingers of one hand (Fig. 132) (the tip is wider than is apparent in the illustration). By squeezing the bulb I can irrigate, and by releasing the bulb I get a suction effect. A new rubber bulb is important. This frees the other hand to hold the flap or rotate the eye. I myself favor Dr. Scheie's technic over the aspiration technic with the Fuchs two-way syringe. I have found the Fuchs syringe a bit more awkward to handle.

KARA'S TECHNIC. The technic described by Gerald B. Kara is an aspiration or suction technic utilizing motor-driven suction. Unlike the Fuchs or the Scheie technic, irrigation does not follow the suction. For mature cataracts it is done as a one-stage procedure. For other forms of cataract, such as the zonular, it may be preceded by measures that will soften the lens matter. This procedure is not used in adults where a standard form of procedure is recommended.

Essentially, the operation, which is a one-stage procedure, is done in the 12 o'clock position through an incision made with a narrow keratome penetrating the anterior capsule. An iridectomy may be performed in the 12 o'clock position. Motor-driven suction follows, and the incision is closed with one or two absorbable sutures. The needle used is a No. 17 gauge needle with a dull tip. The internal bore is that of a No. 18 needle.

Whereas in the adult the suction on the motor-driven erisophake is about 20 units when alpha-chymotrypsin is used and 30 units for the ordinary adult cataract where alpha-chymotrypsin is not used, more suction is required in mature congenital cataracts, usually about 40 units.

The needle is kept in constant motion and is applied in the area of lens matter. Suction is started or broken by foot control.

The method described above is not used for calcified plaques or for polar-type cataracts, especially those of the posterior type. In these cases, Dr. Kara feels that sooner or later one will have to remove this capsule to obtain a clear central area. In these cases the suction is reduced from 40 units to 30 units, and the plaque or the posterior capsule becomes attached to the needle and is pulled out.

One of the advantages of this operation is that it is a short procedure—as little as 30 seconds. Dr. Kara does not see any real advantage in slowing down the time required to perform the operation. Although some of these cases have been followed for 2 or 3 years, he does not know the long-range results.

In the case of bilateral cataracts, Dr. Kara will operate when the patient is 6 months old if the lens is hypermature. If the cataract is unilateral and hypermature, he will wait until the patient is 1 or 1½ years of age. In the unilateral cataract where the lens is not mature, i.e., the vision is 20/100 or better, he will leave the lens alone.[22]

Combined Procedures. DISCISSION AND LINEAR EXTRACTION. My present choice of operation might be called a combined discission and linear extraction of the Barkan type. This consists of a discission followed a few days later by washing the swollen lens material out through an opening into the anterior chamber. The

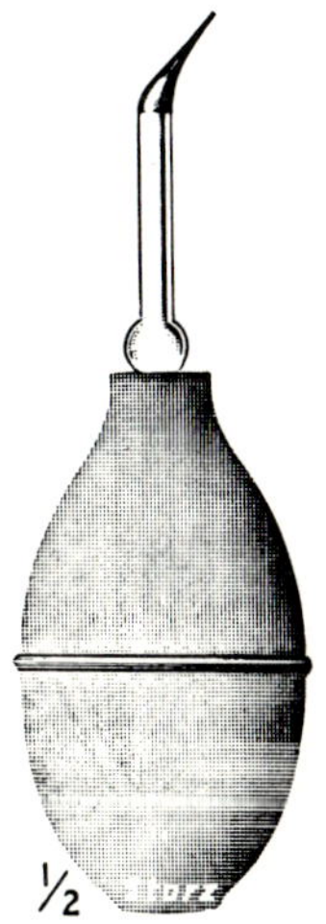

FIG. 132. Storz instrument No. E-4914.

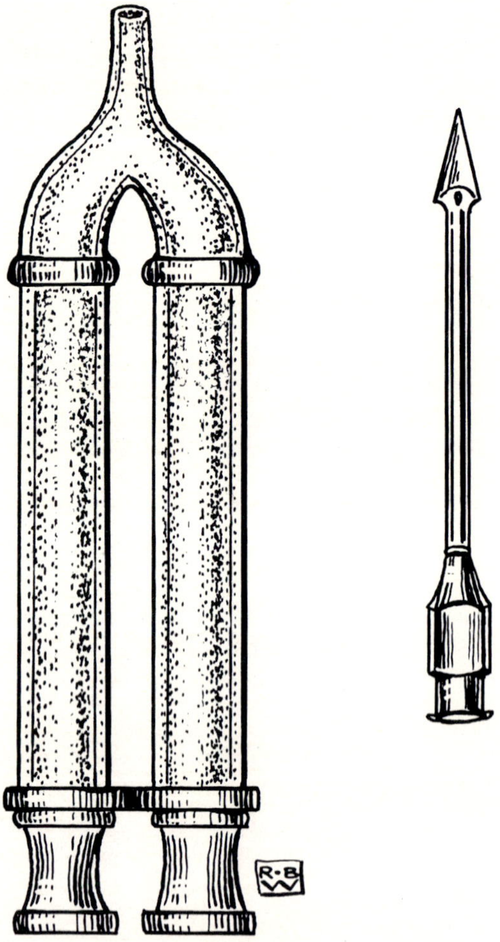

FIG. 133. Double-barreled syringe and the Rodriquez Barrios needle for suction of congenital cataracts. A regular, one-barreled syringe also may be used. The Fuchs two-way syringe cannot be used with this needle. (Modified from Boyd, B. F.: Highlights of Ophthalmology *4*:255)

major disadvantage of this operation is the need for two operations and two periods of anesthesia. However, the first period of anesthesia is brief. The major advantages are that the results are excellent and the complications are minimal.

The incision is usually made through the cornea at the limbus and closed with one or two chromic sutures. I find that I can wash out more lens matter by this planned two-stage procedure in a higher percentage of cases, and I rarely have to do a third stage. In accordance with present-day feelings the needle-knife avoids the posterior capsule in discission. I prefer a fairly extensive discission of the anterior capsule so that excessive swelling of the lens material and the associated secondary glaucoma, if present, are relieved by the second procedure. To date I have not had to resort to using urea or acetazolamide (Diamox) to control any secondary glaucomas because the second stage of surgery follows in a few days. The behavior and "feel" of the lens in the first stage of surgery lessens the chance of misjudging the type of cataract and helps to outline my course in the second stage. It is not always possible, especially in children, to tell whether the cataract is going to be liquid which can be aspirated or hard and rubbery.[7] Although a modification of the slit lamp and other aids for identifying the details of the lens are recommended, from a practical standpoint, I have not found them to be very helpful.

As a rule, I prefer to develop a conjunctival flap and make a keratome incision parallel to the iris; if the pupil has not dilated well with atropine preoperatively, I will add one or two vertical iridotomies below. Chromic sutures and adequate closure of the wound are used by me routinely. The prolonged use of atropine and phenylephrine (10% Neo-Synephrine) is an absolute necessity. Local cortisone is used, and systemic cortisone is ordered if indicated.

DISCISSION AND ASPIRATION (SUCTION). *Barrios' Technic.* The technic described by Rodriquez Barrios is essentially a discission followed by an aspiration using a modified Amsler needle manufactured by Grieshaber. The needle has sharp cutting edges to facilitate discission of the anterior capsule, has one

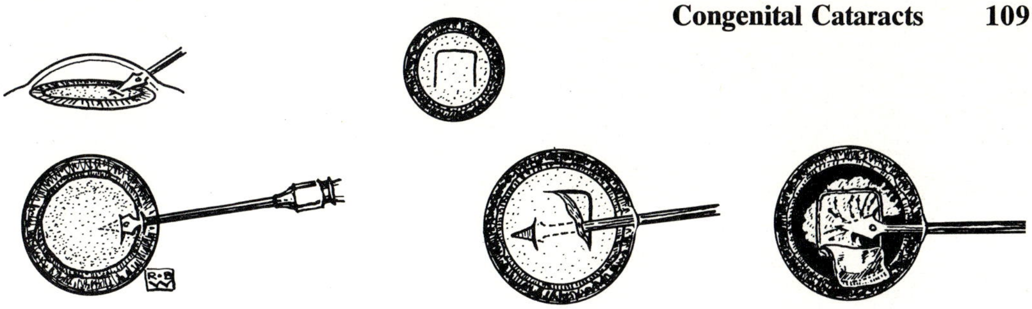

FIG. 134. (*Left*) The needle enters the anterior chamber through the cornea 1 mm. from the limbus. The keratome-shaped point of the needle perforates the anterior capsule for a wide capsulotomy. (*Center*) The classic anterior capsulotomies may be "x" or cross-shaped. Rodriquez Barrios prefers to do one with the shape of an inverted "U" (inset). The point of the needle is introduced behind the anterior capsule, and the inverted "U" shaped capsulotomy is obtained as shown. (*Right*) After the anterior capsulotomy, the opaque lens matter is removed by suction and irrigation. (Modified from Boyd, B. F.: Highlights of Ophthalmology *4*:255)

opening which should be pointed downward so as to avoid aspirating the iris and is attached to either an ordinary 2-ml. syringe partly filled with a balanced solution or a special double-barreled syringe to permit both aspiration and irrigation. The needle is introduced through the cornea 1 mm. from the limbus, and a large capsulotomy—preferably of the inverted "U" type—is made, taking care to keep the needle flat and away from the iris and the posterior capsule. Keeping the anterior chamber deep by irrigation as the needle enters and is withdrawn into the chamber helps to avoid complications. Aspiration and irrigation are continued until the pupillary area is clear, but excessive manipulation is to be avoided. A balanced solution or a small amount of air is left in the anterior chamber.

It is usual to wait 2 or 3 weeks before considering a second aspiration. If this is indicated, the same technic is used. If a secondary membrane forms, the management is as outlined in Chapter 5 under "Capsulotomies and Capsulectomies" (Figs. 133-135).[7]

Vargas' technic is still another discission-suction operation which destroys the anterior capsule by multiple thrusts with a

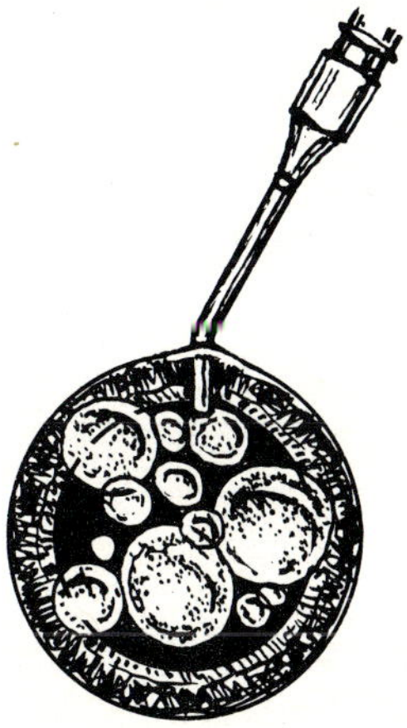

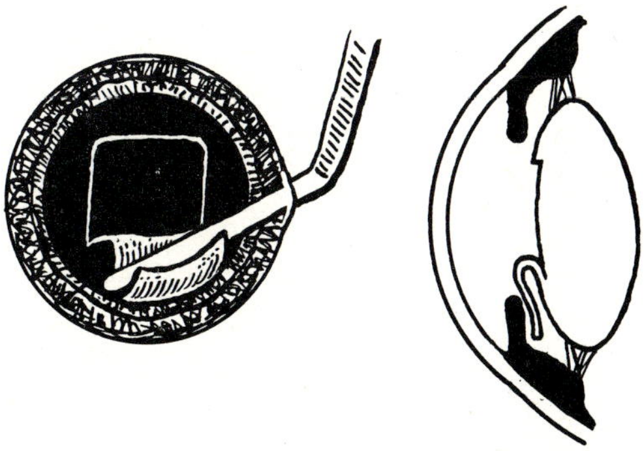

FIG. 135. (*Left*) Utilizing a Castroviejo spatula the flap remaining in the anterior capsule is placed behind the iris. (*Right*) Air is introduced in the anterior chamber. (Modified from Boyd, B. F.: Highlights of Ophthalmology *4*:255)

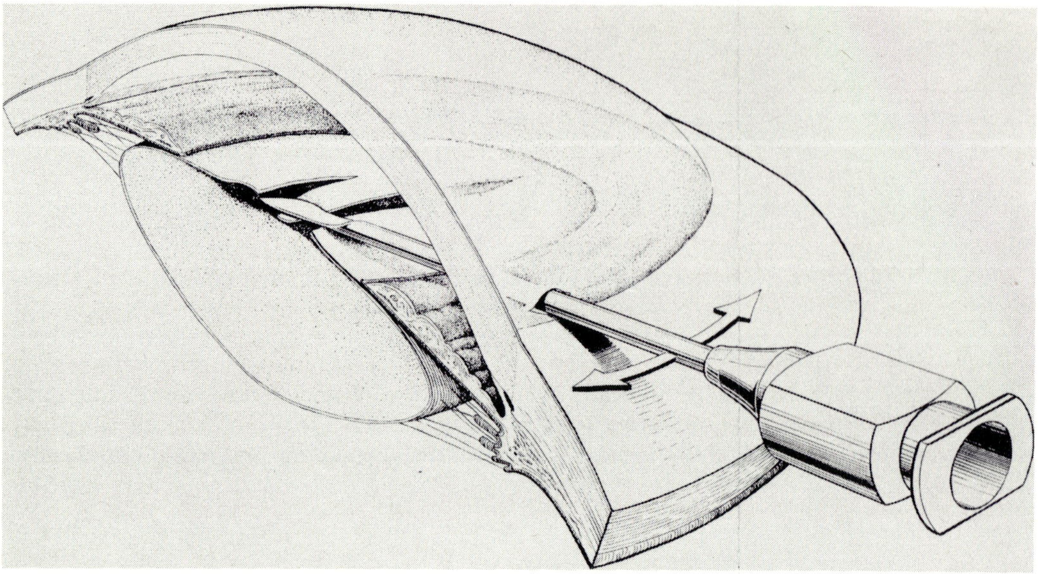

FIG. 136. Maumenee's technic for aspiration of congenital cataracts. The goniotomy needle enters through the cornea very close to the limbus. It is kept flat in order to avoid damage of the posterior capsule. The arrow shows the movement of the needle as the surgeon lacerates the anterior capsule. The needle is attached to a regular syringe and not to the Fuchs two-way syringe. (Boyd, B. F.: Highlights of Ophthalmology *4*:255)

20-gauge needle attached to a 5-cc. syringe. The needle is thrust in multiple places before sucking out the lens cortex.[10]

Maumenee's technic is essentially the same as that described by Rodriquez Barrios except that Maumenee utilizes a special goniotomy-like needle manufactured by Storz. A regular syringe is used to aspirate and irrigate the lens matter. The same precautions are used to avoid the iris and the posterior capsule (Figs. 136-138).[7]

Troutman's technic is a modification of

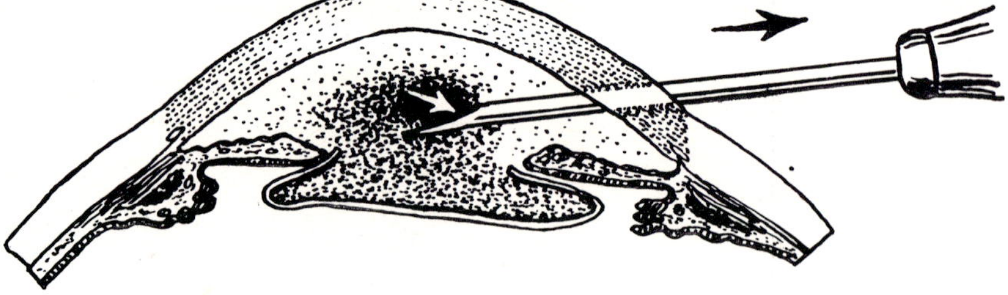

FIG. 137. Suction of lens material, Maumenee's technic. Lens material present in the anterior chamber following a wide anterior capsulotomy. Arrows show the direction of flow of the opaque lens material when suction is performed through a goniotomy needle and a regular syringe. The anterior chamber flattens moderately. Notice the very slight inclination of the needle, the opening held face up, and the relation of its tip to the posterior capsule. (Modified from Boyd, B. F.: Highlights of Ophthalmology *4*:255)

that described by Fuchs. The modification helps to solve the problem of management of the iris.

If the lens is totally opaque the technic is as follows:

Four-plane incision: A razor blade holder (Barraquer) fixes a piece of cracked blade so that 0.5 mm. of the sharp tip protrudes beyond its end. A 4 mm. limbus-based conjunctival flap is cut. Holding the instrument vertically, a scleral groove is made 1 mm. posterior to the surgical limbus. Bleeding is controlled with cautery [Fig. 139]. A fine serrated-edged spatula is introduced to the depth of the groove and the cornea is split in plane anteriorly for 2 mm. [Fig. 140]. The anterior chamber is entered by making a vertical incision at the junction of the anterior flap with a razor blade. A very fine scissors is introduced into the anterior chamber and the vertical internal incision is completed for a length of 1 cm. in congenital cataracts. (Scissors corneal section, Troutman, with stop to prevent closure of blades at tip.) This allows sufficient room for introduction of capsulotomy instruments and for performance or peripheral or full iridectomy. The extreme limits of the external razor incision must be extended 2 mm. further than the desired length of the internal incision; otherwise the external flap obscures the extreme ends of the internal incision [Fig. 141]. When the iris appears normal a peripheral iridectomy is performed with "colibri" forceps and Barraquer scissors. If there is a tonic pupil or synechiae, a full iridectomy and/or a radial iridotomy may be performed [Fig. 142]. The anterior capsulotomy is made with a Nieto knife or Cystotome. . . . Fine, modified, Schweiger forceps are utilized to remove a large portion of the anterior capsule [Fig. 143]. If [the] lens is totally opaque aspiration and irrigation are performed at once with Fuchs' two-way syringe, before

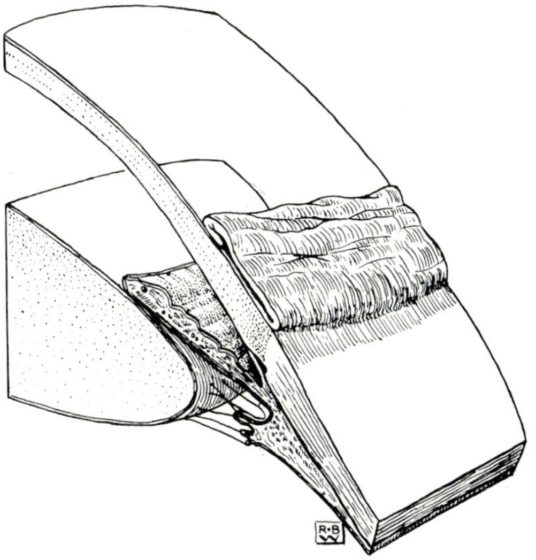

FIG. 139. Troutman's suction technic for congenital cataracts. (Modified from Troutman, R. C.: Highlights of Ophthalmology *4*:293)

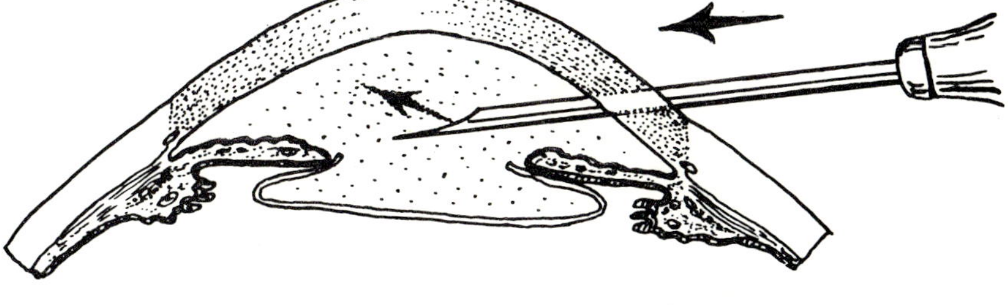

FIG. 138. Maumenee's technic for suction of congenital cataract. Anterior chamber refilled. The anterior chamber is being irrigated with saline from the syringe after part of the lens material has been aspirated. The density of the opaque material in the chamber is definitely diminished. The anterior chamber is completely re-formed. The sharp point of the needle is kept away from the posterior capsule. Aspiration and irrigation are continued until the pupillary area is clear. (Modified from Boyd, B. F.: Highlights of Ophthalmology *4*:255)

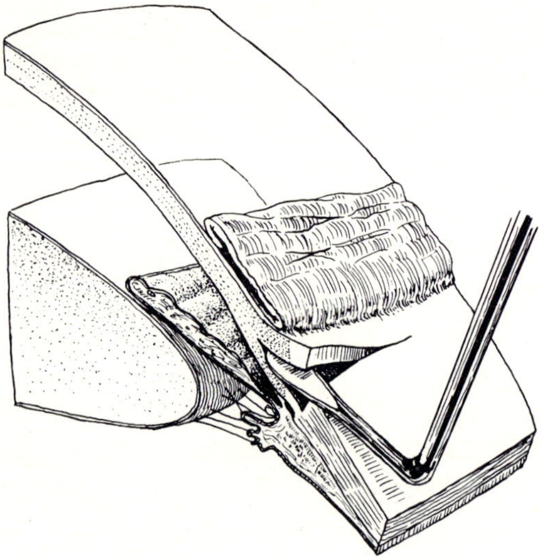

FIG. 140. Troutman's technic. The incision. Splitting of the cornea. (Modified from Troutman, R. C.: Highlights of Ophthalmology *4*:293)

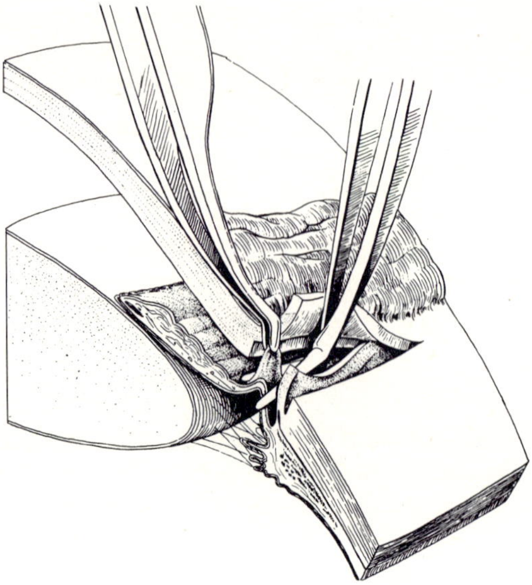

FIG. 142. Troutman's technic. Peripheral iridectomy. (Troutman, R. C.: Highlights of Ophthalmology *4*:293)

wound closure. If [the] lens is not totally opaque, as in lamellar cataracts, the wound is closed and suction performed later. The eye remains as shown [in Fig. 144] with lens material in [the] anterior chamber [and] the four step incision closed with suture and peripheral iridectomy.[48]

However, if the lens substance is not mature, only an anterior capsulotomy is performed and the wound is closed. Several days or weeks later when the lens matter flocculates, an incision in the cor-

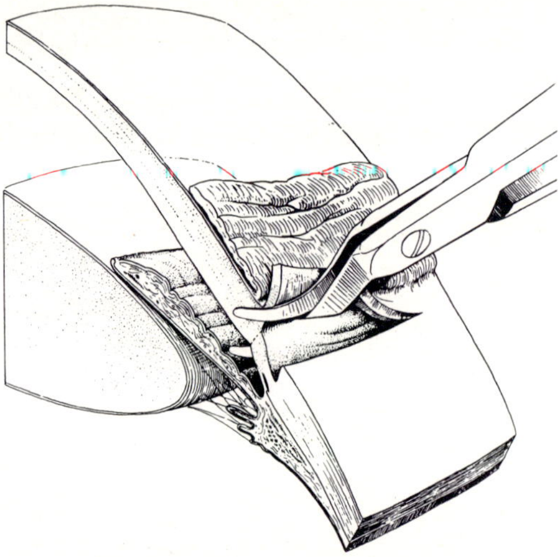

FIG. 141. Troutman's technic. Final step of the incision. (Troutman, R. C.: Highlights of Ophthalmology *4*:293)

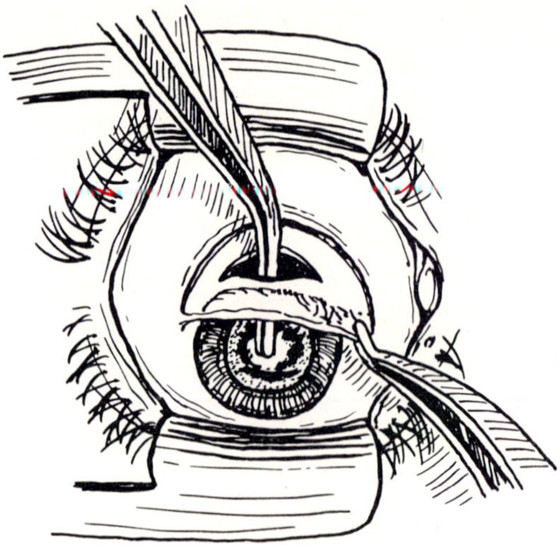

FIG. 143. Large bite in the anterior capsule. (Modified from Troutman, R. C.: Highlights of Ophthalmology *4*:293)

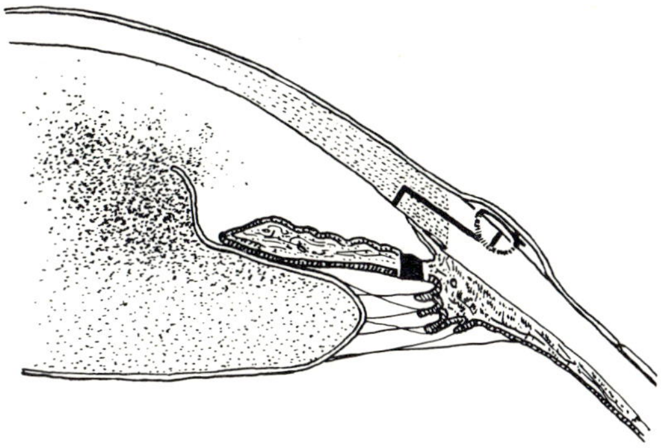

FIG. 144. Lens material in the anterior chamber. Wound closure. Iridectomy. (Modified from Troutman, R. C.: Highlights of Ophthalmology *4*:293)

nea is made about 2 mm. from the limbus with a narrow keratome or a razor blade. The 3-mm. opening here is made on the temporal side to permit the entrance of preferably the largest Fuchs cannula. If the incision is slightly shelved and is not made too obliquely, the scar will not obstruct the pupillary area and the wound usually will close itself (Figs. 145 & 146). Sutures should be used if the shelf is insufficient or if the incision is too wide.

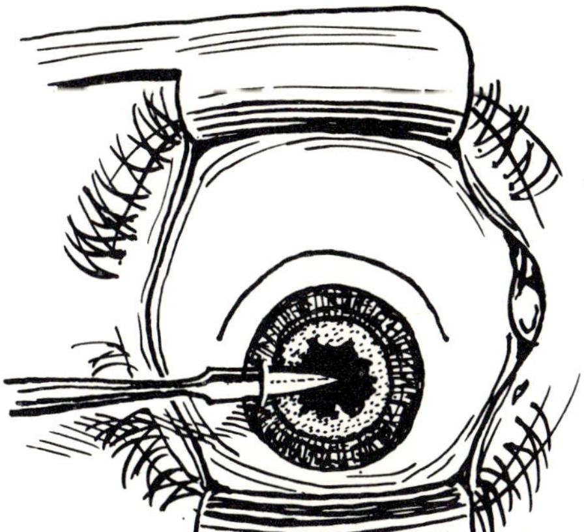

FIG. 145. Troutman's technic. Second operation. (Modified from Troutman, R. C.: Highlights of Ophthalmology *4*:293)

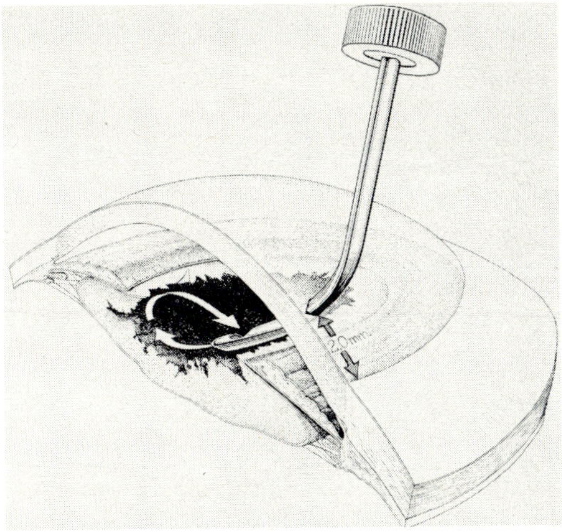

FIG. 146. Troutman's technic. Second operation, final stage. (Troutman, R. C.: Highlights of Ophthalmology *4*:293)

To avoid complications in using the Fuchs syringe, the cannula should be parallel to the posterior capsule.[7]

ASPIRATION (SUCTION) AND DISCISSION. *Carbajal's technic* as outlined below is to be done only in soft cataracts—those included under Types I, II, III or VII.

In his first technic,[10] Dr. Carbajal uses a short-beveled 19-gauge needle on an empty 2-ml. syringe, which is thrust into the lens at one point for the suction (Fig. 147, A & B). Following this the needle is withdrawn carefully and the anterior chamber is re-formed with saline, using a 28-gauge needle on a 2-cc. syringe. Then, under ultraviolet illumination for visualization, the anterior capsule of the lens is sliced with a fine Ziegler 3 mm. needle-knife in a fan-shaped fashion along three planes (Fig. 147, C). The anterior chamber may have to be re-formed before each discission to prevent injury to the vitreous face and the corneal endothelium. Finally, the needle-knife is withdrawn, and the anterior chamber is re-formed with either saline solution or air.

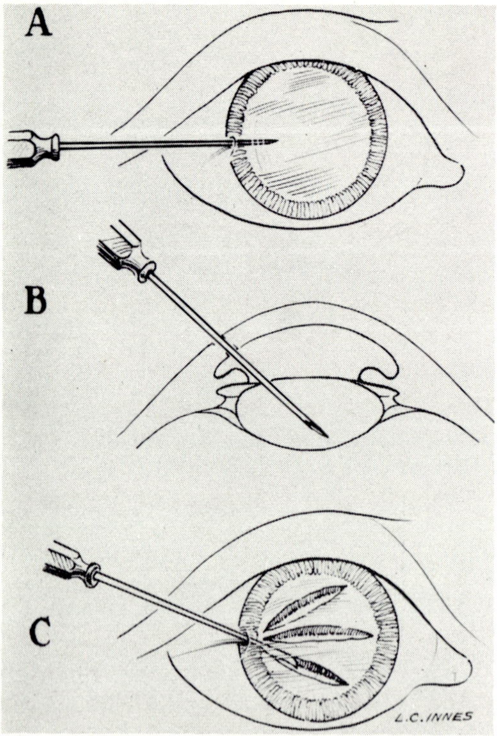

FIG. 147. Procedure for congenital cataract. (A) The needle is introduced through a scratch incision at the 9 o'clock position and enters the center of the proximal half of the lens. (B) The needle tip must not penetrate the posterior capsule, or the vitreous will be injured. (C) The anterior lens capsule is cut in a fan-shaped fashion. (Carbajal, U. M.: Am. J. Ophthal. *52*:361)

In his more recent modified technic,[11] Dr. Carbajal makes use of a special needle-knife (made from a 19-gauge needle by the Storz Instrument Company) which can be adapted to a 2-cc. syringe or to a Maumenee handle. This procedure is similar to the one just described, except that the anterior chamber is entered just once. Since the tip and the blade of this needle-knife are razor sharp and have a gentle curve, the anterior capsule can be cut into shreds and aspirated easily. If the opacity is located on the posterior capsule, great care should be exercised in making the discission to avoid rupturing the vitreous face. If the first two attempts to slice the posterior capsule opacity fail, no further attempt should be made. The membrane or after-cataract can be cut with Vannas scissors more effectively a month or two later.

Intracapsular Extraction

In intracapsular extraction in children or those patients under 20 years of age, alpha-chymotrypsin has little to offer at this time. The problems encountered both at the time of surgery and postoperatively are serious.

Operative problems are related to lenticulovitreal adhesions (see p. 3), increased scleral pliancy, incomplete chemical zonulolysis at times, increased intraocular pressure under general anesthesia, tendency for immediate and delayed iris prolapse or later synechia formation, delayed wound separation and staphyloma formation.

In children the scleral sac is much less rigid than it is in an adult. This is seen best if one compares the adult sclera with the infant's sclera after an evisceration (Fig. 148). The over-all strength of the adult scleral sac is approximately four times that of the infant's scleral sac. The scleral sac in infants can collapse even under its own weight. Therefore, the lack of rigidity and the very pliant sclera account for a major cause of vitreous loss in children. It is known that to record an intraocular pressure in infants and children a deep general anesthesia is necessary, and, probably because of the difference in the size of the globes of the infants, the value of the reading of the standard Schiotz tonometer may be questionable. The use of d-Tubocurarine or retrobulbar anesthesia in children may give unpredictable results in lowering the intraocular pressure—even with massage—partly because of the small orbital size. In fact, some feel that retrobulbar local anesthesia will cause an elevation of intraocular pressure in children.

Girard recommends the use of acetazolamide (Diamox) and urea as giving the most predictable results in lowering intraocular pressure in children. At surgery, approximately ½ hour before opening the eye, an intravenous infusion of 100 mg. of acetazolamide (Diamox) and a 30 per cent solution of urea in 10 per cent invert sugar is started. The total dosage is 1.5 Gm. per Kg. of body weight.[19] However, the true value of acetazolamide (Diamox) in reducing the intraocular pressure in children or in normal eyes has been questioned because Diamox does not have the same dehydrating effect under these conditions; here its value, which is considered to be minimal, is only to decrease the formation of aqueous.[7]

The chief postoperative problem is poor patient control combined with overzealous postoperative examination of an eye in which the wound is not healing well. The four-step incisions and closures, scleral rings and modifications, improved anesthesia, intravenous carbonic inhibitors and urea, postoperative sedation, head bandages and arm splints are only partial answers to cataract surgery in infants. The lens of infants sometimes will deliver spontaneously even without the use of an erisophake. However, the Flieringa-Bonaccolto ring may partly overcome the increased structural pliancy of the infant's sclera. If this ring is used, it is the present feeling that it should be applied after the rectus muscles have been exposed at the level of the equator. Since Girard's study indicates that in infants it works best if there is a 1 mm. clearance, one should have a selection of these rings handy at the time of surgery. Excessive bulging forward of the lens-zonular membrane indicates that the retrolental pressure is too high; if this is not controlled, the extent of corneal opening and the intended procedure should be modified. At present newer zonulolytic agents have no effect on the lens-vitreous adhesions.

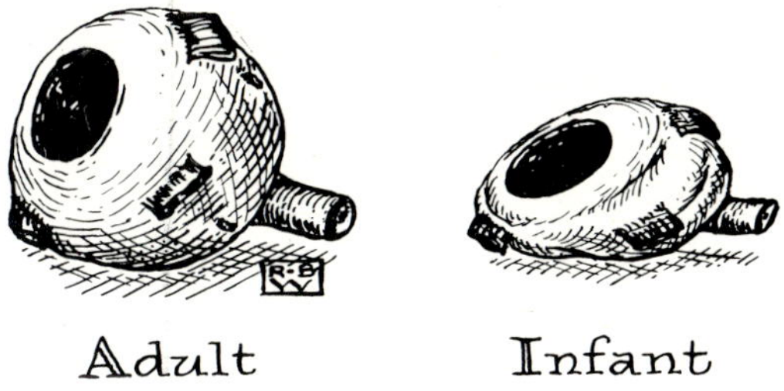

FIG. 148. In children the scleral sac is not as rigid as it is in an adult. This is seen best if one compares the adult sclera with the infant's sclera after an evisceration.

COMPLICATIONS OF CONGENITAL CATARACTS: FURTHER COMMENTS

Many of the complications of congenital cataract surgery and preventive measures have already been discussed. Since blindness may be the end-result of these complications, a partial review seems to be justified.

The most common and most feared complications are related to vitreous loss, inadequate pupillary opening, glaucoma and detachment of the retina. Both the glaucoma and the detachment of the retina are often related to vitreous disturbance.

Vitreous loss is a problem in intracapsular extractions and, to a lesser extent, in linear extractions. Retrobulbar anesthesia including hyaluronidase followed by digital massage is a routine that I follow, although some surgeons feel that because of the small orbital size it should not be used. Following this procedure I take a reading of the ocular pressure with a sterile tonometer despite the questionable value of such a procedure in children in whom a deep anesthesia is needed and where the shape of the cornea itself might affect such a reading with an instrument more suitable for adult-sized corneas. If the pressure of the eye is high, I will continue with massage until I record a pressure that is within normal limits. Capsulotomy in linear extraction is done with toothed forceps. However, only one application of the forceps should be made; otherwise, vitreous can be lost. When a linear extraction follows preliminary discission, capsule forceps should never be used. In some patients the anterior capsule can be very strong. If after the capsule is grasped reasonable traction does not tear it, it should be ruptured with the cystotome or some other sharp instrument. This can be done without releasing the grasp of the capsule forceps. Since vitreous loss can occur as a result of overvigorous expression, only gentle stroking of the cornea rather than pressure on the globe should be used. For the same reason, one should not attempt to irrigate too strongly. This also can result in vitreous loss.

Inadequate Pupillary Opening and Glaucoma. If the pupil does not dilate preoperatively, a vertical iridotomy below and a full iridectomy above are mandatory. These measures can prevent an inadequate pupillary opening or an updrawn pupil and a secondary glaucoma. Pupillary block is the most common cause of glaucoma in congenital cataract and the principal cause of blindness after operation. Prophylactically it is essential to keep the pupil dilated with atropine even for as long as a year following surgery. If an atropine sensitivity develops, scopolamine or cyclopentolate hydrochloride (Cyclogyl) and phenylephrine (10% Neo-Synephrine) are indicated. Phenylephrine alone is not sufficient.

Signs of pupillary block following cataract surgery in children differ from those in an adult. In children there may be an obvious iris bombé, but as a rule gross peripheral synechiae on clear cornea in even one area and, most commonly, an unevenness in the depth of the anterior chamber indicate the diagnosis.

An updrawn pupil can be avoided by doing an inferior iridotomy in all cases in which the pupil does not dilate well preoperatively. Since another serious complication is iridocyclitis, which in turn can create a cyclytic membrane and pupillary and angle block with a secondary glaucoma, cortisone preparations should be used if the postoperative reaction is severe. If a final discission has to be done in the presence of a small pupil that dilates poorly, vitreous may block the pupil and cause glaucoma. When the final discission is done peripheral iridotomies should be done at the same time as a safeguard against pupillary block with ensuing glaucoma. If pupillary block is not promptly recognized and relieved (preferably with a complete or a peripheral iridectomy), a severe glaucoma due to the peripheral synechiae results. In these cases medical treatment and surgical maneuvers such as cyclodialysis or cyclodiathermy may be tried, but they usually fail and the eye is lost.

Retinal detachment may occur without surgery in congenital cataracts. However, doing too much at surgery, especially to the vitreous, can set the stage for detachments. Therefore, it is important to do the least possible damage to the vitreous. The possibility of retinal detachment demands the best possible control of postoperative inflammation with cycloplegics, mydriatics and steroids. The prognosis of detachment surgery is unfavorable. In a personal communication Dr. Cordes mentioned that "while the prognosis for successful retinal detachment operation is very poor in these cases, Pischel has found that enough of them have been successful that surgery should be tried."[16]

SUMMARY AND CONCLUSIONS

Congenital cataracts in children present many problems preoperatively and postoperatively. Since no method of cataract extraction in children is without complication, there is still no "best approach." The answers to some of the hazards and problems in cataract surgery have been found, while other problems remain unsolved.

Although there is no unanimity of opinion and while there is a group who feel that early surgery may overcome some forms of amblyopia and nystagmus, the consensus still favors delaying surgery until 1 year of age in cases with total bilateral congenital cataracts. At this time the child can tolerate general anesthesia better, and the eye itself responds more satisfactorily to surgery. I am totally in accord with this approach.

The surgeon has a wide choice of surgical procedures for managing congenital cataracts. Today iridectomy for optical purposes is not frequently used. Many surgeons still prefer discission, while an equal number—or perhaps a slightly larger number—prefer linear extractions. A few of the many approaches to surgery of congenital cataracts are summarized in Table 1, p. 95. It cannot be emphasized too strongly that in many cases of Types I, II, III, IV and VII, no surgery is indicated if it is felt that there is or might be a vision of 20/60 or better.

Even with the new advances in cataract surgery, intracapsular extractions should not be used in infants. As a rule, my personal preference is a combined procedure —a discission, avoiding the posterior capsule, followed by a linear extraction. Although this two-stage procedure, which is the choice of many surgeons besides myself, requires two anesthesias, the results are among the best.

Since glaucoma and retinal detachment are two of the most serious complications following congenital cataract surgery, a complete iridectomy is most important in all cases where the iris will not dilate well preoperatively. Atropine and mydriatics should be used for a long time postoperatively.

As. Dr. Cordes pointed out, it bears emphasis that

> When entering the vitreous, it is important to do the least possible amount of damage to the vitreous as clinical experience and laboratory findings show that the more the vitreous is damaged the greater is the danger of late detachment of the retina occurring 10 to 35 years after the surgery.[16]

TRAUMATIC CATARACT

In traumatic cataract where there is a subluxated lens in the anterior chamber, the removal is comparatively simple. The lens is removed with the usual incision after the cataract has been trapped in the anterior chamber. Sometimes lenses of this nature can be pulled into the anterior chamber and the same procedure followed. The use of urea or mannitol is helpful in these cases. With its use one may not need the Flieringa-Bonaccolto ring.

Where there is a contusion in traumatic cataract, if there is a small opening in the peripheral portion of the lens, the most widely accepted form of management is to avoid the use of atropine or cortisone preparations which would hinder the sealing off of this small penetration. Constriction with drugs such as pilocarpine might help to seal the opening in the capsule. Miosis facilitates the formation of posterior synechiae between the iris and the lens-capsular wound, possibly inhibiting aqueous from penetrating into the lens stroma. However, some report spontaneous closure of the capsular wound without progression of localized cataractous changes even with the use of atropine.[18] However, if the opening is central and especially if it is large, it is wise to use atropine and cortisone. If the patient is under 30 years of age, one can wait in that there is a good possibility that this type of lens may absorb of itself. If the lens matter does not absorb, an extracapsular extraction or anterior capsular discission can be used. If the patient is over the age of 20, occasionally one can do an intracapsular extraction. As a rule, it is best to operate when the cataract becomes mature.

Intralenticular Foreign Bodies

Lenticular foreign bodies, especially metallic ones, may be removed if the foreign body is small and the injury is not too extensive. Satisfactory phakic vision may be preserved with no apparent increase in lenticular changes in some cases. Certain small nonmagnetic intralenticular foreign bodies may safely be watched if the damage seems to be localized to the lens.

Magnetic foreign bodies, especially iron, should be removed from the lens as rapidly as possible to avoid siderosis bulbi. If neither siderosis nor ocular irritation is present, the foreign body may be considered to be walled off or composed of an inert alloy and may be left undisturbed. If there is a delay of weeks or months following injury and if the capsular wound is closed and the cataract is localized, observation is recommended.[18] If lens extraction is indicated, an intracapsular extraction sometimes may be attempted with the use of alpha-chymotrypsin if the patient is over 20 years of age. It is best to wait for 6 months after the foreign body surgery before performing the lens extraction unless circumstances warrant earlier interference.

In adults with traumatic cataracts, I find that the prognosis is somewhat better than it is in children. On occasions I have used alpha-chymotrypsin and have noted, as others have, that this makes the removal of the lens, or the capsule, easier. However, the surgeon must consider carefully whether or not he will use alpha-chymotrypsin in adults with traumatic cataracts, since the enzyme can, in some cases, reach the interior vitreous with possible damage to the retina.

If there is a traumatic cataract with vitreous in the anterior chamber, it seems wise to remove the lens as early as possible before other complications set in. Urea and/or the Flieringa-Bonaccolto ring may be used. Some prefer to preserve the round pupil, feeling that it will keep the vitreous back from the cornea, thus preventing dystrophy, detachment and secondary glaucoma. I prefer a full iridectomy with one or two vertical iridotomies below. It is important to attempt an intracapsular extraction. A balanced solution and air at the time of surgery are also most important.

Urea and/or the Flieringa-Bonaccolto ring help the problem of immediate vitreous loss. A balanced solution and air keep the vitreous from the back of the cornea. Acetazolamide (Diamox) and bed rest with binocular dressings are important.

Steroids and antibiotics can be used prophylactically.

Traumatic Cataract in Children: Prognosis

To date very little has been written on the management of traumatic cataract in children.

In 1900 Baudry wrote, "Beware of traumatic cataracts. In general, every injury to the crystalline lens should be considered as a serious menace to the existence of the eye." This statement made over half a century ago might be revised today to read, "every injury to the crystalline lens should be considered as a serious menace to *useful vision* in that eye."

In 1938 a review of 90 cases of traumatic cataract at the Wilmer Institute in Baltimore showed that approximately one third of these patients retained "useful vision." However, the average age was listed as 26 so that, obviously, these were not all in children.[27]

In 1943 Black reviewed 100 cases of traumatic cataract before the Ophthalmological Society of the United Kingdom. These cases represented all age groups, and it was concluded that more than 50 per cent had vision enabling them to see no more than "hand movements."[27]

In 1961 McKinna[27] reported the results of treatment of traumatic cataract in 52 children seen at the teaching hospitals of McGill University, Montreal, and the University of California Medical Center, San Francisco. In summarizing the results of patients 6 years of age and *under,* McKinna concludes:

> 1) Visual acuity: Only one patient had vision of 20/30 or better with correction. This patient had intermittent occlusion and aphakic correction postoperatively until the acuity in the injured eye had improved to 20/30+. . . .
>
> 2) Deviation: At least nine patients developed deviations about equally divided between esotropia and exotropia. . . .
>
> 3) Operative procedure: Nine patients underwent two or more operative procedures and four patients underwent three or more procedures. Three patients developed retinal detachment; two of these had two or more operative procedures and the other a linear extraction. . . .
>
> One patient developed glaucoma and one eye was lost following a surgical procedure in 1937 (pre-antibiotic era). . . .

As for the patients *over* the age of 6 years, McKinna concludes:

> 1) Visual acuity: Seven patients have corrected vision of 20/20 or 20/30; two patients have 20/70; the remainder, counting fingers, hand movements or light perception. One of the patients with corrected vision of 20/30 was treated in Hawaii with postoperative intermittent occlusion and aphakic correction at the age of seven years.
>
> 2) Deviation: Seven patients developed deviations; four exotropias and three esotropias.
>
> 3) Operative procedures: Nine patients underwent two or more operative procedures. Two patients (one from each center) developed glaucoma postoperatively and rerequired further surgery to control the glaucoma. One patient developed retinal detachment after four needlings. This occurred six years after the last needling.

In summarizing the results of the *total group* of 52 patients, McKinna notes the following:

Visual acuity: The visual acuity obtained in both groups is uniformly poor. Only 1 patient under the age of 6 years had vision of 20/30 and 7 patients over this age had 20/30 or better.

Deviation: In the total group, deviations occurred whether or not clear pupillary areas were obtained.

Surgery: As far as surgery is concerned, the results, particularly in children under the age of 6, have been uniformly poor regardless of the procedure used. The impression is gained that one cannot emphatically recommend either discission or linear extraction on the basis of these results but that a linear extraction, when possible, may be a more desirable procedure than discission.

Complications: Among the complications, glaucoma was noted in 2 patients, and 4 patients developed retinal detachments 3 to 20 years after the cataract procedure.

In summing up, Dr. McKinna quotes Dr. Cordes' statement that, "if you are not sure what to do, you had better not do it."

I have also found through personal experience that the prognosis for traumatic cataracts in children is very poor. In children under the age of 6, I favor a discission followed by a linear type of extraction and have used an aphakic correction in the injured eye plus occlusion of the uninjured eye. This is followed by the use of a contact lens when the child is able to tolerate one. Except for the amblyopia of disuse and because of the poor visual results, one wonders whether it might be better to wait, when possible, until the child reaches adult years. Of course, with glaucoma or a known detachment, one cannot wait.

In future years new zonulolytic agents, better anesthesia and methods for overcoming the elasticity of the child's eye may make it possible to obtain better visual results following surgery for traumatic cataracts in children.

CATARACT SURGERY IN DIABETICS

Diabetes, like glaucoma, may be undiagnosed in some patients. Today the prognosis for diabetics undergoing cataract surgery is somewhat better, but it is still guarded. Thanks to better control of the diabetes and to antibiotics, infection plays only a small part in the production of complications.

Multiple complications, such as hyphema and uveitis, are common following cataract surgery in the diabetic. Needless to say, the ophthalmic surgeon must work closely with the patient's internist prior to, during and following surgery. General anesthesia should be avoided in diabetics.

Preoperatively the entire eye should be studied, careful attention being given to the cornea, the angle and the iris, especially in regard to blood vessels, in anticipation of the tendency to bleed. This tendency is noted particularly in diabetics, and the areas noted should be avoided when possible.

If one uses a conjunctival flap as I do, especially when using alpha-chymotrypsin, the incision should be slightly corneal but not short. While the larger incision invites more bleeding, especially in the 3 to 9 o'clock area, it also facilitates the extraction. In these cases especially, some favor a pure corneal incision with no conjunctival flap. There is less tendency for bleeding when the incision is corneal. The difficulty is further increased when one is forced to operate on a mature or a hypermature lens in the presence of rubeosis. The prognosis is especially guarded in this type of case but one may occasionally be surprised by a patient who has obtained some useful vision for 1 or 2 years following surgery. The use of the light coagulator over the iris where an intended iridectomy is planned may help to reduce bleeding. Some surgeons will not do an iridectomy. A sphincterotomy in an uninvolved portion and the removal of the lens might be tried. Others have reported that occasionally there will be no bleeding even with a complete iridectomy in patients with rubeosis.

Poor dilatation is often seen in diabetics with cataracts even when phenylephrine (10% Neo-Synephrine) is given preoperatively. Iris pigmentation is seen more frequently even without the use of alpha-chymotrypsin. Fortunately, the pigment is innocuous.

Alpha-chymotrypsin is of great value in these cases and may account for the reduced incidence of anterior uveitis. Part of the decrease is related to the reduced incidence of extracapsular extractions.

With the use of a conjunctival flap, additional sutures and careful technic, today there is not the problem of wound healing that there used to be. The proper use of alpha-chymotrypsin with irrigation of the wound edge and later the anterior chamber has not resulted in poorer wound healing even in diabetics. Of course, the prognosis for vision in the diabetic is not as good as it is in the nondiabetic. No real advances have been made in treating diabetic retinopathy and the associated changes in the media.

MYOPIA AND DETACHMENT

The presence of high myopia and potential retinal detachment in patients with cataracts always present a serious problem in management. One study of the complications and the final results of cataract operations performed on patients with high myopia showed that detachment of the retina was the most formidable complication encountered. It is recommended that the surgeon wait 1 year before operating on the fellow eye because a possible retinal detachment will most likely appear in the first year after cataract surgery.

Prophylactic Steps

A study of the incidence of retinal detachment in aphakia emphasizes two points that are often overlooked; these are the possibility of perforating the globe with either (1) the superior rectus suture, or (2) the retrobulbar injection.[50] I know of two cases in which a hole was created in the area where a superior rectus suture had been applied. Therefore, every effort should be made to avoid these pitfalls.

In the presence of a high myopia, some surgeons recommend an extracapsular extraction with a complete iridectomy so that the fundus can be examined more easily in case a detachment of the retina occurs.[40] However, even with a complete iridectomy, capsular remains often make it difficult to locate holes.[25] I do not favor this approach, and at present my thoughts on this matter are as follows:

If one anticipates a cataract extraction in a patient with high myopia, the light coagulator of Meyer-Schwickerath, scleral diathermy and/or scleral shortening procedures may be considered prophylactically when the cataract is still small and central. However, in this particular field there is the greatest disagreement as to the advisability of such treatment either by internal or external procedures. Many specialists feel that light coagulation is a safe and easy way of sealing and strengthening degenerated areas. It has been pointed out that diathermy or photocoagulation to the flat retina is uncomplicated and exact. If repair is withheld until detachment occurs, damage to the retina can be aggravated after the cataract extraction. Small tears increase in size, degenerated areas fragment, and cystic areas either become more cystic or perforate. Others feel that light coagulation especially is dangerous in that it may produce retinal contraction.

Possible Indications and Therapy

There are no definite indications for prophylactic external surgery or internal light coagulation on which all will agree. Since patients who have had a retinal detachment in one eye show an increased frequency of retinal detachment in the fellow eye, these eyes would seem to furnish good cases for prophylactic treatment before the cataract in the fellow eye becomes too dense to permit visualization of details. Many feel that eyes showing areas of degeneration should not be treated until a detachment actually occurs. Some feel that treatment is indicated in a patient who has had a retinal detachment in the other eye, especially if the degeneration is above the horizontal meridian. However, retinal breaks without elevation that are below the meridian are less likely to cause retinal detachments and can be watched with a greater degree of safety if the lens changes are not too rapid. These lower breaks without elevation can be treated if there is no evidence of spontaneous pigmentation. Light coagulation seems to be helpful as an adjunct in those cases that have many retinal breaks without detachment in different areas of the globe. If this method is used, it is wise to allow pigment formation in the treated quadrants before applying the next stage of light coagulation. Usually an interval of 2 to 3 weeks is satisfactory.

In examining and treating these eyes, good dilatation is important. With scleral indentation and the direct and indirect ophthalmoscope one may visualize the involved areas in the far periphery. If the area of the holes shows no retinal elevation or if it settles with bed rest, the Zeiss light coagulator can be used. Areas of degeneration can be surrounded by the light coagulator or prophylactic scleral diathermy. In treating these eyes showing degeneration, it is important that either the light coagulator or prophylactic scleral diathermy should be applied to the areas of normal retina surrounding the areas of degeneration. This is especially true of areas of lattice degeneration because the areas of degeneration proper are too stiff to seal the retina adequately. In that retinal contraction may follow, it is felt that light coagulation or external diathermy should not be used prophylactically completely around the eye. Certainly the use of the light coagulator or diathermy in large areas as a prophylactic measure makes it difficult to find holes in detached retina over these treated areas should retinal separation occur at a later date. It has been pointed out that a barrage of light coagulation completely around the periphery of the retina can be done in three or four stages with intervals of 2 to 3 weeks between barrages. The treatment should always be minimal. Unfortunately, it provides no guarantee that detachment will not occur. The use of scleral diathermy in the upper and the lower quadrants of the eye, done in stages prior to cataract extraction, is another method advocated for trying to prevent retinal detachment (Fig. 149).

In the Barraquer Clinic, a prophylactic lamellar scleral resection was being used prior to cataract extraction in patients with high myopia who previously had shown advanced fundal pathology or who gave the history of detachment in the other eye and also when a complete cataract was present, making visualization of the fundus impossible. However, I question whether this much surgery is necessary or helpful. When one is presented with the problem of a complete cataract and the possibility of a detached retina, a most important aid is a good history. Of course, the usual procedures such as determination of light projection are also important.

Electroretinograms, if one is fortunate

enough to have them available, may be of some help where there is a complete cataract and one suspects a retinal detachment. Dr. Burian states,

As we might expect, the ERG is subnormal or even extinguished in retinal detachment. Some authors feel that there is a definite relationship between the height of the b-wave and the extent and duration of the detachment and that the chances for reattachment of the retina by surgery can be predicted from the height of the b-wave. Other authors do not attribute a prognostic value to the b-wave in this respect. They have found an improvement of the b-wave of the ERG after successful surgery, in some cases even if the ERG was extinguished before surgery. In retinal detachment, as in some other conditions, the a-wave would seem to be the last to disappear and the first to reappear in successful cases, sometimes being at first exaggerated in amplitude.

An important finding in patients with unilateral detachment is the reduction of the ERG in the nondetached fellow eye. This is quite regularly observed and justifies the close attention given to these eyes.[8]

Work by another group of investigators on electroretinography in the presence of detachments shows not only a subnormal ERG but also a reduced oscillatory potential; the decrease in the ERG was proportional to the extent of the retinal detachment. There was some correlation between the decrease in ERG potentials and the duration of the detachment. As to the effect of operation on the ERG, most patients with a normal ERG had a good operative prognosis; provided that an oscillatory potential was seen, even patients having a subnormal ERG also showed a good operative result. Cases showing no response, so-called extinguished ERG, frequently had poor operative results. These studies suggest that a successful operation produces an increased ERG giving rise to a decreased oscillating potential for a few months after the operation.

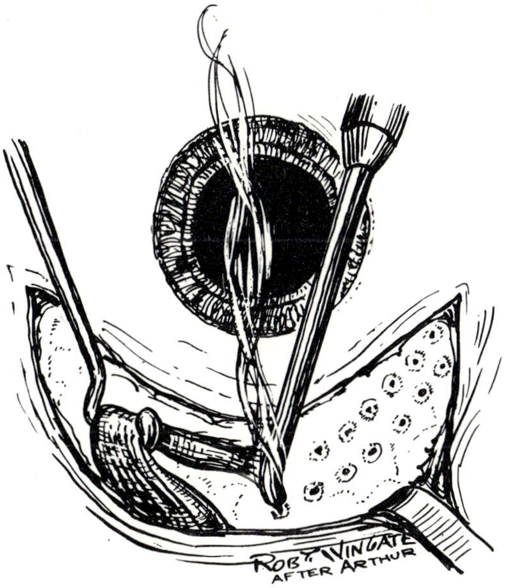

FIG. 149. Cyclodiathermy. (Modified from Callahan, Alston: Surgery of the Eye: Diseases, Springfield, Ill., Thomas)

The absence of the oscillating potential predicts a poor prognosis without regard to the amplitudes of the a- and b-waves.[49]

Another method that is reported to be useful and reliable for diagnosing retinal detachment in the presence of cataracts is intensity-modulated ultrasonography.[2]

Since time-amplitude ultrasonography yields only a graph while modulation ultrasonography permits permanent recording of high-resolution cross-section views of the light-opaque portions of the eye and the orbit, only intensity-modulated ultrasonography is reported to be suitable for general clinical use.[20]

Yet, from a practical standpoint, Dr. Morton Rosenthal points out that at this time he has found that in the case of most cataracts, when the pupil can be maximally dilated, he can get some impression of the retina prior to surgery. At this time he feels that the electroretinogram has not been too helpful to him; in addition, he finds that the ultrasonographic system is not readily available or suitable for general clinical use.[36]

If the cataract is complete and I cannot visualize the fundus, I will proceed as follows: In order to visualize the fundal details better at a later date, I will do a vertical iridotomy below and a complete iridectomy above. My personal preference in these cases is an intracapsular cataract extraction. At present I am using a small amount of alpha-chymotrypsin which is carefully washed out prior to the extraction of the lens.

At the Wills meeting in 1960, I was asked to comment on Dr. Spaeth's paper concerning the greater incidence of detachment in myopia. I asked whether the use of alpha-chymotrypsin might possibly reduce the number of detachments because of the need for less pulling in removing the lens. Dr. Spaeth felt that its use would not but jokingly questioned whether the alpha-chymotrypsin might not increase the number of detachments following cataract surgery in patients with high myopia. Surgeons who use alpha-chymotrypsin agree that it should be used in cases of high myopia; however, many of these eyes show liquid vitreous, and alpha-chymotrypsin may possibly damage the retina in these particular cases. Therefore, only a small amount of alpha-chymotrypsin should be used, and an attempt should be made to remove the excess prior to the actual extraction.

Dr. Pischel stated that

> From statistics available at present, there does not seem to be an increase in the number of detachments of the retina following cataract extraction when the enzyme is used in comparison to extractions without its use.[33]

Joaquin Barraquer noted a decrease in retinal detachments in 1959. Without the enzyme there were 10 cases of detached retina following 262 cataract extractions or an incidence of 3.8 per cent. With the enzyme, there were 3 cases following 219 cataract extractions or an incidence of 1.3 per cent.[4]

In summary, when the cataract is complete and I suspect a retinal detachment, I prefer to remove the cataract and treat the detachment, if there is one present, after I can study the location of the holes in the retina.

Optimal Time for Repairing Retinal Detachment Following Cataract Surgery

If one suspects the possibility of a retinal detachment in an eye that has just been operated for cataract, the patient should be kept in bed and binocular dressings should be used. On the 4th or the 5th day one can safely examine the fundus for evidence of detachment. If a detachment is noted, the patient should wear pinhole glasses for 6 weeks. One should wait at least 6 weeks before doing scleral buckling procedures following cataract extractions complicated by a retinal detachment. Prior to this time the corneal wound does not heal well enough to withstand the stress and strain of a scleral buckling procedure. A prime indication for a scleral buckling procedure is a retinal detachment following a cataract extraction. As a rule, ordinary diathermy presents a very poor prognosis. Vitreous implants may be a helpful adjunct in the treatment of these difficult cases.[40]

SUMMARY AND CONCLUSIONS

Present-day considerations in reference to cataracts, high myopia and detachment have been reviewed. Since there are no definite indications for prophylactic detachment surgery, recent ideas on this subject have been outlined. I have indicated my present choice of the management of this problem and have included Dr. Morton Rosenthal's views on this subject because of his special interest in retinal detachments.

From a practical standpoint Dr. Rosenthal questions the value of the suggestion made by one group that one should wait 1 year following cataract extraction in the first eye before operating the second eye, especially if the cataract in the fellow eye is mature. I agree with him. In this situation a detachment may occur in the second eye and may not be detected. He, too, strongly favors an intracapsular cataract extraction, preferably with a complete iridectomy, in patients with high myopia. He also favors using alpha-chymotrypsin in patients with high myopia and cataracts. He agrees that it should be used in a small amount and should be carefully washed out. Because it is possible to treat large areas and miss completely the small but very significant lesions, he questions the value of using external encircling diathermy or buckling, even when done in stages, in the eye that has a complete cataract or may potentially show a detachment. Concerning eyes showing a partial cataract and a hole with retinal elevation that settles with bed rest, it is Dr. Rosenthal's feeling that these cases are not helped by the use of the light coagulator prophylactically. However, cases with holes but no elevation do respond. As to treatment of large areas of lattice degeneration with the light coagulator, it is his feeling, and I agree, that this is a situation in which the "cure" is worse than the disease because the treatment can lead to irreversible vitreous retraction and inoperable detachments.

If a cataract is complete and he suspects a detachment, he, too, removes the cataract and treats the detachment 4 to 6 weeks later. He points out that if he detects a detachment in the immediate postoperative period, he does not immobilize the patients or use pinholes.

I myself feel that every effort to preserve the macula with bed rest when possible and pinholes should be tried until corneoscleral healing of this cataract wound permits a scleral-shortening procedure.

CORNEAL DYSTROPHIES, CATARACTS AND THE USE OF ALPHA-CHYMOTRYPSIN

Dystrophy and cataract is a very serious combination in that the operation for cataract often will make the corneal problem worse, especially if the dystrophy is of the Fuchs type. It is said that a well-known eye surgeon who performs every type of major eye surgery will not operate cases of cataract with Fuchs' dystrophy because of the poor prognosis. In the presence of Fuchs' dystrophy it is absolutely essential to remove the cataract with extreme gentleness and a minimum of manipulation. Preliminary to cataract extraction, corneal transplantation should be considered.

Hughes feels that in Fuchs' endothelial-epithelial dystrophy there need be no hurry to operate on patients with relatively good vision and central changes limited to the endothelium without overlying epithelial edema. The risk of operation in these early cases probably outweighs the disadvantage of later operation which often results in clear grafts. It is probably best to wait until there is definite epithelial edema with reduction of vision below reading level (e.g., 20/70) before corneal transplantation is performed. Over half of 22 cases of this type obtained satisfactory results. He concluded that such cases appear to heal more slowly, probably because of disease in adjacent host stroma.[46]

According to Fine, successful results may be expected in 80 per cent of early or moderately advanced Fuchs' dystrophy but in only about 50 per cent of advanced cases. The margins of the graft should be outside the edematous portion of the cornea.[46]

In cases of cataract and endothelial dystrophy with stromal edema, a therapeutic penetrating keratoplasty should be carried out 6 to 8 months before cataract extraction, but present reports indicate that 30 to 50 per cent of clear transplants will become cloudy after the cataract operation.[46]

Since chemical zonulolysis has reduced manipulation to a minimum, it has been very tempting to the surgeon to use it in cases of Fuchs' dystrophy. Here the problem reduces itself to "would the chemical trauma be less than the mechanical trauma?" Unfortunately, especially in the early stages of dystrophy, it is not easy to make a clear-cut diagnosis of Fuchs' dystrophy. Secondly, the combination of Fuchs' dystrophy and cataract is fortunately not very common, and third, the experience of removing cataracts under these circumstances even without the enzyme has not been completely successful. In terms of damage to the cornea and resultant vision, the scattered reports of surgeons using the enzyme for removing cataracts are discouraging. In terms of the frequency of the combination of Fuchs' dystrophy and cataract, Dr. Sallares, who has had a great deal of experience with corneal transplantation and cataract extraction, so far has not had this combination. Furthermore, in terms of whether the enzyme causes damage to the normal cornea in cataract extraction, he added that in reviewing a series of 100 cataract cases in which alpha-chymotrypsin was not used in contrast to 100 cases in which it was used, he noted no greater incidence of corneal changes in the latter group. In fact, there were fewer corneal changes using chemical zonulolysis.[37] Fuchs' dystrophy, especially in terms of the use of alpha-chymotrypsin, must be distinguished from: (1) the corneal guttata of the Hassal-Henle wart type, and (2) hereditary deep corneal dystrophy.[28] Hassal-Henle bodies are seen chiefly in the periphery of the cornea and do not contraindicate the use of alpha-chymotrypsin. Hereditary deep corneal dystrophy can be mistaken for Fuchs' epithelial and endothelial dystrophy. At this time it seems that alpha-chymotrypsin can be used safely in hereditary deep corneal dystrophy. Berliner has stated that Fuchs' epithelial dystrophy, senile type, begins with endothelial changes.[6]

Management of Dystrophy Prior to Cataract Extraction

Corneal Transplantation. If the dystrophy is of the Fuchs type and if the area is small and central, a corneal transplant of the involved area followed by a cataract extraction 6 months later is the procedure of choice. Some feel that even this may not work because Fuchs' dystrophy is a disease of the entire endothelium. Dr. Castroviejo will first treat the dystrophy by a corneal transplant, provided that the dystrophy is not too extensive and the graft can be placed in contact with healthy cornea. It is his feeling that Fuchs' dystrophy does not have to involve the entire cornea and that the far periphery can show Hassal-Henle warts which are sometimes mistaken for part of Fuchs' dystrophy. These Hassal-

Henle warts are seen chiefly in the periphery of the cornea.

If the graft remains clear, Dr. Castroviejo will wait 6 months or longer before attempting the removal of the cataract;

> Otherwise the transplant which has not had time to cicatrize at the edge, closing the gap by endothelium and a new Descemet's membrane, may become cloudy.[12]

In cases with very advanced Fuchs' dystrophy, Dr. Castroviejo will perform

> . . . a total penetrating keratoplasty with extraction of the lens whether the lens is transparent or cataractous and a large iridectomy from 10 to 2 o'clock to minimize the postoperative incidence of increased tension. This operation is performed to improve the eye functionally, if the transplant remains clear. If the transplant becomes cloudy, a final attempt to improve the eye functionally can be made with a partial penetrating keratoplasty.[12]

Cataract Surgery

In Fuchs' dystrophy the prognosis should always be guarded, and surgery should be performed when the patient requires it, provided that he understands the risks involved. In general, if the Fuchs' dystrophy is old and advanced, surgery of the cataract should be delayed as long as possible.

Technic of Cataract Surgery

As to the technic of cataract surgery, key words in each surgical maneuver are *gentleness* and *minimal manipulation*. The type of conjunctival flap is relatively unimportant in Fuchs' dystrophy. I prefer a limbus-based flap instead of a fornix-based flap.

One might avoid further endothelial damage by taking the following precautions:

1. The incision should be scleral and at least 180° to 200°. McLean feels that a truly scleral incision is indicated in the presence of Fuchs' dystrophy and cataract. The opening must be started over the anterior portion of the ciliary body and must not enter the anterior chamber directly. He feels that the incision should not be any wider than is necessary for a sliding delivery of the lens.[29] Personally, although I like to consider my wound a scleral-scleral one, I avoid going "too scleral" because of the increased hemorrhage in the more posterior portion of the wound. I feel that hemorrhage requires more irrigation and that this in turn adds more trauma. Some feel that the incision can be done in the regular fashion.

2. If a balanced solution such as Ringer's or Gey's is necessary, it must be used cautiously. Some feel that no solution of any kind should enter the eye.

3. I myself prefer a complete sector iridectomy for all age groups in these cases because I feel that the lens can be slid out more easily in this fashion and the iridectomy may serve as a partial safety valve for borderline or future glaucoma such as that due to pupillary block. (If glaucoma should follow despite this, I would prefer to treat it medically, turning to repeated cyclodiathermies only if necessary.) Occasionally, if the area of dystrophy is small and central, I will cautiously make one radial iridotomy below under clear cornea with special curved scissors, avoiding the endothelium.

4. One should use air injected into the anterior chamber. Some feel that, in addition, binocular dressings with the patient almost flat for 2 to 3 days until the air is absorbed will help to keep the vitreous away from the cornea. If vitreous should follow later and corneal edema result, air should be reinjected, and vitreous should be removed through a posterior sclerotomy if necessary.

5. Anterior chamber lenses definitely should not be used. Contact lenses also are avoided because of added damage to a sick cornea.

Dr. W. E. Fry pointed out at the 1962 Wills Conference that he is fully aware that it has been stated in the literature that alpha-chymotrypsin should not be used in Fuchs' dystrophy, but he feels that in this type of dystrophy minimal trauma is indicated in the surgical procedure. At present, he feels that alpha-chymotrypsin, if used correctly, will help to minimize trauma.

Dr. Fry's suggested technic is as follows: He will make a corneoscleral incision, not exaggerating the scleral incision which he feels would invite more bleeding. After gently lifting the cornea and after irrigating a small amount of alpha-chymotrypsin between the iris in three quadrants, being sure not to touch the endothelium, he will do a complete iridectomy. With slight pressure and counterpressure the lens will become loosened and almost "walk out" on its own.

Hereditary Deep Corneal Dystrophy

Hereditary deep corneal dystrophy can be confused with the more common posterior corneal changes of corneal guttata, endothelial dystrophy and with the endothelial dystrophy of the senile type spoken of as the endothelial-epithelial dystrophy of Fuchs. In 1921, Vogt described "corneal guttata." This entity and endothelial dystrophy occasionally may be a forerunner of the endothelial-epithelial dystrophy of Fuchs. The Vogt type and the endothelial-epithelial dystrophy occur late in life and tend to progress in severity; they have little hereditary basis. Hereditary deep corneal dystrophy can be confused with endothelial dystrophy of the senile type because of the similar anatomic location and the similiarity of the lesions. The senile type of endothelial dystrophy appears later in life and has little hereditary basis. It tends to progress and occasionally produces anterior changes. Trauma is a frequent cause of exacerbation of these lesions. Hereditary deep corneal dystrophy appears earlier in life and is transmitted as a mendelian dominant. As a rule, it does not seem to progress significantly and has never been reported to produce anterior changes. The corneal endothelial changes include bedewing together with scattered discrete circular areas which appear to be denuded of endothelium and to have a curved surface with the convexity anteriorly. The anterior stroma and the epithelium are normal (Fig. 150). This type of dystrophy is rare, and only 9 kinships with fewer than 20 cases have thus far been described in the literature. It might be possible that there is a relationship to the syndrome hypophosphatasia, an inborn error of metabolism consisting of abnormal mineralization of bone, decreased serum alkaline phosphatase and increased phosphorylethanolamine in the urine. The case described by Magruder[30] of a 38-year-old white male illustrates other points of dissimilarity in the two entities. Surgical trauma in the form of lens extraction in two eyes in this case had no untoward effect on the lesions over the follow-up period of 24 months for the right eye and 22 months for the left eye. It is particularly interesting to note the absence of noxious effects from the use of alpha-chymotrypsin in the two eyes. Tumbling and the use of the erisophake also caused no problems. Bilateral corneal contact lenses were used successfully without untoward effects. In contrast, in the

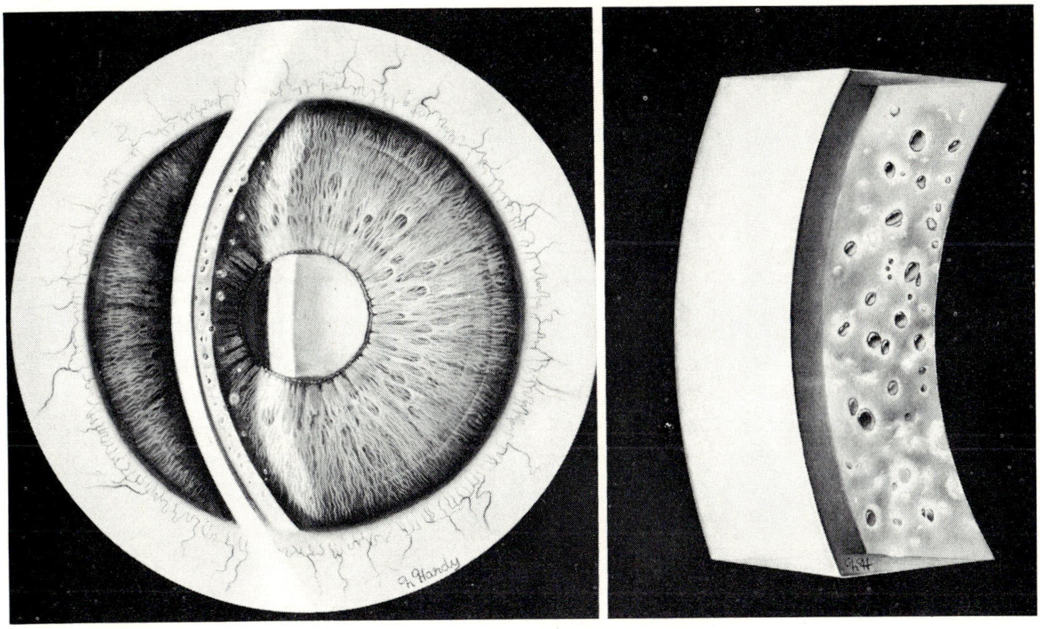

FIG. 150. Slit-lamp appearance of corneal lesions. (*Left*) Low-power view. (*Right*) High-power view. (Magruder, G. B.: Am. J. Ophthal. *52*:677)

endothelial-epithelial dystrophy of Fuchs and occasionally in corneal guttata described by Vogt, it is a well-known clinical observation that trauma—whether in the form of cataract surgery, keratoplasty or other forms of mechanical insult—frequently causes exacerbation and a rapid downhill course.[30]

Recently an ophthalmologist consulted me regarding a problem in a patient with a definite Fuchs' dystrophy who had gained no useful vision following a cataract extraction. This surgeon had followed all the currently recognized steps in the extraction of the cataract for an eye showing Fuchs' dystrophy. The lens was extracted by the use of a scleral incision, the capsule forceps and a sliding technic. No useful vision resulted, and the surgeon's question was whether or not alpha-chymotrypsin should be used in the second eye which also showed a cataract and an advanced dystrophy.

Following this, in January 1962, I wrote to Drs. Harvey Thorpe, Saul Sugar and Alston Callahan asking their current ideas on the use of alpha-chymotrypsin and specifically in the presence of Fuchs' dystrophy. (My feelings on this have already been outlined in the foregoing pages.) I received the following answers to my question and have been given permission to quote directly:

> It would be my own thought that alpha-chymotrypsin should not be used in the second eye . . . I have seen cases with only 20/200 vision that I am certain would have had almost normal vision had the enzyme not been used. To sum up, I fear alpha-chymotrypsin with a subnormal cornea regardless of the type of dystrophy and specifically Fuchs' dystrophy.
> —Alston Callahan, M. D., Birmingham, Ala.

> I've used chymotrypsin routinely since the Brussels meeting in everyone from age 20 to 80 . . . except in cases of endothelial dystrophy, especially if the epithelium shows

bedewing. I have seen no complication that I could attribute directly to the use of chymotrypsin. I have not used chymotrypsin in Fuchs' dystrophy.

—H. Saul Sugar, M. D., Detroit, Mich.

I do not use alpha-chymotrypsin for zonulolysis in routine cataract extraction as a rule after 65 years of age unless I run into a tough zonule. It is my opinion that its use is contraindicated in the presence of a degenerating endothelium, particularly in those cases which show secondary epithelial degeneration of the Fuchs type. In Fuchs' dystrophy with cataract, I prefer to do a penetrating corneal transplant 6-12 months prior to contemplated cataract surgery.

—Harvey Thorpe, M. D., Pittsburgh, Pa.

In 1961, Barraquer said,

In adults corneal dystrophies do not seem to result from the use of alpha-chymotrypsin, but if dystrophy is already present the enzyme may hasten its progress.[3]

At the Wills 1962 conference, it was concluded that corneal grafts tended to remain clear more often after unplanned extracapsulars and definitely remained clear in well-planned extracapsular extractions[34] (see p. 146).

Because of the same problems a similar approach might be considered in extractions of cataracts from eyes showing minimal signs of Fuchs' dystrophy.

The late stages of Fuchs' dystrophy resemble bullous keratopathy following surgical injury to the endothelium epithelialization of the anterior chamber or, most commonly, endothelial damage produced by long-standing glaucoma. For treatment of a late Fuchs' dystrophy, see p. 152.

SUMMARY

Dystrophies and cataracts present a very difficult problem. Prognosis as to useful vision following cataract extraction, especially with the dystrophy of Fuchs, should be extremely guarded. Currently, it is felt by most surgeons that although alpha-chymotrypsin may be used safely in hereditary deep corneal dystrophy, the enzyme should not be used in Fuchs' dystrophy.

GLAUCOMA AND CATARACTS

The correct management of the combination of glaucoma and cataracts can present a difficult problem. Even in cataract surgery uncomplicated by glaucoma, the perfect solution has not been evolved yet. The correct management must be individualized and tailored to meet the specific case.

It is beyond the scope of this text to consider in detail all the problems related to the present concepts of glaucoma. For this the reader is referred to excellent current general and specific references.*

For the most part, broad general principles (rather than a detailed analysis) stressing the *management* of the combined problem will be outlined.

Today glaucoma is classified into primary and secondary types. Primary glaucoma is further subdivided into open-angle and angle-closure types.

In both the primary and the secondary types there can be combined or mixed varieties. Mixed types of glaucoma can be noted between the open-angle and the angle-closure types. Mixed glaucomas with a primary and a secondary component can occur in instances such as lens intumescence with narrow-angle glau-

* Suggested books on this subject include:

1. Becker, B., and Shaffer, R.: Diagnosis and Therapy of the Glaucomas, St. Louis, Mosby, 1961.
2. Lerman, Sidney: Glaucoma: Chemistry, Mechanics and Therapy, Springfield, Ill., Thomas, 1961.
3. Sugar, H. S.: The Glaucomas, New York, Hoeber-Harper, 1957.

Other references will be found at the end of the chapter.

coma or secondary glaucoma due to uveitis in an open-angle glaucoma. In both the primary and the secondary glaucomas, a clearly defined set of findings is not always present.

As to the treatment of cataracts associated with glaucoma in terms of modern advances in cataract surgery there is still no unanimity of opinion.

In the broadest of terms with reference to this problem, Reese stated,

> Cataract and glaucoma frequently go hand in hand. Patients with glaucoma have a higher incidence of cataract, and patients with cataract have a higher incidence of glaucoma . . . It is important to appreciate incipient cataractous changes before surgery for primary glaucoma is done. This is advisable because the glaucoma surgery itself usually hastens the progression of previously existing cataractous changes. Thus, following the glaucoma surgery in the course of six months to a year, a cataract develops. Therefore, if a glaucoma patient does have incipient cataractous changes, it is well to know it before the glaucoma surgery, and to so inform the patient of the possibility that such changes may progress.[35]

Dr. Spaeth, Dr. Berliner and others will, as a rule, operate the glaucoma first if operation is necessary and at a later date will remove the cataract. Still, in the broadest terms, my own approach, shared by others such as Dr. W. E. Fry and Dr. Castroviejo, is that if the glaucoma is controlled by 1 per cent pilocarpine—and depending on the appearance of the angle and outflow studies, an iridectomy (a full one preferably) plus extraction of the cataract intracapsularly is sufficient. It was pointed out by Teng and Katzin that nature is often kind in borderline cases, and small grossly invisible filtering blebs may result and control the pressure.[45] I always forewarn my patients about the possible need for controlling the glaucoma with medications postoperatively or by further surgery. If carbonic anhydrase inhibitors, miotics and epinephrinelike compounds *must* be used to control the pressure, my second choice would be to do the glaucoma operation first and remove the cataract at a later date. My third choice is simultaneously performed glaucoma surgery of the external filtering type and cataract extraction. I have seldom used this type of surgery, but in those selected cases in which I have, the results have been good.

Among the arguments cited against simultaneous glaucoma and cataract surgery are:

1. Many cases will be controlled satisfactorily by the cataract extraction with iridectomy.

2. If this fails the patient can be better treated medically or surgically by operations such as a cyclodialysis, repeated if necessary, than by simultaneous glaucoma and cataract surgery.

3. The greatest danger is that filtering operations done at the same time as the cataract extraction may lead to serious complications such as flat chamber, more synechiae and eventual blindness.

An example of a case that might be ideal for simultaneous glaucoma and cataract surgery is a neglected glaucoma with an intumescent lens where the pressure has been elevated.

Among the benefits cited for simultaneous surgery for glaucoma and cataract are:

1. Decrease in the terms of total disability to the patient including the time required for the restoration of vision. Simultaneous surgery may be especially indicated in patients with poor general health in order to avoid two operations.

2. Possibly fewer complications such as postoperative corneal disease and less total trauma to the eye

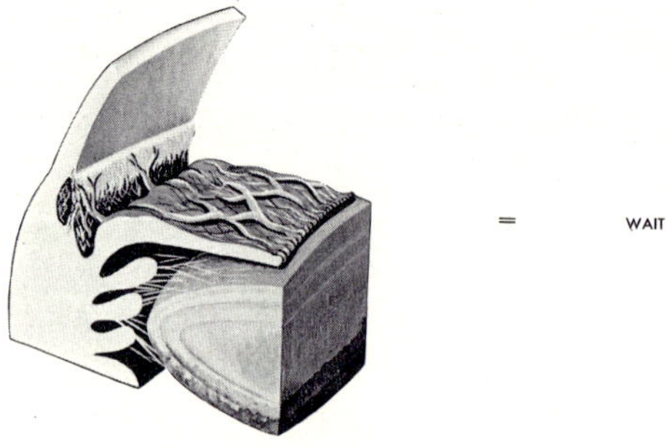

FIGURE 151

(Drs. R. Cordero Moreno and H. Van Den Beld C.)

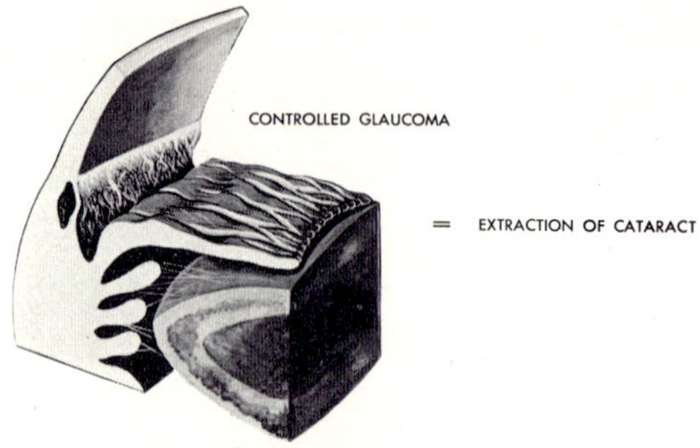

FIGURE 152

(Drs. R. Cordero Moreno and H. Van Den Beld C.)

3. One period of apprehension for the patient and the surgeon

4. Avoidance of "malignant glaucoma" which is benefited by lens extraction

5. Reduction in the period of hospitalization and the cost

Among present-day advances that help to make all glaucoma surgery and perhaps simultaneous surgery more successful are: (1) carbonic anhydrase inhibitors, urea and mannitol; (2) retrobulbar anesthesia with hyaluronidase and digital massage; and (3) alpha-chymotrypsin—by increasing the number of intracapsular extractions and thereby decreasing the factors related to lens-matter retention in extracapsular extractions and the associated secondary types of glaucoma.

All agree that the intracapsular extraction is indicated in the combination of cataracts with glaucoma. Since each case should be judged on its own merits, it is difficult to classify the type of surgery indicated in each case.

An excellent summary on the management of the problems related to glaucoma and cataracts was shown in an exhibit at the 1962 Interim Meeting of the Pan-American Congress by Drs. R. Cordero Moreno and H. Van Den Beld C. (Catedra de Oftalmologia, Universidad C. de Venezuela). They have granted me permission to use their drawings and to combine under one drawing rather than three, the phacoanaphylactic reaction "phacotoxic" and "phacogenetic," pointing out to me that there is some confusion and overlapping of the nomenclature and the classification. This total group might best be classified under lens-induced uveitis and glaucoma and phacolytic glaucoma. They stress that in all of these forms of glaucoma the important therapy is the removal of the lens or the washing out of as much of the lens material as is possible.

The illustrations are almost self-explanatory. The primary glaucomas are subdivided into the open-angle and the angle-closure types.* In these charts the secondary glaucomas include only the intumescent cataract, cataract plus capsular exfoliation (pseudoexfoliation), phacoanaphylactic reaction† and cataract plus uveitis.

* Dr. Moreno suggests that in these charts the secondary glaucomas include only the intumescent cataracts, cataract plus capsular pseudoexfoliation, lens-induced glaucoma (phacoanaphylactic, phacotoxic, phacolytic) and cataract plus uveitis. He also makes the suggestion that the term pseudoexfoliation should be used throughout this chapter.

† A discussion of other names for this will follow.

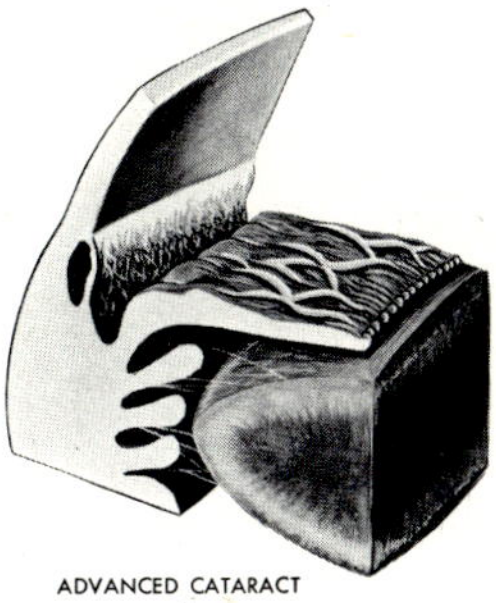

FIGURE 153

(Drs. R. Cordero Moreno and H. Van Den Beld C.)

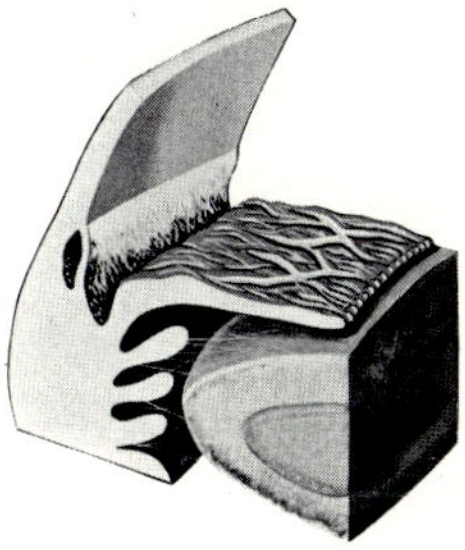

FIGURE 154

(Drs. R. Cordero Moreno and H. Van Den Beld C.)

I have expanded somewhat on these ideas, adding my own comments with which Drs. Moreno and Van Den Beld C. may or may not agree.

PRIMARY GLAUCOMA— OPEN-ANGLE TYPE

1. If there is an incipient cataract plus controlled glaucoma, watchful waiting is the best course (Fig. 151).

2. If the opacities in an incipient cataract are such that the miosis results in poor vision despite the control of the glaucoma, extraction of the cataract should be considered. Here, of course, one should have tried epinephrinelike compounds to see if the mydriatic effect can offset the blurring of the miotics and at the same time help to control the glaucoma. I would include in this consideration the use of systemic carbonic anhydrase inhibitors plus the results of outflow studies, careful field studies and gonioscopic examinations (Fig. 152).

3. If the cataract is advanced, despite the fact that the glaucoma can be controlled, it is wisest to do an iridectomy and extract the cataract. By doing so the patient may be cured with one operation rather than with two (Fig. 153).

4. As a rule, if there is a glaucoma that is not controlled, regardless of whatever state the cataract is in, the emphasis should be placed on the control of the glaucoma (Fig. 154).

PRIMARY GLAUCOMA— ANGLE-CLOSURE TYPE

1. In an acute attack of glaucoma with an incipient cataract, R. Cordero Moreno and H. Van Den Beld C. recommend treating the glaucoma (Fig. 155).

Saul Sugar says.

> In a case of cataract in which miotic controlled angle-closure glaucoma is present (without angle block), lens extraction cures both cataract and the potential angle-closure

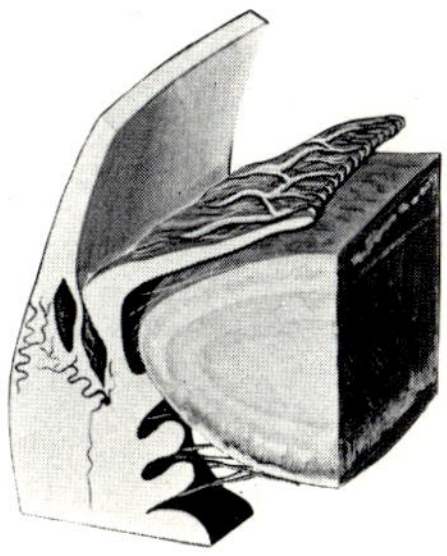

FIGURE 155

(Drs. R. Cordero Moreno and H. Van Den Beld C.)

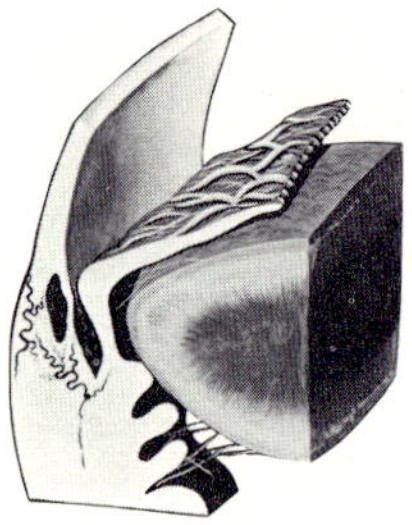

FIGURE 156

(Drs. R. Cordero Moreno and H. Van Den Beld C.)

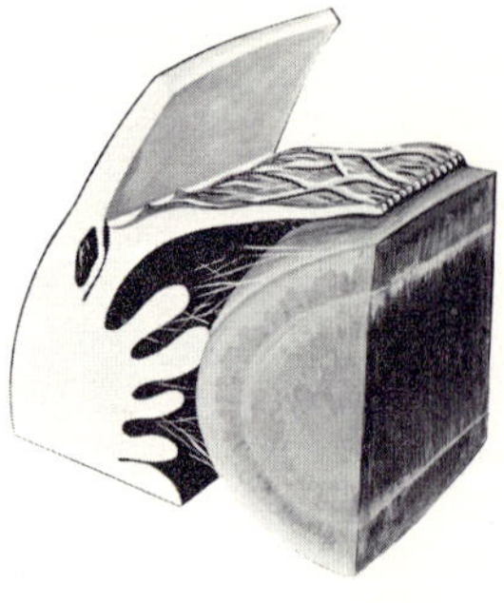

FIGURE 157

(Drs. R. Cordero Moreno and H. Van Den Beld C.)

glaucoma. This is not true in acute angle closure with angle block.[43]

2. If there is an advanced cataract and an acute attack of glaucoma, extraction of the lens plus an iridectomy is indicated. Medical treatment such as local miotics and carbonic anhydrase inhibitors should be used to lower the tension and whiten the eye if possible. Since surgical removal of the lens is safer when the eye is softer and white, 2 per cent pilocarpine should be used during the interim. If the ocular pressures do not respond to these measures, retrobulbar injections, massage and intravenous urea or mannitol ½ hour before operation should be used (Fig. 156).

SECONDARY GLAUCOMA

1. **An intumescent cataract showing a secondary glaucoma** necessitates extraction of the lens. Since an intumescent or advanced cataract presents the same clinical picture and the same mechanism as does an angle-closure glaucoma, the differential diagnosis is important.

In advanced cataract:

1. An intumescent cataract is present.

2. Usually only one eye is involved.

3. Any refractive error can be present, even a high myopia.

4. The fellow eye may show a normal anterior chamber depth. (It is rare to have an angle-closure glaucoma in one eye with a deep anterior chamber in the other eye.) (See Fig. 157.)

2. **When there is a cataract, capsular exfoliation (or pseudoexfoliation) plus glaucoma,** the treatment should be essentially the same as that outlined under glaucoma of the open-angle type. (See descriptions in Figs. 151-154.) One must distinguish pseudoexfoliation from the true splitting of the lens capsule seen in "glass blowers' " cataract where there usually is no associated glaucoma.

The usual medical treatment for open-angle glaucoma is indicated. However, it is best to hold the pupil fixed and rigid. In the surgical treatment of the glaucoma, cyclodialysis and filtering operations have been used but should be followed by the constant use of miotics to prevent further exfoliation from the capsule.

In the surgical treatment of the lens, it is interesting that the actual lens removal has no great effect on the elevated tension. During surgery one should be pre-

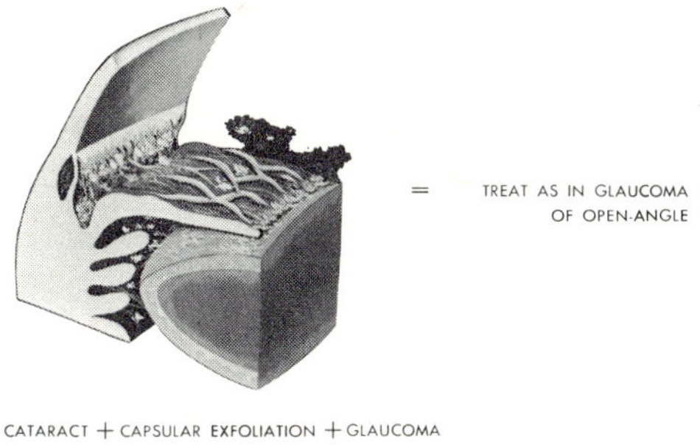

FIGURE 158

(Drs. R. Cordero Moreno and H. Van Den Beld C.)

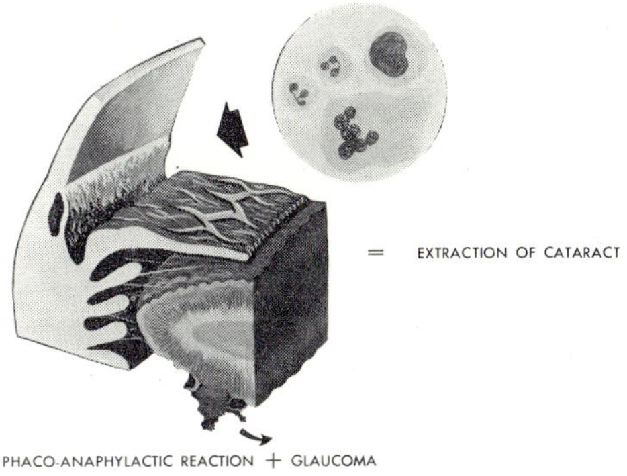

FIGURE 159

(Drs. R. Cordero Moreno and H. Van Den Beld C.)

pared to see a dislocated lens and to expect the loss of fluid vitreous. After surgery of the lens one can expect a rise in pressure which is treated first medically and later surgically as indicated.

In pseudoexfoliation associated with glaucoma, sometimes called glaucoma capsulare, it is impossible to be certain whether the capsular debris or the pigment granules deposited in the trabecular spaces, or both, are the cause of the glaucoma. There can be exfoliation without glaucoma. The differential diagnosis between open-angle glaucoma and capsular exfoliation must be made by slit lamp and gonioscopic appearance. Both conditions are insidious in nature. Visual acuity, field changes and provocative tests are essentially the same. In capsular exfoliation, slit-lamp examination shows exfoliated shreds on the cornea, in the anterior chamber, on the iris and on the lens. The gonioscope shows an open angle or one of normal depth in both capsular exfoliation and open-angle glaucoma. In capsular exfoliation there is a characteristic slight veiling and dense trabecular pigmentation in the angle (Fig. 158).

3. **Lens-induced Glaucoma** (Fig. 159). Secondary glaucoma can be caused by the lens, either mechanically or by uveitis. Today the terms used most commonly to describe the inflammatory reaction and the glaucoma resulting from the presence of free lens material in the eye cavities are lens-induced uveitis with glaucoma and phacolytic glaucoma.*

Formerly, subdivisions of lens-induced uveitis with glaucoma were phacoanaphylactic and "phacotoxic" reaction; however, the clinical and the histologic pictures of these reactions are so similar that I feel it unnecessary to give detailed descriptions of them individually in this text.

Finally, I feel justified in including subluxated lenses in this grouping as a lens mechanically obstructing the angle or irritating the ciliary body sometimes may cause a glaucoma; also, a uveitis component may be added which confuses the picture.

LENS-INDUCED UVEITIS AND GLAUCOMA. *Clinical Picture.* Lens-induced uveitis results from reactions to lens material either through the intact capsule, by trauma, or following extracapsular extraction of a mature or a hypermature lens. It occurs rarely after spontaneous rupture

* Formerly referred to as "phacogenetic" or "phacogenic."

of the capsule. The eyes are often soft at the time of the acute reaction, but glaucoma may develop following the development of synechiae, scarring and membranes, at which time the condition is called lens-induced uveitis with glaucoma.

Pathologic Picture. Broadly speaking, the pathologic picture is characterized by marked exudation of giant cells, plasma cells, lymphocytes and other forms of white blood cells, much reaction in the anterior chamber and large precipitates on the back of the cornea spoken of as "lardaceous" or "mutton-fat" precipitates.

Treatment (see "Treatment of Phacolytic Glaucoma," p. 137). Removal of the lens or lens material will often cure the uveitis and the glaucoma.

A further subdivision of lens-induced uveitis is *lens-induced uveitis in the second untraumatized eye.* Clinically, the differentiating diagnostic feature is that while the second eye is inflamed, the so-called exciting eye is quiescent, whereas in sympathetic ophthalmitis there are exacerbations and remissions in both eyes simultaneously. Unfortunately, following injuries, sometimes sympathetic ophthalmitis and lens-induced uveitis may exist simultaneously! If lens-induced uveitis is suspected in the second, untraumatized eye and the originally affected eye has become blind, enucleation of this blind eye for purposes of confirming the diagnosis is warranted.

Pathologically, the presence of epithelioid cells in the choroid in sympathetic ophthalmitis differentiates sympathetic ophthalmitis from lens-induced uveitis in the second, untraumatized eye. Sympathetic ophthalmitis is characterized by massive lymphocytic infiltration with nests of epithelioid cells superimposed on the lymphocytic infiltrate. Giant cells are commonly present among the epithelioid cells.

PHACOLYTIC GLAUCOMA. This type of glaucoma is sometimes listed under secondary glaucoma due to spontaneous rupture of the lens capsule. Lenticular intumescence (swelling) leads to thinning of the capsule with leaks through the anterior and, more frequently, the posterior capsule and then spontaneous rupture of the lens capsule or spontaneous absorption of the lens. The possible causes of the glaucoma include chemical irritation of the lens substance, an increased protein of the aqueous, and obstruction in the trabecular spaces by particles of lens substance or phagocytes.

Clinical Picture. The glaucoma in these cases is of sudden onset. The clinical picture is typical of a patient with a *hypermature* cataract. This condition is often seen in elderly patients who have had successful cataract surgery on the other eye and have neglected the now involved eye. Occasionally it may complicate an uninfected, traumatic cataract. There is often faulty light projection, possibly related to the diffusion of the light by the hypermature cataract or by the reduced function of the retina because of the increase in intraocular pressure or toxic effect on the retina. The anterior chamber shows a dense flare, possibly related to the liquefied cortex which leaks anteriorly, posteriorly or both. This dense flare may obscure the other details of the anterior segment of the eye. The angle, when it is seen, is that of a wide one, and the chamber, when seen, is deep. The anterior segment is otherwise relatively normal. There are no "mutton-fat" keratitic precipitates. In the early stages there is an impaired facility of outflow. Phacolytic glaucoma can be distinguished by gonioscopy from a swollen (intumescent) cataractous lens that has induced angle closure.

Pathologic Picture. Large mononuclear phagocytes filled with lens material are seen at the site of the leak in the anterior or the posterior capsule or both and in the trabecular meshwork. There are no "mutton-fat" keratitic precipitates, and the posterior segment of the eye is otherwise relatively normal.

Treatment of lens-induced uveitis and its subdivisions is essentially the same. This consists of removal of the lens or lens material in spite of the glaucoma. Beforehand, one should try to lower the intraocular pressure. Steroids may be used to decrease the inflammatory process, while epinephrine compounds, carbonic anhydrase inhibitors and urea should be used to lower the intraocular pressure.

The ideal procedure is an intracapsular extraction. Theoretically, one might fear performing an extracapsular extraction in this type of eye; however in these eyes the capsule is often very weak and friable and, therefore, an extracapsular may result. On the other hand, the surgeon must remember that the zonule may be very weak, and the lens can be dislocated easily. However, occasionally the capsule can be thickened by inflammation, and in these cases one cannot plan for but can hope and try for an intracapsular cataract extraction. Despite the fact that preoperatively the light projection may have been poor, postoperatively the vision may be good. With the removal of the lens the glaucoma may be cured without further therapy.

SUBLUXATED LENS. Spontaneous or traumatic subluxation of the lens can result in glaucoma with angle closure. In those cases without angle closure but with decreased outflow facility, the glaucoma

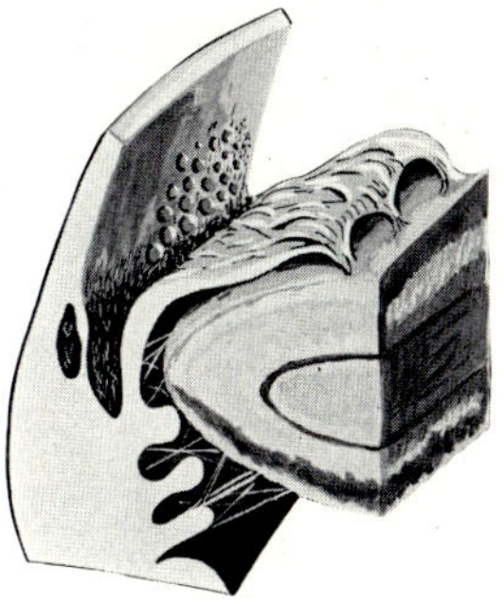

FIGURE 160

(Drs. R. Cordero Moreno and H. Van Den Beld C.)

may also be explained by congenital anomalies of the angle. (See Marfan's syndrome, p. 138.) However, wide open, normal-appearing angles can appear with posteriorly subluxated lenses and show impaired outflow facilities for unknown causes.

Treatment. (See Chap. 10.)

4. **When there is a cataract, a uveitis and a secondary glaucoma,** extraction of the lens is the procedure of choice. However, every effort should be made to control the uveitis before the extraction. If the uveitis is active, it should be treated with local as well as systemic cortisone or ACTH. If present, foci of infection should be eliminated. If the uveitis is tubercular, isoniazid, para-aminosalicylic acid and streptomycin should be used. Miotics can be of help temporarily. Atropine should be used cautiously. Surgically, iridectomy and possibly cyclodialysis should be used for pupillary or angle block (Fig. 160).

FUCHS' HETEROCHROMIC CYCLITIS. A special variety of uveitis and secondary glaucoma can be seen in Fuchs' heterochromic cyclitis.

In terms of the glaucoma, in the early stages the course is similar to that of chronic simple glaucoma. By gonioscopy the angle is normal or open except for membranous vessels originating from the root of the iris and proceeding to the trabecular region. The main cause of the secondary glaucoma is a decreased facility of outflow as shown by tonography. It is probable that the trabecular spaces are filled by cellular deposits from the aqueous. In histologic sections, fibrosis or sclerosis of the trabecular network can be found. Spontaneous subluxation of the lens or phakolysis of a hypermature complicated cataract must be considered as secondary causes. Medically, the glaucoma should be treated with epinephrine-like compounds or systemic carbonic anhydrase inhibitors and miotics. Surgically, a filtering operation such as a trephine procedure or a sclerotomy with cautery and iridectomy is suggested.

It has been pointed out that in Fuchs' heterochromic cyclitis laboratory work-up is fruitless and that therapy is not very effective.

In terms of the cataract, generally speaking the patient with heterochromic cataract withstands surgery well. Neither extracapsular nor intracapsular extraction offers special difficulty. In these cases no special change in the operative technic is indicated. The extraction of the lens may tend to make the uveitis less chronically active. It is possible that the cataract in one eye may act as a foreign body. However, in some cases uveitis and glaucoma may flare up after the operation.

5. **Dislocated Lens and Glaucoma.** MARFAN'S ECTOPIA LENTIS AND GLAUCOMA. In these cases the glaucoma may be due to trabecular anomaly, pupillary block or a posterior lens dislocation. The glaucoma should be treated medically if possible. Surgically, if there is a pupillary block, an iridectomy is the procedure of choice. Often an iridectomy will prevent the lens from moving in and out of the anterior chamber. Some feel that cyclodialysis is the surgical procedure of choice, and the use of goniotomy also has been suggested.

Since the prognosis for removal of the lens in these cases is very poor, surgery should be delayed until maximal corrective vision is determined to be sure that the patient really needs the operation. Many of these cases are followed by retinal detachment even without surgery, and the chances are greater following surgery. In my experience, alpha-chymotrypsin does not seem to help to dissolve the remaining zonules without the loss of vitreous. For vision, optical iridectomy has been suggested in cases of this type.[23] If lens extraction is indicated in the young, fixating the lens with a needle-knife from one side and scratching the lens in the pupillary area with another needle-knife is the most conservative and the indicated approach. Grieshaber-Haab needle-knives are excellent for this maneuver. Dr. José Barraquer uses a 3-pronged needle inserted at the pars plana to trap such a lens (Fig. 161). (See Chap. 10.)

6. **Congenital Cataract and Glaucoma.** For cataracts in children, I favor a needling (discission) in most cases, followed in a few days by a linear type of extraction (see p. 107).

If the pupil does not dilate preoperatively, a vertical iridotomy below and a full iridectomy above is mandatory. These measures can help to prevent a secondary glaucoma.

A secondary glaucoma can follow a traumatic cataract or lens discission. In a lens discission a wide opening in the anterior capsule is a preventive as a rule. Rarely is the meshwork so blocked by lens material that the glaucoma cannot be controlled by local medications and carbonic-anhydraselike drugs. On the other hand, if the glaucoma is not controlled, the treatment is to open the anterior chamber and wash out part (or preferably all) of the lens matter.

Pupillary block following cataract surgery in children is the main cause of the glaucoma. Prophylactically it is essential to keep the pupil dilated with atropine for even as long as a year following surgery. If an atropine sensitivity develops, scopolamine or cyclopentolate hydrochloride (Cyclogyl) and phenylephrine (10% Neo-Synephrine) are indicated. Phenylephrine alone is not sufficient.

Signs of pupillary block following cataract surgery in children differ from those in an adult. In children, as in adults, there can be both angle block and pupillary block. As a rule an inflammatory membrane behind the iris prevents an iris bombé except in the extreme periphery where presumably there is no inflammatory membrane. Unevenness in the depth of the anterior chamber and, commonly, gross peripheral synechiae on a clear cornea in even one area are seen. If the chamber is shallow on one side and wide on the other, the diagnosis is certain. Treatment here consists of iridectomy and discission of any pupillary membrane. If there is an angle block, cyclodialysis is indicated.

7. **Spherophakia With Microcornea and Glaucoma.** Because at times the lens must be removed even though it does not show cataractous changes, this condition is listed here.

The cause is classified as a congenital systemic affection of the mesenchymal tissue.

Marchesani's syndrome is a familial condition characterized by spherophakia, brachydactyly, brachycephaly and a short pyknic build. In a high proportion of these cases the glaucoma is probably due to spherophakia.

In spherophakia with glaucoma, the glaucoma is usually due to pupillary block, but secondary angle block or decreased facility of outflow may supervene.

TREATMENT. If the glaucoma is due to angle closure, a peripheral iridectomy is indicated. Miotics can be used after surgery. When the glaucoma in spherophakia is due to lack of communication between the anterior and the posterior chambers, the tension is lowered when the pupil is dilated because the circumference of the lens becomes free. Therefore, the treatment in this condition is at first the use of mydriatics; eventually, intracapsular extraction with full iridectomy is indicated. In the removal of these lenses a selection of loops, small and large with guards so that the lens cannot fall through the loop, is important. José Barraquer's 3-pronged needle offers another approach to this problem (Fig. 161, *top*). (See Chap. 10.)

8. **Glaucoma in the Patient With Diabetes and Cataract.** Glaucoma in the dia-

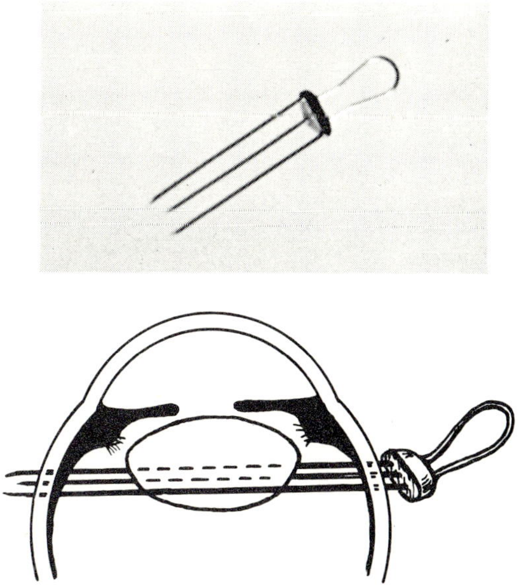

FIG. 161. The position of the triple needle for subluxated lenses. (Modified from Barraquer, Joaquin: Trans. Am. Acad. Ophthal. Oto-laryng. *66*:46)

betic is most often associated with rubeosis extending into the angle of the eye. The prognosis is very poor. Attempts to control the glaucoma should be made medically and then surgically. Cataract extraction is rarely successful in these cases and most often is disastrous.

When asked what he would do in an individual of 30 years of age with diabetic rubeosis, a mature cataract, some light projection and a history of having lost the other eye when nothing was done, Dr. Edmund Spaeth replied: "Whatever you do, you will be wrong. However, I would try doing the cataract under these circumstances provided the patient knew the problems involved. I might even try removing the lens without an iridectomy."[41] Dr. W. E. Fry said that under these circumstances he, too, would attempt to remove the lens with a sphincterotomy in an area relatively free of vessels.[17]

For the glaucoma the medical treatment includes the administration of local epinephrinelike drugs combined with carbonic anhydrase inhibitors or a trial of miotics.

Surgically, cyclodiathermy may be the safest and best procedure for the glaucoma. A second approach is thermal sclerectomy with iridectomy.[5] When I asked Dr. Bietti about this procedure he said, ". . . To perform the incision of the iris, I am using a simple long non-protected diathermic needle, as it is used to remove single hairs or cilia." A modified Scheie procedure using the Hildreth coagulator to make an opening through the sclera and also to burn a hole into the iris to produce an iridectomy can be tried also. For operations of this nature or for operations prior to cataract extraction, drugs such as urea cannot be expected to help appreciably in those patients with a secondary glaucoma and a damaged blood-aqueous barrier.

Surgery for the cataract may be attempted if: (1) the pressure is controlled beforehand; (2) the patient has less than 20/200 vision with light projection and some indication of macular function; (3) the complications of a maturing lens are anticipated; (4) there is a reasonable life expectancy; and (5) the patient and his family are fully aware of the poor prognosis.

With the use of alpha-chymotrypsin, I favor a limbus-based flap for better wound healing. However, to minimize bleeding on making the cataract section, the incision should be extended as far to the corneal side as possible. A corneal incision without any flap may be used even though alpha-chymotrypsin is used. As a rule, when using alpha-chymotrypsin it is better to use a flap.

If an iridectomy has not been done, light coagulation of the iris in the 12 o'clock position and in the lower iris should be used a few days or weeks prior to the lens extraction if an iridectomy below is anticipated. If the tension does not rise following this treatment, a combined iridectomy and lens extraction using alpha-chymotrypsin should follow. Some favor a small sphincterotomy in a relatively rubeosis-free area; others might attempt no iridectomy at all, and still others feel that even with an iridectomy the iris bleeding will stop.

9. **Glaucoma Secondary to Implant.** For glaucoma secondary to lens implants after cataract extraction, removal of the implant is necessary. In the removal of these implants an adequate corneal incision has been recommended as most important.

10. **Aphakic glaucoma** occurs most frequently as a result of complications

associated with or following the lens extraction.* There has not been a greater incidence of aphakic glaucoma with the use of alpha-chymotrypsin. (See also "Flat Chamber," p. 153.)

The differential diagnosis is principally that of: (1) primary glaucoma undiagnosed preoperatively; (2) pupillary-block glaucoma; (3) angle-block glaucoma; and (4) a combination of pupillary-block and angle-block glaucoma.

1. PRIMARY GLAUCOMA UNDIAGNOSED PREOPERATIVELY. A number of glaucomas considered to be secondary to cataract extraction are in reality primary glaucoma which becomes manifest following a cataract extraction. Perhaps the operation of choice in the aphakic eye is a cyclodialysis with or without an iridectomy. The cyclodialysis should be repeated if necessary.

2. ANGLE-BLOCK GLAUCOMA. Medically, miotics such as 2 per cent pilocarpine or strong anticholinesterase drugs should be tried. Surgically, when synechiae are present, a cyclodialysis is the operation of choice.

3. PUPILLARY-BLOCK GLAUCOMA, often seen with a vitreous block, occurs most frequently after round pupils; however, it may occur even with a full iridectomy in aphakia. Dr. Paul Chandler states that pupillary block in aphakia with a full iridectomy occurs only in those cases where there has been a flat chamber with choroidal separation. Diagnosis is on the basis of an over-all shallowing of the anterior chamber with elevated tension.[26]

Medically, one should first try acetazolamide (Diamox) and dilate the pupil with drugs such as phenylephrine (10% Neo-Synephrine).

* It must be remembered that in both normal and glaucomatous patients there is often a period of hyposecretion.

Surgically, transfixion of the iris, iridotomy or, preferably, an iridectomy are the operations of choice. In pupillary block with a full iridectomy, treatment must include not only the freeing of the hyaloid if it is adherent to the cornea and the injection of air or balanced solution into the anterior chamber but also peripheral iridectomy for a new opening into the iris.[26] (See "Flat Chamber," p. 156.)

After pupillary block, simple incision of the hyaloid may relieve the block in some cases, especially if the hyaloid is considerably thickened. However, since a new hyaloid may form, it seems best to do an iridectomy. Cyclodialysis alone is valueless.

4. A COMBINATION OF PUPILLARY-BLOCK AND ANGLE-BLOCK GLAUCOMA. The glaucoma associated with retained lens matter most frequently follows an unplanned extracapsular extraction and is related to an iridocyclitis following the retention of lens matter. Therefore, the best prophylactic treatment is an intracapsular or a planned extracapsular extraction where more of the lens matter may be washed out under better controlled conditions. Postoperatively, if the reaction is severe, mydriatics and heat assist the absorption. I would wash out the excess lens material if the absorption were prolonged.

Especially after intracapsular extraction this pitfall can be avoided if one remembers Dr. Saul Sugar's feeling that when a glaucoma develops following cataract surgery, iridectomies are better than iridotomies and two iridectomies are better than a single one. He suggests that perhaps sector iridectomy might be wiser than peripheral iridectomy if pupil-block glaucoma alone were to be considered.[43]

This combined type of glaucoma, which is secondary to pupillary-block and angle-block synechiae, must be treated medically or surgically. Medically, for the pupillary-block component, drugs to dilate the pupil, such as phenylephrine (10% Neo-Synephrine), should be tried first. Then, if successful, DFP-like drugs should be tried for the angle-block component. Acetazolamide (Diamox) or similar drugs can serve as an adjunct.

As for the surgical treatment, a cyclodialysis performed in the same operation with an iridectomy at the limbus is the procedure of choice. This can be done in two steps, making the cyclodialysis in one upper quadrant and following this with an iridectomy using a keratome in the same quadrant.[47] Another possibility is a cyclodialysis and an iridectomy in the same quadrant at the same time; this can be made by using an inverted "L" incision; that is, after the cyclodialysis has been performed, the wound can be extended in the form of an "L" to the limbus, and an iridectomy performed.[47]

In 1949, Drs. Allen and Lee described a procedure for cyclodialysis in which a scleral incision was made 3 mm. back from and parallel to the limbus.[24]

In 1951, Dr. Allen described a simplified cyclodialysis technic which consisted of a radial incision through the sclera at the limbus, with or without a combined iridectomy or iridotomy.[1] In reply to my questions concerning aphakic glaucoma and a combined cyclodialysis and iridectomy, Dr. Allen stated,

> I prefer to use a scratch incision parallel to the limbus. I have used this type of incision and converted it into an "L" or "T" type of incision in order to obtain more room for such things as an iridectomy for biopsy or extraction of a foreign body in the chamber angle. Because of this, I suppose the use of a similar procedure in an iris bombé would not be too illogical.[1]

Following aphakia complicated by glaucoma, Dr. Castroviejo considers cyclodialysis to be the operation of choice. He will use a cyclodialysis if the angle closure cannot be relieved by strong miotics and if the angle closure is comparatively recent.[12]

11. **Air-Block Glaucoma.** In this type of glaucoma the most important preventive is avoiding the use of an excess amount of air. The second most important measure is to use a balanced solution instead of air or a balanced solution plus a smaller amount of air.

Air can cause pupillary block as in air blockade following cyclodialysis in phakic and aphakic eyes as well as after cat-

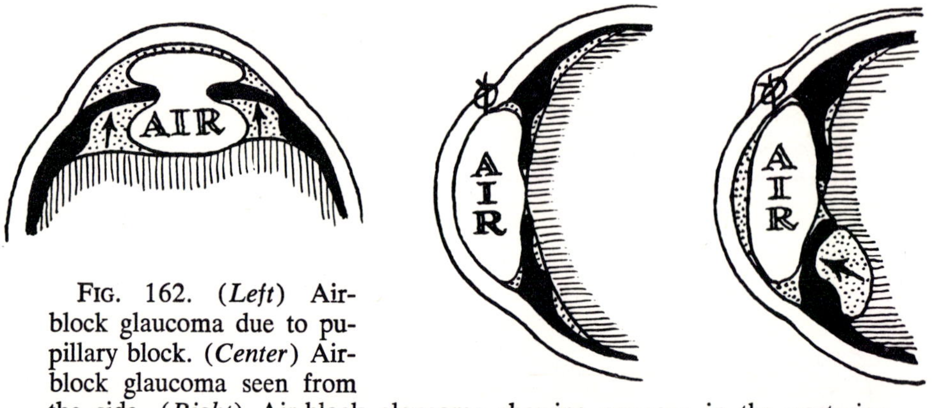

FIG. 162. (*Left*) Air-block glaucoma due to pupillary block. (*Center*) Air-block glaucoma seen from the side. (*Right*) Air-block glaucoma showing aqueous in the posterior chamber pressing the iris forward and causing angle closure. (Modified from Barraquer, Joaquin: Trans. Am. Acad. Ophthal. Oto-laryng. *66*:46)

aract extraction (Fig. 162). It can also cause angle block by entering the posterior chamber and forcing the iris forward.

If the mydriasis, carbonic anhydrase inhibitors (Diamox) and urea and positioning the patient do not break up the block, removal of the air and an iridectomy, preferably away from the original section, should be used (Fig. 163).

12. **Secondary Glaucoma Following Glaucoma Operations (Malignant Glaucoma).** Malignant glaucoma has been defined as a complication of glaucoma surgery in which the anterior chamber fails to form or collapses shortly after surgery and tension elevation recurs.

This complication occurs especially following external filtering operations such as trephining, sclerectomy or iridencleisis. The most susceptible eyes are those with chronic angle closure that cannot be brought back to normal with miotics alone.

The exact cause of malignant glaucoma is unknown, but following glaucoma surgery there may be a forward prolapse of the lens and the vitreous, followed by a trapping of aqueous from behind and then a pupillary block. The chamber then becomes flat, and the pressure rises. Two other possible causes of malignant glaucoma are thought to be: (1) a subchoroidal hemorrhage, and (2) stretching or incomplete tearing of the zonule fibers so that the lens comes forward.[43]

PROPHYLAXIS. If angle-closure glaucoma is secondary to a swollen cataractous lens, it is preferable to remove the lens and do an iridectomy. A peripheral iridectomy alone for the glaucoma is insufficient. Primary lens extraction is the operation of choice.

If malignant glaucoma has occurred in one eye, it can occur in the other. Therefore, if the other eye is glaucomatous, prophylactic glaucoma surgery should be done before the tension rises to a point at which it cannot be controlled by miotics alone.

If a filtering operation of one type precipitated the malignant glaucoma in the first eye, another type of glaucoma surgery should be tried in the second eye.

The need for carbonic anhydrase inhibitors and osmotic agents to control the pressure and the presence of an extremely shallow chamber with a history of malignant glaucoma in the first eye are the indications for lens removal in cases in which there are any significant lens changes.

MEDICAL TREATMENT. Miotics, carbonic anhydrase inhibitors, urea or mannitol and retrobulbar injections should be used to reduce the tension to normal and whiten the eye if possible. Surgery then should follow.

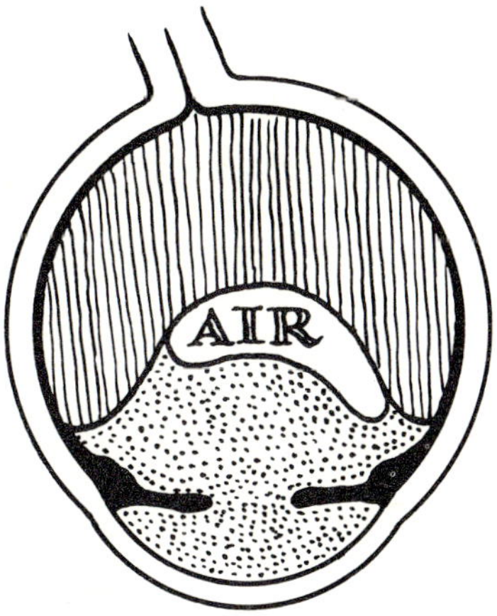

FIG. 163. A method used when the air block is due to air behind the iris is to position the patient face downward so that the air moves toward the posterior pole of the eye and away from the iris. (Modified from Barraquer, Joaquin: Trans. Am. Acad. Ophthal. Otolaryng. *66*:46)

SURGICAL TREATMENT. *Aspiration of the vitreous* through the pars plana with or without the injection of air or saline into the anterior chamber has been tried and reported to be helpful.[5] An iridectomy is sometimes added. However, I have known these measures to fail.

Still another conservative variation of this approach for the management of malignant glaucoma has been proposed. This consists of preparing a conjunctival flap 4 mm. from the limbus and then using light surface scleral diathermy for 2 mm. to each side of the scleral incision. Then, 4 mm. from and parallel to the limbus, a cyclodialysis incision is made through the sclera and a preplaced suture is used, and separating the wound, a perforation with cautery is made to release aqueous from the retrolental space.

Following this a cyclodialysis is performed, and air is injected into the anterior chamber. The sclera and the conjunctiva are then sutured.[39]

Surgical removal of the lens is the procedure of choice.

Dr. Sugar feels that if a broad iridectomy has not already been done, then two or three small peripheral iridectomies done at the time of the lens extraction may avoid the need for excising the hyaloid or the vitreous at a later time.

TECHNIC. With the use of the steps outlined under medical treatment, posterior sclerotomy and vitreous aspiration are usually not necessary to lower the pressure prior to opening the eye. Since it is safer, the incision should be made, in part at least, *ab externo* and finished with scissors. Multiple preplaced or postplaced "hard" sutures are advised. Intracapsular extraction should be attempted and in these cases usually results. Chandler stated that in these cases vitreous loss is not only acceptable but might even be advisable. If vitreous is not lost, the eye may continue to show malignant glaucoma. If one succeeds in removing the lens without loss of vitreous, it is probably advisable to rupture the hyaloid after the sutures have been tied.[13]

After tying the sutures, the surgeon should fill the anterior chamber with a balanced salt solution.

Vitreous Incision. For those cases in which, after the chamber is formed, the chamber again collapses and the pressure again becomes elevated, it is necessary to make an incision into the vitreous. In these instances the mechanism of the glaucoma is probably that of another pupillary block caused by a vitreous detachment and aqueous humor collecting in or behind the vitreous body. Prior to these incisions the pressure again must be lowered by acetazolamide (Diamox), urea or mannitol; if necessary, a posterior sclerotomy should be performed.

Tapping this collection of fluid or breaking vitreous condensation as for a secondary cataract operation is necessary. Occasionally the tap must be made with a Wheeler knife to the middle of the vitreous cavity.

I have watched the anterior chamber form spontaneously after such a tap. Injection of a balanced salt solution should be made if the chamber does not form.

Usually miotics will be needed postoperatively and, surgically, a cyclodialysis may be necessary.

TYPES OF GLAUCOMA SURGERY

In regard to glaucoma surgery for angle-closure glaucoma, it is generally agreed that a peripheral iridectomy is the operation of choice. Today, in open-angle glaucoma one operates only when all medications (carbonic anhydrase inhibitors, miotics and epinephrinelike compounds) given in the highest concentrations possible and as frequently as possible fail to preserve the acuity and the field. When surgery is indicated, each surgeon still will follow the old rule of performing that surgery which, in his hands, works best. One of the finest glaucoma surgeons I have known used, almost exclusively, a sclerecto-iridectomy, reopening the same area when necessary. I know also of a group of surgeons who used a cyclodialysis almost equally frequently, repeating this as indicated. It is interesting that Dr. Edmund Spaeth, whose broad surgical experience is well known, said at the Wills Conference of 1962,

> For many years my operation of choice in open-angle glaucoma has been the trephine. I have not used the trephine in three years and now favor iridencleisis because it has fewer of the immediate or late complications seen with the trephine.

Simultaneous Glaucoma and Cataract Surgery

Among the type of one-stage operations that have been proposed are:

1. Iris inclusion operations such as iridencleisis, incarcerating one or two pillars, combined with a lens extraction.
2. Anterior sclerotomy or its equivalent, such as trephining or sclerectomy with cautery, often with complete iridectomy and lens extraction
3. Cyclodialysis followed by lens extraction
4. Combinations of the above, such as sclerectomy and iridencleisis

Some General Considerations Related to the Technic of Simultaneous Glaucoma and Cataract Surgery*

It is important in doing this type of one-stage operation that one have a good strong Tenon's capsule to avoid flat chambers following the operation. Some surgeons stress the need for suturing Tenon's capsule and the conjunctiva as separate layers in the external filtering procedures, especially those of the trephine type. In the simultaneous iridencleisis and cataract extraction, if the pupil appears to be updrawn at the time of surgery, Hughes adds a vertical iridotomy below. Others feel that they can avoid an updrawn pupil and obtain equal success by incarcerating a tongue above rather than a single wick of iris. Because cyclodialysis possibly works by internal drainage, and since a thick conjunctiva and Tenon's capsule is not necessary, this might be the simultaneous operation of choice where the conjunctiva is thin. I myself have had no experience with this type of operation. In using a cyclodialysis combined with a cataract extraction the lower temporal quadrant is recommended for the cyclodialysis.[26] Air is injected into the anterior chamber, and then the lens is extracted from above. The one objection to making a cyclodialysis in this lower quadrant is that blood may plug the opening. The objection to making a cyclodialysis above is that it is technically more difficult to proceed with the next steps. Some surgeons will object seriously to combining the sclerectomy with an iridencleisis, feeling that this combination will certainly lead to a flat chamber.

* See also pp. 29-30.

Summary and Conclusions

The combination of glaucoma and cataracts presents a difficult problem. In the case of cataract in which miotic-controlled angle-closure glaucoma is present (i.e., without angle block), lens extraction cures both the cataract and the potential angle-closure glaucoma. This is not true in acute angle closure with angle block.

In open-angle glaucoma, some surgeons will always operate the glaucoma first if there is a cataract and the ocular pressure is not controlled by the medications, systemic and local, given frequently and in the highest concentrations possible. I feel that if the glaucoma can be controlled with 1 per cent pilocarpine alone, and if there is a cataract, very often an iridectomy and removal of the lens will be sufficient. Some surgeons prefer to combine simultaneous glaucoma surgery such as an iris inclusion or sclerectomy with the extraction of the lens.

Among present-day advances that help to make all glaucoma surgery and perhaps simultaneous surgery more successful are: (1) carbonic anhydrase inhibitors and urea; (2) retrobulbar anesthesia with hyaluronidase and digital massage; and (3) alpha-chymotrypsin which increases the number of intracapsular extractions and therefore decreases the factors related to lens-matter retention in extracapsular extraction and the associated secondary types of glaucoma.

Dr. Edmund Spaeth pointed out that we must emphasize the use of urea as a most valuable agent in related cataract-glaucoma surgery.

UVEITIS AND CATARACT

One should suspect latent uveitis in one-eyed patients.

Hypermature cataracts which can show iritis and a secondary glaucoma will cause trouble if not operated on early. Even in the face of an active uveitis one should extract the cataract, since that may be the cure.

In those cases in which there is a bilateral old uveitis without posterior synechiae but with subnormal vision, hypotony is evidence of a sick eye; these eyes do not tolerate operation well. Intracapsular extraction is imperative in cases with uveitis; extracapsular extraction might lead to phthisis bulbi. Even minute amounts of retained lens matter may be more than the eye can tolerate. A full iridectomy should be done, posterior synechiae freed with a spatula and an inferior iridotomy performed before delivering the lens. An inferior iridotomy widens the pupil and lessens the chances of a postoperative inflammatory membrane. It is also a safeguard against postoperative updrawn pupils.

Steroids are a boon to ophthalmology. The use of cortisone preparations preoperatively and postoperatively should be considered when removing cataracts in the presence of uveitis. Formerly, when a patient had uveitis, cataract surgery normally would not be considered; today, surgery can be carried out despite uveitis.

CATARACT EXTRACTION FOLLOWING CORNEAL-GRAFT SURGERY

At the 1962 Wills Conference, Dr. James Purnell discussed 18 cases of cataract extraction following corneal-graft surgery. In each case the corneas were clear prior to the removal of the lens. Six to 12 months had elapsed before cataract extraction. In 6 of the cases, the removal of the lens was successful. In 12, the graft became opaque or semi-opaque. The opacity began 2 to 4 weeks following the removal of the lens. In all these cases, a round-pupil intracapsular extraction with no trauma to the cornea was attempted. In those cases in which the haze could be seen to develop, it was noted that the vitreous touched the back of the cornea. The pressure in each of these cases was normal. Air was injected in an attempt to prevent the corneal haze, and the graft cleared. So long as the air remained, the graft stayed clear, and vision was satisfactory. As the air was absorbed, the graft became edematous. Air injections were repeated, and each time the edema disappeared. In the successful clear corneas it was noted that the vitreous was held backward and did not touch the back of the endothelium. Because it was noted that in 3 cases of unintentional extracapsulars the graft remained clear, it was decided to extract the lenses as planned extracapsulars. Four cases were operated in this fashion, and all the grafts remained clear. In these cases, the anterior capsule was removed carefully, and the nucleus and the cortex were expressed, leaving the posterior capsule intact. In these cases the vitreous face did not touch the back of the eye. These cases in which a well-planned extracapsular was done following successful corneal transplantation suggest that a well-planned extracapsular is the method of choice in order to retain the permanent clear grafts following the cataract extractions.

In a personal communication regarding cataract surgery following corneal transplants Dr. A. Benedict Rizzuti stated,

It is advisable not to remove the cataract until the eye has become completely quiet. This usually requires a minimum of about six months. In cases where a traumatic cataract has occurred at time of corneal surgery, one could remove the cataract at the same time or wait one week and then carry on with the extraction.

I have used alpha-chymotrypsin in six cases of keratoplasties. None of the grafts has become cloudy. The method of extractions was five intra-capsular and one extra-capsular. In all of the six cases a complete penetrating keratoplasty was performed . . .

Vitreous in direct contact with the posterior surface of the cornea is a definite cause in my mind in setting up a bullous keratopathy. In this type of case the injection of air is mandatory and should be performed very early so as to prevent the spread of the keratopathy. In the corneal clinic at the Brooklyn Eye and Ear Hospital, I have seen a fairly large number of cases of this type but cannot give you an exact figure.

Dr. Castroviejo states,

. . . in eyes previously operated for keratoplasty, if the transplant was performed over six months previously, the cataract surgery is as uncomplicated as if the cornea was entirely normal. I have not one or two but several dozen of such cases. In most of these cases the cataract extraction has been intracapsular and if the operation resulted in an extracapsular extraction, it was due to an accidental rupture of the capsule but not voluntary. Therefore, my experiences do not agree with that reported at the Will's conference. Maybe there were other factors in the cases treated at Will's which had nothing to do with the successful performance of keratoplasty and cataract surgery.

I personally use alpha-chymotrypsin very rarely, only in young patients from twenty to forty years of age when the lens is swollen and cannot be grasped with capsule forceps. This criterion is the same whether the patient has had corneal surgery or not.[12]

I have performed intracapsular extractions following corneal transplants and have not encountered the clouding of the cornea. This was done in six eyes. In my cases, no alpha-chymotrypsin was used inasmuch as, at the time I feared that the enzyme might possibly injure the corneal graft. The grafts remained clear.

Lamellar Transplants and Cataract Surgery

Dr. Jorge Buxton pointed out that cataract extractions following lamellar grafts may be performed sooner than in penetrating grafts but preferably 6 months later. Extreme gentleness, a corneoscleral incision favoring the scleral cut, a sliding technic and minimal contact with the endothelium are important in order to avoid changes in the graft.

There is always danger that a lamellar graft may become detached and lost, be it following suture removal after grafting or, very infrequently, after cataract extraction. "Fortunately," Dr. Buxton continues, "it is not imperative that a new graft be replaced immediately. The eye can be patched; measures can be taken to lower intraocular pressure; even four or five days later, the membrane that fills the defect can be peeled off easily with forceps or scraped with a razor blade and a new lamellar graft applied." Dr. Buxton prefers fresh tissue to preserved material for lamellar or penetrating grafts.[9]

Summary and Conclusions

Cataracts may be extracted 6 to 12 months following corneal surgery of the lamellar or penetrating type. Since clear grafts can cloud over and since lamellar grafts can re-detach, maximal gentleness and precautions outlined for removing a graft in the presence of a dystrophy seem to be indicated, especially since the original corneal surgery may have been done for a dystrophy. In penetrating grafts some advise a well-planned extracapsular while others perform a planned intracapsular. Clear grafts have been reported following the use of alphachymotrypsin in the removal of the lens.

If a lamellar graft is lost following cataract surgery, a delay of even 4 or 5 days until one can obtain fresh corneal tissue to replace this graft seems to be the procedure of choice.

REFERENCES

1. Allen, J. H.: Cyclodialysis, Southern M. J. *44*:931, 1951.
2. Araki, Minour: Diagnostic of retinal detachment by ultrasonic examination, Societas Ophthalmologica Japonica *66*: 46, 1962.
3. Barraquer, Joaquin: Advances in the surgery of the crystalline lens, Lecture presented at the American Academy of Ophthalmology and Otolaryngology Meeting, Chicago, 1961.
4. ——: Personal communication.
5. Becker, B., and Shaffer, R.: Diagnosis and Therapy of the Glaucomas, p. 259, St. Louis, Mosby, 1961.
6. Berliner, M. L.: Biomicroscopy of the Eye, vol. 1, New York, Hoeber, 1949.
7. Boyd, B. F.: Congenital cataracts: modern concepts, Highlights Ophthal. *4*:255, 1961.
8. Burian, H. M.: Clinical retinography, Inter. Ophth. Clinics *2*:21, 1962.
9. Buxton, Jorge: Symposium: Surgical management of cataracts, New York Eye and Ear Infirmary Alumni Association, April 10, 1962.
10. Carbajal, U. M.: A safe approach in surgery of congenital cataracts, Am. J. Ophthal. *52*:361, 1961.
11. ——: A new needle knife for congenital cataract surgery, Annual meeting of the Philippine Ophth. Soc., Oct., 1961.
12. Castroviejo, Ramon: Personal communication.
13. Chandler, P. A.: Surgery of complicated cataracts *in* Haik, G. M. (ed.): Symposium on Diseases and Surgery of the Lens, p. 132, St. Louis, Mosby, 1957.
14. Cordes, F. C.: Surgery of congenital cataracts *in* Haik, G. M. (ed.): Symposium on Diseases and Surgery of the Lens, St. Louis, Mosby, 1957.
15. ——: Linear extraction in congenital cataract surgery, Am. J. Ophthal. *52*: 355, 1961.
16. ——: Personal communication.
17. Fry, W. E.: Personal communication.
18. Galin, M. A., Taylor, A., and McLean, J. M.: Intralenticular foreign bodies, A.M.A. Arch. Ophth. *66*:830, 1961.
19. Girard, L. J., *et al.*: The problems of intracapsular cataract extraction in infants and children, Am. J. Ophthal. *54*: 1064, 1962.
20. Irvine, A. R.: Annual review: lens and vitreous, A.M.A. Arch. Ophth. *67*:151, 1962.

21. Jones, I. S.: The treatment of congenital cataracts by needling, Am. J. Ophthal. *52*:347, 1961.
22. Kara, G.: Symposium: Surgical management of cataracts, New York Eye and Ear Infirmary Alumni Association, April 10, 1962.
23. Krewson, W., and Spaeth, P.: Thirteenth Annual Clinical Conference of Wills Eye Hospital, Philadelphia, Feb. 9-11, 1961.
24. Lee, O. S., and Allen, J. H.: Cyclodialysis, Am. J. Ophthal. *32*:1713, 1949.
25. Lincoff, H.: Retinal detachment (round table discussion), Pan American Association of Ophthalmology, Lima, Peru, Feb. 1, 1962.
26. McGarry, H. I.: Annual review: glaucoma, A.M.A. Arch. Ophth. *66*:871, 1961.
27. McKinna, A. J.: Results of treatment of traumatic cataract in children, Am. J. Ophthal. *52*:43, 1961.
28. McLean, J. M.: Alpha-chymotrypsin extraction in corneal dystrophy, III Curso Inter. Oftalmol., p. 103, May, 1961.
29. ——: The Collected Letters of the International Correspondence Soc. of Ophthal. and Otolaryng., Series VII, p. 8, New Orleans, La., January 15, 1962.
30. Magruder, G. B.: Lens extraction in hereditary deep corneal dystrophy, Am. J. Ophthal. *52*:677, 1961.
31. Newell, F. W.: Symposium on Congenital Cataract, An. Inst. Barraquer *3*:355, 1962.
32. Newton, F. H.: Congenital cataracts: a review of 84 cases, Am. J. Ophthal. *52*:368, 1961.
33. Pischel, Dohrmann: Questions and answers, J.A.M.A. *176*:477, 1961.
34. Purnell, J. E.: Cataract extraction following corneal graft surgery, Lecture presented at the Fourteenth Annual Clinical Conference of Wills Eye Hospital, Philadelphia, Feb. 16, 1962.
35. Reese, A. B.: An appraisal of the current trend in cataract surgery, Montgomery Lecture, Ireland, 1962.
36. Rosenthal, Morton: Personal communication.
37. Salleras, Alejandro: Personal communication.
38. Scheie, H. G.: Aspiration of congenital or soft cataracts: a new technique, Am. J. Ophthal. *50*:1048, 1960.
39. Scott, A. S., and Smith, V. H.: Retrolental decompression for malignant glaucoma, Brit. J. Ophthal. *45*:654, 1961.
40. Shapland, C. D.: Detachment of the retina in the aphakic eye, III Curso Inter. Oftalmol., p. 215, May, 1961.
41. Spaeth, E. B.: Personal communication.
42. Sugar, H. S.: Secondary glaucoma, (Lecture) Yale University School of Medicine Postgraduate Course in Ophthalmology, New Haven, March 11, 1960.
43. ——: Personal communication.
44. Symposium on Congenital Cataracts, Third International Course of Ophthalmology, Barraquer Institute, May, 1961.
45. Teng, C. C., and Katzin, H. M.: Personal communication.
46. Thomas, C. I.: Annual review: cornea and sclera, A.M.A. Arch. Ophth. *67*: 171, 1962
47. Thorpe, H. E.: Symposium: Complications of Cataract Surgery, New York Eye and Ear Infirmary Alumni Association, April 9-12, 1962.
48. Troutman, R. C.: Surgery of congenital cataracts, Fuchs' irrigation, Highlights Ophthal. *4*:293, 1961.
49. Tsuzuki, Kosai: Clinical importance of the oscillatory potential in the human ERG. Report II. Observation of the oscillatory potential in retinal detachment, Soc. Ophthal. Japonica *66*:69, 1962.
50. Valenzuela, R.: Aphakia and retinal detachment, Arch. Chil. Oftal. *17*:84, 1960.

5

Postoperative Complications

STRIATE KERATITIS

Postoperative striate keratitis may be partially explained by hypotony, excessive irrigation, instrumentation or manipulation of the cornea. A small incision or poorly placed sutures also may play a part. Damage following the extra manipulations required by the use of alpha-chymotrypsin also can be a cause. Dr. Edmund Spaeth does not feel that alpha-chymotrypsin "plays any role" in striate keratitis.

Prophylactic steps include a large corneal incision, the use of Ringer's or a balanced solution, careful and minimal instrumentation. Today, if alpha-chymotrypsin is used, most surgeons favor the capsule forceps rather than the erisophake and use a sliding rather than a tumbling technic. However, in most cases, I will use the erisophake and the tumbling technic.

With the exception of the striate keratitis noted in Fuchs' dystrophy, most cases of striate keratitis clear up spontaneously.

Infrared rays and Dionin are not of any real help.

CORNEAL EDEMA AND BULLOUS KERATOPATHY

Persisting postoperative corneal edema, which can go on to a bullous keratopathy, presents a very serious problem.

Differential Diagnosis and Prophylaxis

1. See striate keratitis. In certain cases there may be a relationship.

2. Epithelial ingrowth. This can be avoided by a limbus-based conjunctival flap correctly prepared and closed. To avoid an epithelial ingrowth chromic sutures are preferable as there is an increased ingrowth with the use of silk sutures. Estrada noted that epithelial ingrowth is not seen in corneal transplants and for this reason feels that a pure corneal incision may avoid epithelial ingrowth. (See p. 160.)

3. Glaucoma. As a rule, the edema in glaucoma is diffuse. To rule this out a pressure may be taken with an applanation tonometer shortly following surgery.[8] Preoperatively a complete diagnostic workup will rule out a primary glaucoma. A known glaucoma should be controlled, preferably prior to the cataract surgery. Secondary glaucomas, especially following vitreous loss, pupillary block or vitreous adhesions that plug up the angle, must be considered. (See p. 141.)

4. Unrecognized dystrophy

5. Endothelial trauma from the erisophake, the capsule forceps, the irrigating syringe or the solution itself. There should be no more than minimal trauma to the cornea. Especially with the use of alpha-chymotrypsin, some surgeons favor the use of the capsule forceps and sliding,

feeling that the incidence of corneal damage is smaller. In known or suspected dystrophy, I prefer this combination.

6. Impaired metabolism of the cornea

7. Rupture or laceration of Descemet's membrane can produce an opacity in the involved area. If the membrane curls on itself, it can be resutured.[22]

8. Defective corneal incision or suturing may cause edema because of the associated trauma.

9. Vitreous, iris, capsule or other lens material against the cornea

Prophylactic Considerations

The best treatment is prevention.

1. Ideally the incision should be scleral and large, i.e., 180° to 200° or more.

2. The site of the incision may be important (see p. 26).

3. Alpha-chymotrypsin. There is no real proof that the use of alpha-chymotrypsin will cause an increased corneal edema. It has been pointed out that there is an increased striate keratitis with the use of alpha-chymotrypsin, but this can be avoided if proper precautions are taken.

4. Balanced solutions. Many feel that these are important in preventing corneal changes. However, if one does not want to prolong the action of alpha-chymotrypsin, those balanced solutions containing calcium should be avoided. It is felt that those solutions containing saline and methylcellulose cause more corneal damage; however, it is also felt that the saline component is responsible.

Early Treatment of Corneal Edema

As to the early treatment in the corneal edema stage when there are vitreous corneal adhesions at the end of 1 week and the adhesion of the vitreous is small and recent, pupillary dilatation sometimes is sufficient to separate the adhesion. Dr. Reese advocates this approach, keeping the patient flat on his back and then trapping the vitreous with constrictorlike drugs. However, this does not always work; when it does not, the following steps can be taken.

1. At this time air injection into the anterior chamber is the best solution. Using a needle-knife (I feel that this is preferable to an Amsler needle) a small tract is made horizontally below in the area of 6 o'clock. The tract is made with a fluorescein strip to stain the needle blade. A No. 27 or 29 blunt needle then is used to inject air into the anterior chamber. A sterile Q-tip or spatula can be used to tap the air bubble and to push the vitreous away from the damaged endothelium. This is perhaps the most important single step; therefore, one must not delay. When air is injected into the anterior chamber, it is preferable that a single bubble of air fill the chamber. Vitreous strands may be indicated by three or four small air bubbles instead of the single large one. If the vitreous still touches the endothelium, mechanical separation with a cyclodialysis spatula is necessary. Two days of bed rest with the patient flat on his back—ideally, with both eyes closed—will help the air to hold back the vitreous from the endothelium. Acetazolamide (Diamox) should be included in the postoperative treatment.

2. Air injection plus a posterior sclerotomy is my second choice. If the amount of air injected is fairly large or one does not trust his suture line, a posterior sclerotomy certainly should be done beforehand. If it is not done, the air may

cause an iris prolapse or partially open the wound. Some surgeons feel that the vitreous aspiration is more important than the air injection. Others feel that a trial of urea, acetazolamide (Diamox) and bed rest may be used as a conservative substitute for sclerotomy for 24 to 48 hours more if the corneal edema is minimal and the eye is quiet. The decision to do a sclerotomy is easier to make if there is a choroidal detachment, but the method is the same with or without a choroidal detachment. The opening through the sclera is usually at the pars plana in the temporal lower quadrant. The area of the incision is surrounded by diathermy, and fluid is released cautiously.

3. An operation consisting of opening the wound, doing an iridectomy, mechanically breaking any adhesions and purposely losing some of the vitreous through an anterior approach has been proposed. This is followed by an air injection into the lower portion of the cornea through a preplaced tract. It is felt that in many of these cases showing corneal edema, the edema will slowly disappear. (At this time, I would prefer to lose vitreous through a posterior route because I feel that the eye would respond better.)

Late Treatment or the Bullous Keratopathy Stage

The prognosis here is always poor because recurrences are common. The most important consideration is the control of pain. The following treatment is recommended at this stage:

1. The simplest method is the use of methylcellulose incorporated in drops. This keeps the cornea lubricated and reduces the pain somewhat.

2. A hair dryer applied over the cornea may remove some of the fluid and temporarily improve vision.[21]

3. Hypertonic solutions or ointments such as 5 per cent sodium chloride gradually increased to 15 per cent may be applied. This draws out fluid from the edematous corneal stroma, but the effects do not last long. Glycerin in the form of an ointment is also recommended.[1]

4. A local neurectomy of the greater superficial petrosal nerve performed by a neurosurgeon may be helpful.

5. It has been suggested that irradiation of the lacrimal gland or its extirpation may be helpful in that the bullous keratopathy may come about following the imbibition of tears by the cornea.[12]

6. A Bard-Parker knife applied at a right angle to the cornea is used to scrape the epithelium off. This is followed by the use of silver nitrate, tincture of iodine or 25 per cent trichloracetic acid. A gray corneal haze may result, but pain in the bullous keratopathy is decreased. This may be repeated again.[4]

7. If the pain is controlled, a radial iridotomy under the clear area of the cornea in an eye that is quiet is practical and worth trying. Occasionally it helps to restore vision, especially if the bullae or the resultant scars are limited. The use of the light coagulator applied from the side of the clear cornea to create a pupil is another consideration, provided, of course, that capsular or other opacities behind the pupil are not anticipated.

8. A retrobulbar injection of procain followed by alcohol is also helpful for control of pain.

9. A thin conjunctival flap, sometimes combined with a lamellar corneal transplant, is considered by some to be the most satisfactory solution.[9] Dr. Dunnington has modified the Gundersen technic somewhat. He mobilizes a thin layer of conjunctiva from above and below and ties the sutures in the episcleral tissues

lateral to the limbus and then runs a continuous suture to unite the upper and the lower folds. The attachments of the upper and the lower folds are further supported by sutures above and below the limbus. To mobilize the conjunctiva, he does not make slits above and below. Dr. Dunnington reported that all of the 8 to 10 patients on whom he has used this technic were more comfortable, although their vision is poor—in the range of 20/100 or 20/200. To date, only 1 of these cases has had a separation at the junction of the upper and the lower folds.[6]

10. Dr. Castroviejo feels that, "For a bullous keratopathy (total) after a cataract extraction there are two choices, a total lamellar graft to improve the cornea structurally and make the eye more comfortable, hoping that the bullous keratopathy will not recur."[3]

11. The second choice, Dr. Castroviejo feels, for functional improvement is the use of a "keratoprosthesis . . . a small plastic cylinder 2 mm. in diameter, held in place in the cornea by an intralamellar plate of 4 mm."[3]

12. The use of a special knife to free the vitreous from the back of the endothelium can be tried. Of course, further damage to the endothelium and a scar will result from this maneuver.[20]

13. If the pressure is elevated, cyclodiathermy is the operation of choice.

14. Finally, enucleation may be the end-result.

FLAT CHAMBER FOLLOWING CATARACT EXTRACTION

In many instances a flat chamber, early or late, means an imperfect wound closure. Therefore, one must look for a leak in the wound. Failure to find a leak does not mean that one does not exist. One theory that is still held by many is that a wound leak or the obvious leak from the anterior chamber after filtering operations causes a continuing hypotony resulting in extravasation of fluid from the choroidal vessels, separation of the choroid and the ciliary body and flattening of the anterior chamber. There is considerable clinical evidence to support this theory. Repair of the wound leak, if it is found, often results in prompt re-formation of the chamber.[5]

In regard to failure of the chamber to re-form Dunnington says, "In my experience, persistent failure of the anterior chamber to re-form has been the result of external fistulization which can be remedied only by wound repair."[5]

Among the many causes for imperfect wound closure may be the tissues themselves, excessive thermal cautery and problems related to the surgical technic. In the late type of flat chamber, around the 10th to the 14th postoperative day when supposedly the wound has to withstand for the first time the normal and perhaps somewhat elevated intraocular pressure, the chamber becomes shallow.[18]

Preventive Treatment

A flat chamber can be avoided by:

1. A mitred, step or "half-lap" incision covered by conjunctiva. However, one need not use this type of incision but may use direct edge-to-edge sutures, postplacing them in the fashion I have described previously (see p. 39). Regardless of the type of flap, if alpha-chymotrypsin is used, it is important to wash the excess from the wound edge and from the inside of the eye.

2. Proper suturing. I use at least 5 chromic sutures. Some feel that 3 sutures are sufficient. I feel that more sutures are important if alpha-chymotrypsin is used.

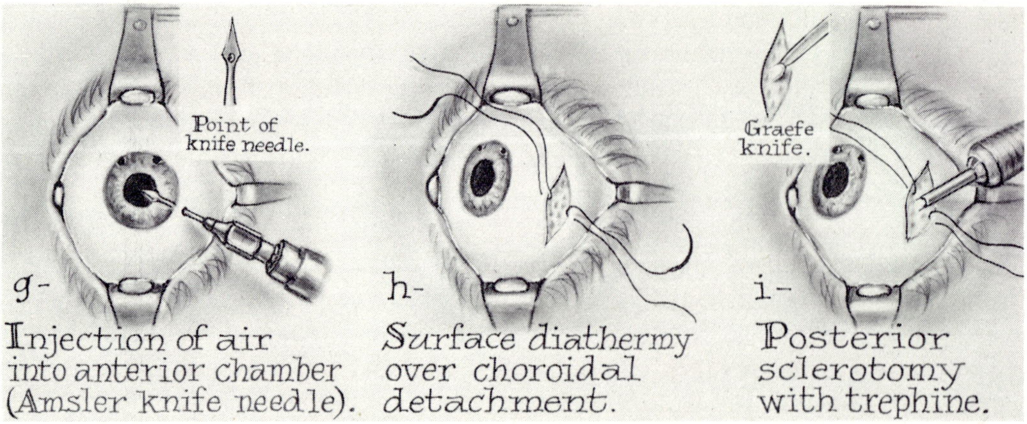

FIG. 164. (A) Injection of air into the anterior chamber (Amsler needle-knife). (B) Surface diathermy over choroidal detachment. (C) Posterior sclerotomy with trephine. (Berens, C., and King, J. H.: An Atlas of Ophthalmic Surgery, Philadelphia, Lippincott)

Silk or chromic sutures may be used safely with alpha-chymotrypsin, since the enzyme does not decrease the strength of these sutures. I have not found that suture knots are loosened by the enzyme.

If there is any question as to whether a suture is placed accurately, it must be removed at the time of surgery and not 2 or 3 days later when a flat chamber has resulted. One cannot say that the incidence of flat chambers is increased with the use of silk, plain or chromic catgut suture material.

Of course, whether the sutures are preplaced or postplaced, it is important that they be placed correctly. A good needle is also important. A quiet, soft eye makes it possible to make an accurate edge-to-edge closure.

3. An iridectomy that is truly peripheral and open. Some surgeons feel that if the iridectomy is peripheral it definitely must be large. I feel that a vertical iridotomy is safer but that a sector iridectomy is *safest.*

4. The judicious use of drugs. The most effective procedure is to induce paresis of the iris sphincter with atropine or scopolamine further supplemented by phenylephrine (10% Neo-Synephrine) to further dilate the pupil and to prevent adherence of the dilated iris to the vitreous face.[24]

5. Postoperative sedation may play a part in preventing wound separation. Often excessive postoperative activity may be partly responsible for flat chambers.

CONSERVATIVE TREATMENT

In a recently developed shallow chamber, maximal dilatation with phenylephrine (10% Neo-Synephrine) is the most important consideration in the conservative treatment. This breaks pupillary block. It can be alternated with miotics to open an obliterated iridectomy or free peripheral adhesions. Swan feels that if "alternate mydriatic and miotic therapy is used, it is desirable to use cyclogyl or some other cholinergic-blocking drug with shorter duration of action than scopolamine or atropine."[24]

Tight dressings and acetazolamide

(Diamox) are recommended, but I personally do not feel that they are very helpful.

Surgical Treatment

One should not be in too much of a rush—certainly not for at least 24 hours. Often nature will help in these cases, and one can afford to be conservative for 5 days. (Some will wait for 7 to 9 days if the eye is quiet and the cornea is clear.) Observation with the slit lamp will disclose the true depth of a chamber. The ocular tension is important, and one eye should be compared with the other, ideally with an applanation tonometer. If the conservative treatment has proved to be ineffective, the surgeon must admit to himself and to the patient that he must intervene. This is difficult to explain to the patient; however, the longer one waits, the poorer are the chances for a good result because of multiple complications.

If the leak is due to a faulty suture, the suture must be removed. If the leak is due to a fistula, which sometimes can be demonstrated with the use of fluorescein on a cotton Q-tip, this must be repaired. In these patients a thorough search frequently reveals no evidence of a leaking fistula. If there is a localized area of boggy conjunctiva, silver nitrate or Dionin are not helpful as a rule. This area should be left alone and watched. If it does not regress, the patient should be returned to the operating room and the involved area closed tightly.

When the above methods do not succeed and if the pupil is round, a peripheral iridectomy which is basal and adequate is recommended. I feel that a sector iridectomy would be safer because there is less chance of this closing.

If there is an obvious choroidal detachment and especially if there is an area of contact of the vitreous face with the back of the cornea, early injection of air into the anterior chamber—plus or minus the removal of subchoroidal fluid—through a posterior sclerotomy is my next step (Fig. 164). A spatula or a moist cotton Q-tip can be applied to the cornea to help the air dissect the vitreous face away from the cornea. This is not always satisfactory, as the chamber may become flat as soon as it is absorbed or the air may get behind the iris and push it into the wound. Air injection can be used if the wound is tight and shows accurate apposition. Later if the wound has no sutures you cannot trust it.

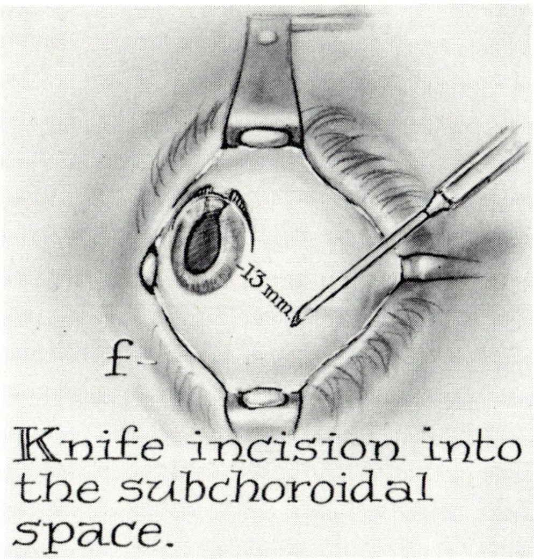

Fig. 165. Knife incision into the subchoroidal space. (Berens, C., and King, J. H.: An Atlas of Ophthalmic Surgery, Philadelphia, Lippincott)

As to the site of drainage, I prefer to make the incision over the area of the choroidal detachment if there is an obvious one. If it cannot be seen, the lower temporal quadrant is still my first choice (Fig. 165). Fluid will often be found here. In a great number of cases, Maumenee feels that it makes no difference—particularly if you can observe a choroidal detachment—if one drains fluid over the ciliary body or over the choroid because the choroidal detachement extends forward over the ciliary body.[5]

As to the sclerotomy, some feel that a trial of urea should be a preliminary step. In performing the sclerotomy it is not recommended that one go deep into the vitreous on the first attempt. Some feel that the posterior sclerotomy is much more important than the injection of air into the anterior chamber. The incision should be made just as is that used for a cyclodialysis. Finally, if these measures fail, a vitreous incision can be considered.

I rarely have seen the late type of flat chamber. This may possibly be explained by the fact that I prefer radial iridotomies and include phenylephrine (10% Neo-Synephrine) as a postoperative medication starting immediately the day following surgery.

In discussing the late type of flat chamber, Dr. Reese states,

> It is well known that the apposition of the hyaloid to the posterior surface of the cornea corrects itself in most instances without surgical intervention but when this opportune time is, it is difficult to know. As a working rule, I believe that three to three-and-a-half weeks after the operation is approximately the time for intervention. It is important to separate the hyaloid from the cornea before permanent adhesions and irreversible changes occur. Such changes may appear as early as ten days to two weeks, and some corneas tolerate the apposition so well the critical time may be longer than three to four weeks.
>
> There are two therapeutic approaches. One is to close the site of the aqueous leak and the other is to inject air into the anterior chamber. I find the injection of air to be the better of the two and resort almost entirely to this measure. The technique of air injection [Fig. 166] seems sufficiently important to warrant its discussion. With a Ziegler knife-needle dipped in methylene blue or on which fluorescein has been allowed to dry, an oblique puncture is made through the cornea into the periphery of the anterior chamber. The fluorescein marks the knife track so that it can be identified later for the air injection. 6 mm. from the limbus, between the superior and external rectus muscles, a 2-3 mm. incision is made into the conjunctiva, and a cataract knife is inserted through the sclera over this site which corresponds to the flat portion of the ciliary body. This incision, therefore, is posterior to the ciliary body, and anterior to the ora serrata. The blade of the knife is directed to the central part of the vitreous, and the blade is rotated 45° until the fluid part of the vitreous escapes and thus until the eye is soft. The vitreous is always fluid in the central part so the knife blade may be adjusted in depth and direction until the fluid vitreous drains. The knife is withdrawn and a 27 gauge needle attached to a syringe filled with air is inserted through the corneal track outlined by fluorescein or methylene blue, and the anterior chamber filled with air. This leaves the anterior chamber from two to three times its normal depth, and the hyaloid far separated from the cornea. It is necessary to perform this sclerotomy in order to get adequate separation of the hyaloid from the cornea, and permit a sufficient amount of air to be injected to remain there, perhaps for a week or more. This maneuver has been done many times, and there have never been any untoward effects from it. As a matter of fact, eyes on which this procedure has been done usually have the same time schedule postoperatively in regard to glasses as eyes on which the procedure has not been necessary. Certainly, I have resorted to air injection on eyes when it was probably not necessary, but on the other hand, I am sure an appreciable number of eyes have been saved by the procedure.[18]

POSTOPERATIVE HYPHEMA

Postoperative hyphema must be differentiated from hemorrhage present at the conclusion of surgery. It is usually related to the dehiscence of the wound, poor suturing, trauma or excessive postoperative activity on the part of the patient.

I feel that I have had less postoperative hyphema since doing an almost routine canthotomy. It seems to me that this leads to less squeezing of the lids.

Usually it is easy to distinguish fresh hemorrhage from that left in the eye at the time of surgery. A small drawing on the chart at the close of surgery is helpful. If hemorrhage is fresh, the color is redder. There is usually a history of pain in the eye. Even with 2 or 3 mm. of blood in the lower anterior chamber the patient may be allowed to get out of bed if the surgeon so desires.

Dr. Dunnington has pointed out that increased sedation is important in these cases. As a rule he makes a point of never mentioning the words blood or hemorrhage to the patient, since the patient may think that this means the loss of his eye. Instead, he will tell the patient that he has squeezed the eye and "bruised it a little bit." If there is a large amount of hemorrhage which will necessitate surgery, he will tell the patient at the time.[6]

Hemorrhage, if it is to occur, often will occur on the 4th to the 5th postoperative day. For this reason it is wise to keep the patient in the hospital for at least this length of time. This is one reason for not doing cataract surgery as an office procedure.

If the hemorrhage increases in amount, I feel that it is wise to keep the patient under close observation at least until the amount is constant or starts to decrease. In the patient with no abnormal bleeding tendencies, I know of no medication at this time which, given preoperatively or postoperatively, will definitely decrease hemorrhage.

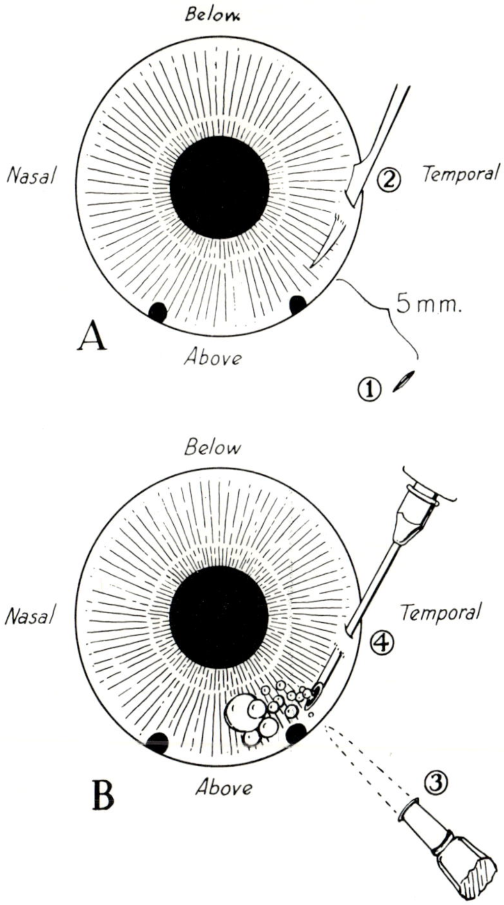

FIG. 166. Air injection into the anterior chamber. (A) 1. A small conjunctival incision 5 mm. from the limbus. 2. An oblique incision through the cornea with a Ziegler needle-knife. (B) 3. Insertion of a cataract knife to the center of the vitreous. 4. Needle inserted with bevel up through corneal tract and air injected. (Dr. A. B. Reese)

FILTERING CYSTIC CICATRIX*

Filtering cystic cicatrix will not occur with more than usual frequency after the

* For further information the reader is referred to the following sources:

1. The Collected Letters of the International Correspondence Society of Ophthalmologists and Otolaryngologists, Series VI, p. 177, Dec. 15, 1961.
2. Dunnington, J.: Hypotony after cataract extraction, Brit. J. Ophthal. *40*:30, 1956.

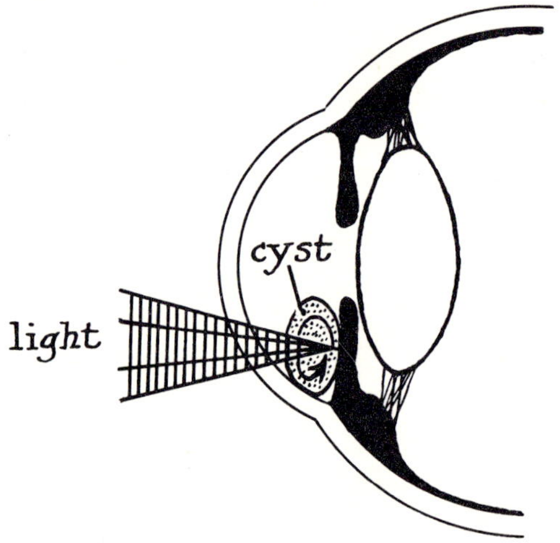

FIG. 167. Photocoagulator is used to destroy the cyst wall. Only low energy is needed to turn the cyst wall white. (Modified from Cibis, P. A.: Trans. Am. Acad. Ophthal. Oto-laryng. *66*: 71)

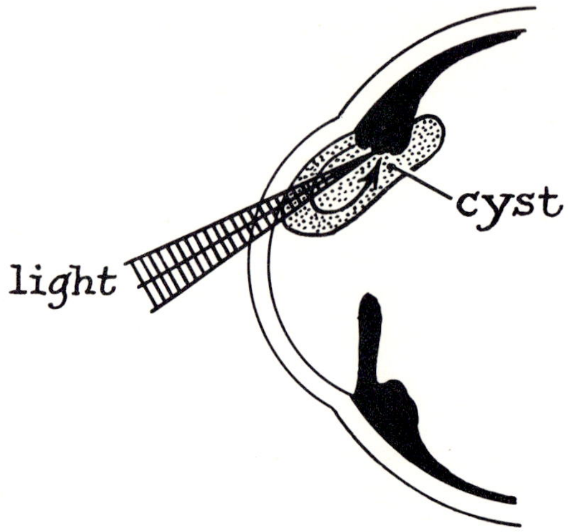

FIG. 168. How the light coagulator is used to destroy a larger cyst after cataract surgery. The coagulator is used only until the cyst wall turns white. (Modified from Cibis, P. A.: Trans. Am. Acad. Ophthal. Oto-laryng. *66*: 71)

use of alpha-chymotrypsin if the wound is opened and closed properly with extra sutures and the excess enzyme is carefully irrigated from the wound edge and the inside of the eye. In filtering cystic cicatrix following cataract surgery, it is important to take an ocular pressure and determine if the angle is closed. If the angle is closed, this cicatrix must be left untouched because it may be a protection against glaucoma. If the cicatrix is small and shows a good conjunctival covering, as a rule nothing need be done. If it is of medium size, thermocautery is the simplest means of eradicating it. Should the thermocautery cause collapse of the anterior chamber, direct suturing must be used immediately.

When the cicatrix is large, one must consider the possibility of epithelial ingrowth or iris or vitreous in the wound. In treating the wound one should take a biopsy and study sections under the microscope. Then the involved areas must be curetted, hard-tissue suture bites used and covered with a conjunctival flap. The treatment of a filtering cicatrix is exactly the same whether or not the enzyme has been used.

TREATMENT OF IRIS CYSTS (TRUE SEROUS) FOLLOWING CATARACT EXTRACTION

Two forms of traumatic implantation cysts must be considered: (1) true serous cysts (translucent), and (2) the "pearl," "solid" or epidermoid cysts[2] (see p. 160).

Since not all iris cysts (true serous, traumatic implantation) are progressive, some need only be watched. There are many ways to manage these cysts, but, unfortunately, they don't always work. These include:

1. Excision
2. Use of half-strength iodine. However, many of these cysts are multilocular,

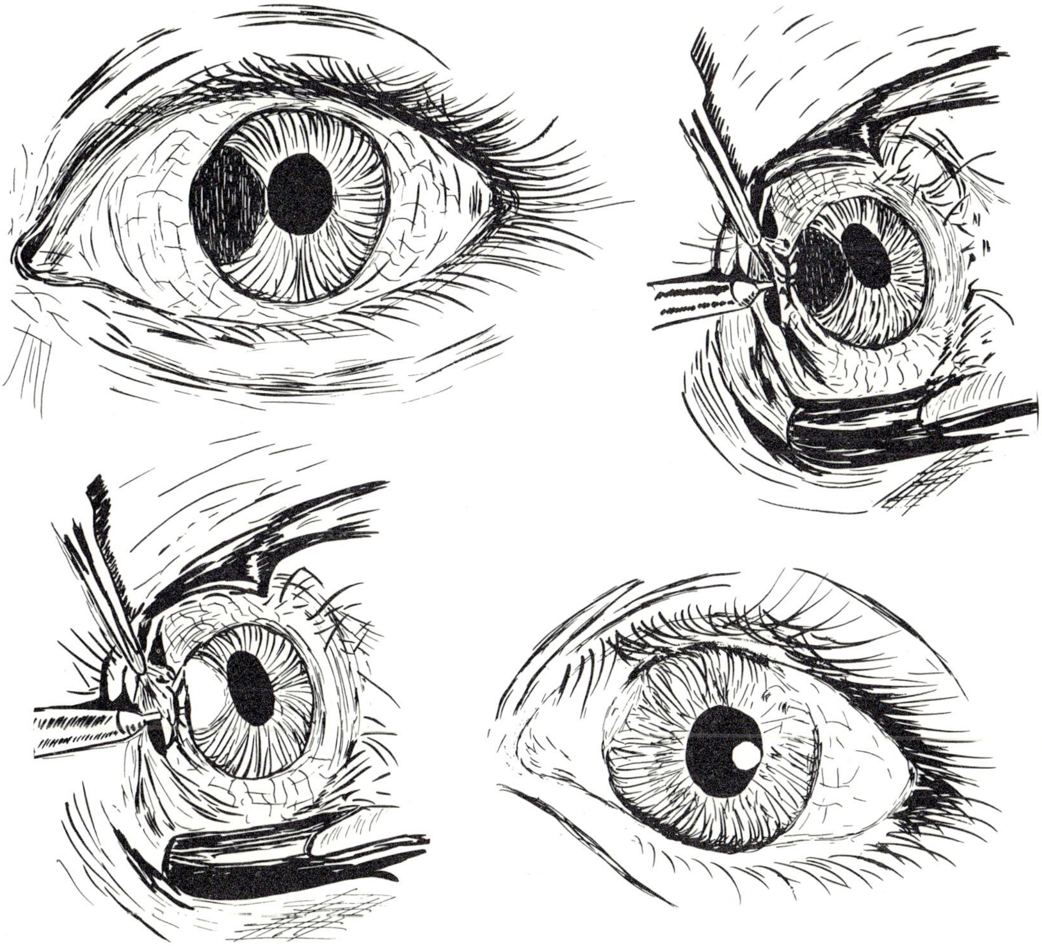

FIG. 169. (*Top, left*) Iris cyst in a 3-year-old boy following linear cataract extraction 1 year previously. (*Top, right*) Electrolysis needle in the center of the cyst. Needle was passed through the limbus into the cyst without entering the chamber. (*Bottom, left*) Needle partially withdrawn and cyst shrinking. (*Bottom, right*) Three weeks postoperatively the eye is white and the cyst is markedly shrunken.

and there is always the danger of damage to the eye proper with the iodine.

3. Diathermy coagulation. An insulated No. 27 to 30 needle is introduced into the cyst, and an electrode is applied.[10]

4. A transfixion may be helpful in some cases.

5. X-ray has been recommended. Sometimes this will shrink the cyst.

6. Light coagulation. Implantation cysts can be destroyed by using the photocoagulator from different angles of exposure. Photocoagulation is used to destroy the cyst wall. Only low energy is needed to turn the cyst wall white (Fig. 167).

Figure 168 shows how the light coagulator is used to destroy a larger cyst after cataract surgery. The coagulator is used only until the cyst wall turns white.

7. My method of handling these cysts is illustrated in Figure 169. This shows an

iris cyst in a 3-year-old boy following a linear cataract extraction which was performed 1 year previously. A shows an electrolysis needle in the center of the cyst. In B the needle extends through the limbus directly into the cyst. C shows the eye 3 weeks postoperatively. The eye is white, and the cyst is markedly shrunken.

If the cyst recurs, additional electrolysis should be performed. If it recurs a third time, the remaining portion of the cyst should be excised.[13] However, I must point out that the ordinary Walker unit is not strong enough with respect to the amount of current necessary for electrolysis. If the cyst is multilocular, it is not always possible to get the hydrogen bubbles into these individual units.

EPITHELIAL INGROWTH

Epithelial ingrowth is produced by delayed or faulty coaptation of wound edges. Surface epithelium in such a wound enters the eye to line the cornea and the angle. This epithelium also can follow and line suture tracks. In cataract surgery, epithelial ingrowth is due to delayed re-formation of the anterior chamber resulting from leaking wounds. Epithelial ingrowth must be differentiated from pearl-like implantation cysts (pearl tumors of the iris) which usually remain small and are confined to the iris. These cysts often result from eyelashes on the iris.[11] Pearl tumors must be further differentiated from the translucent true serous traumatic implantation cysts.

In the early stages of epithelial ingrowth the diagnosis may be extremely difficult, and the condition may be confused with endothelial trauma, rupture or laceration of Descemet's membrane, or vitreous, iris, capsule or other lens material against the cornea (see p. 150).

If one strongly suspects an epithelial ingrowth in the early stages. Dunnington has pointed out that it is justifiable to open the wound and perform a large iridectomy and scrape some of the endothelium *without treating it with alcohol.*[6] Both the iris and the endothelium can be examined for epithelial ingrowth. Since epithelial ingrowth depends on the iris for its nutrition and growth, this procedure may prove to be both diagnostic and therapeutic. Dr. John McLean suggests that removal of the involved iris *without touching the endothelium* is most important.[14a]

Clinical and Pathologic Picture

The typical clinical and pathologic picture in epithelial ingrowth is as follows. On its completion the surgeon usually considers the operation to have been uneventful. A filtering wound, tearing, bulbar injection and a narrow palpebral fissure due to hypotony give a characteristic appearance to these patients. Even though the tension is not elevated, the patients complain of aching pain, chiefly at night. In the second month postoperatively an iris pillar becomes updrawn, or a previously round pupil becomes displaced. With the slit lamp there is noted an increase in aqueous flare with no posterior corneal deposits. Eventually, there is a definite advancing edge along the posterior corneal epithelium. This membrane is usually transparent with waxy edges that are thickened and slightly elevated. Later, as the ingrowth extends toward the center of the cornea, there is a concave advancing edge because the edges are better nourished and grow more rapidly. Usually there is a deep vascularization in the stroma. The membrane grows more rapidly on the surface of the iris than anywhere else. The associated secondary glaucoma which follows hypotony occurs in half of these cases and is due to epithelium growing into the anterior chamber and spreading on the posterior surface of the cornea, resulting in impairment of aqueous flow. Seclusion and occlusion of the pupil by the epithelial lining may produce iris bombé.

Prophylaxis

It has been pointed out that epithelial ingrowth is not seen in a pure corneal type of incision that has not been covered by conjunctiva and is rarely, if ever, seen following a corneal transplantation. Conjunctiva is largely responsible for epithelial ingrowth.[7]

It is the surface epithelium of the conjunctiva that gives rise to the epithelial ingrowth. The best prophylactic measures that one can take against epithelial invasion of the anterior chamber are:

1. The use of a limbus-based conjunctival flap correctly prepared and closed
2. The use of mild chromicized absorbable sutures instead of silk sutures
3. Sutures that do not pass through more than one-half the depth of the incision and which are not kept in too long
4. Steps to prevent a delayed restoration of the anterior chamber; should a flat chamber occur, it should be repaired early.

Since epithelization is extremely difficult to treat successfully, these eyes are often lost. Curetting and treating the epithelization with alcohol is probably still the best treatment.[15] The scrapings must be carefully examined by someone qualified to interpret them. Even as much as half of the iris can be removed. X-ray and other methods have been used but with less success.

A new procedure consisting of a block resection of the inner layers of the cornea and the iris has been reported.[23]

CAPSULOTOMIES AND CAPSULECTOMIES

A capsulotomy is defined as an incision of a secondary cataract, while a capsulectomy refers to the actual removal of a portion of a secondary cataract. Actually, modern surgery has made no striking advances in these technics. However, in adults where the number of intracapsular extractions is continuously increasing because of new technics, including the use of enzymatic zonulolysis, capsulotomies and capsulectomies are being done less frequently. I am amused by the fact that residents are fascinated by capsulotomies and capsulectomies which to them appear to be simpler to perform than a routine cataract extraction. However, I feel that their interest is extremely important, as they seldom see the end-results of their cases during their residency period and therefore cannot fully appreciate the possible complications related to treating secondary membranes such as detached retina, delayed glaucoma and even loss of the eye.

Thin Capsule

For creating an opening through a thin capsule my first choice is a needling or discission. By these terms is meant capsulotomy in respect to incising or dividing the secondary cataractous membrane. Unfortunately, these same terms have been used freely to include cutting the anterior capsule and/or some of the cortex and, on occasion, for cutting all layers of the lens.

For the operative procedure I prefer a small, sharp Ziegler needle-knife with a handle that has been tapered so that the anterior chamber is not lost while one is working in it (Fig. 170). I find that this small knife blade allows greater freedom of movement in the anterior chamber whereas the heel of a large knife blade would limit this free movement. It could also cut and enlarge the corneal incision, thus losing the chamber early in the procedure or creating a larger scar in the cornea later. Losing the chamber early may cause the vitreous to move forward to the back of the cornea, resulting in immediate problems of manipulation and later

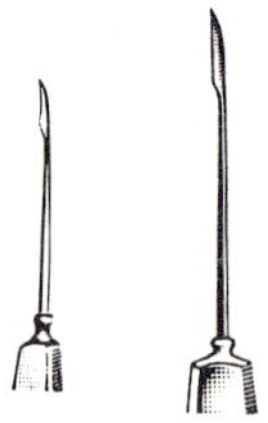

FIG. 170. (*Left*) Needle-knife, Ziegler, 3 mm. (Storz instrument No. E-153). (*Right*) Needle-knife, Ziegler, 5 mm. (Storz instrument No. E-155).

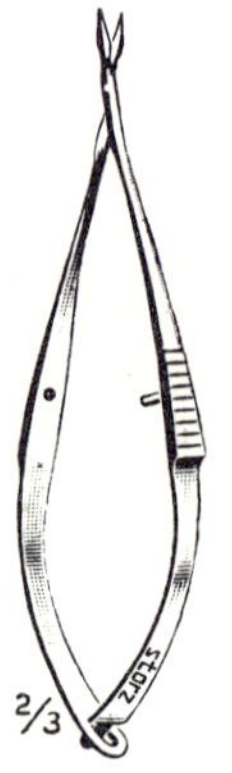

FIG. 172. Capsulotomy scissors, Vannas (Storz instrument No. E-3386).

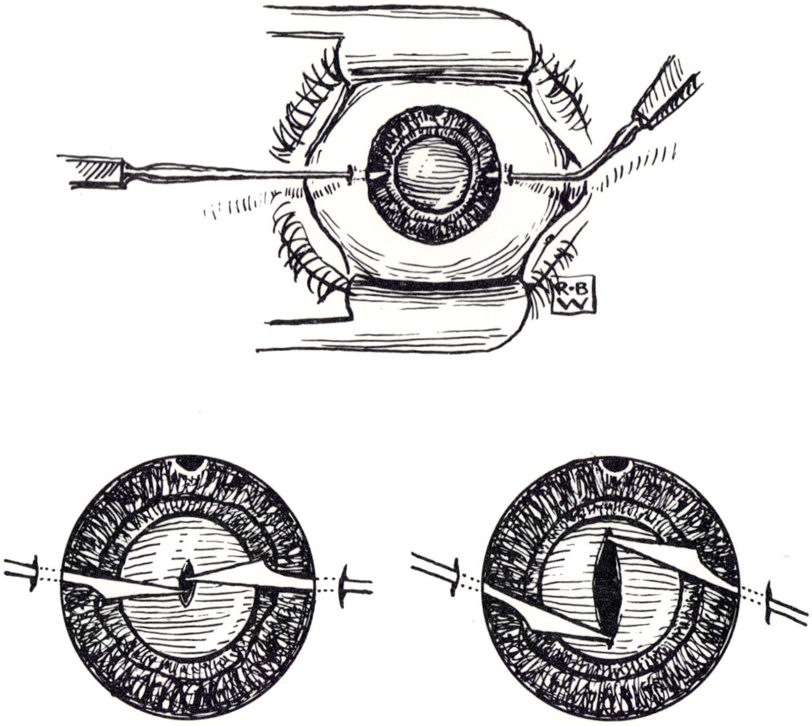

FIG. 171. Severing a secondary cataract with two needle-knives. (Modified from Guillaumat, Louis, *et al.*: Traitement Chirurgical des Affections Oculaires, Paris, Doin)

possibly irreversible endothelial damage, deep corneal scarring and/or synechiae. To ensure sharpness of the blade, I either use a new blade or carefully note on the knife container the date and the degree of sharpness of the blade. When the knife is only moderately sharp it is sent off immediately for sharpening or replacement. I allow no one but myself to handle the knife. Before the operation I place it in a metal container and then into Post's solution to soak. After the operation I return the knife to the metal guard and finally back into the container after I have cleansed and dried it and gently rubbed the tip with Post's solution with my thumb and forefinger. Up until this point I wear gloves after undergoing the usual preliminary scrubbing. It is my impression that the Post's solution mildly lubricates the blade and possibly exerts some antiseptic quality as it dries on the blade.

There are many who advocate a Wheeler type of discission, especially for slightly fibrous membranes (see p. 99). When this technic is used, care must be taken to prevent deep penetration of the knife into the vitreous. I have used this popular maneuver and have had no real problems in executing it correctly; however, I am always concerned that it may stir up the vitreous somewhat more than the method which I have described as my first choice.

I do not precede maneuvering in the anterior chamber with a slanting incision below in the cornea for the purpose of injecting air or a balanced solution postoperatively. My feeling in this respect is based principally on the fact that with my technic I can inject air—if needed—through the corneal incision that I have made without risking the early possible loss of the anterior chamber. I make it almost a rule not to insert the small needle-

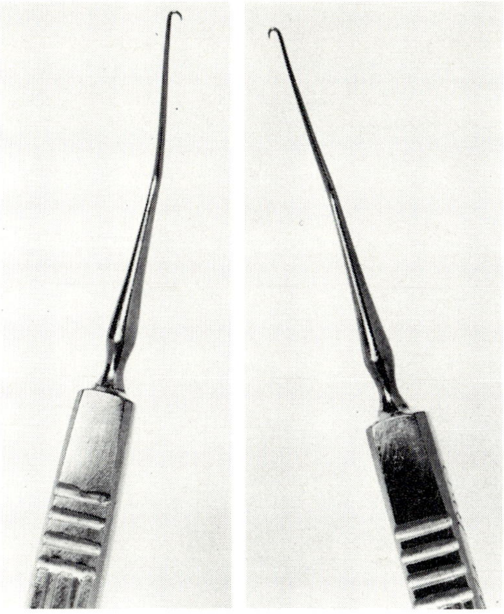

FIG. 173. French hooks (Moria-Dugast Co., Paris, France).

knife through another site at the same operation if my first maneuvers have failed. This is certainly not done if the anterior chamber is lost.

As a second choice for thin membranes, I have utilized two needle-knives or some modification of the Sato method.[20] I have instructed the Storz Company in making special needle-knives with a right and a left bend. With such a knife I am able to fixate from the nasal side while introducing another needle-knife without a bend from the temporal side to sever the capsule (Fig. 171). The fixation of the membrane makes the opening easier and produces less traction on other structures of the eye. This method is not original with me, but so far I have been unable to find the fine bent needle-knives in this country.

MEDIUM CAPSULE

For a medium-sized capsule I prefer the Vannas scissors (Fig. 172) or the "French hooks" (Fig. 173) (see p. 164). Some feel

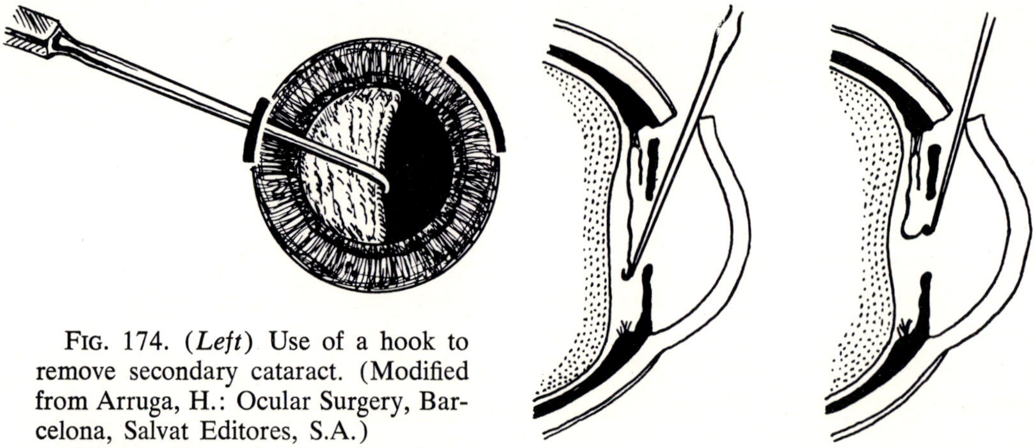

FIG. 174. (*Left*) Use of a hook to remove secondary cataract. (Modified from Arruga, H.: Ocular Surgery, Barcelona, Salvat Editores, S.A.)

(*Right*) Side view of same. (Modified from Guillaumat, Louis, *et al.*: Traitement Chirurgical des Affections Oculaires, Paris, Doin)

that the Wheeler knife is best for this type of case.

Thick Capsule and Cortex

When there is a thick capsule and cortex, my first choice is a capsulectomy using the sharp "French hooks" which have a right and a left angle component (Fig. 174). This method is not new, but in this country it is difficult to find these fine special hooks for doing a capsulectomy in this fashion.

Usually I make a small slanting corneal incision from the 12 o'clock position. The site of incision can be changed depending on preliminary studies with the slit lamp which may indicate that the membrane may be grasped more easily from another position in the cornea. If I feel that an iridectomy is indicated at the 12 o'clock position, a conjunctival flap is developed and the incision is made at the limbus so that it will be easier to work in the plane of the iris. From this 12 o'clock site I can cut synechiae in the lower portion of the iris and at the same time create one or two vertical iridotomies in the lower half of the iris to avoid an updrawn pupil. On occasions, I will scratch in and preplace a suture. However, as a rule, with a good assistant I will dispense with the suture which is a little more trouble than it is worth from the standpoint of its safety factor. I try to keep the incision small so that it might help to create a small iridectomy at the 12 o'clock position. This iridectomy is more appealing in appearance postoperatively. A small incision, especially a slanting one, may not require a suture and will act as a natural barrier to vitreous which usually wants to follow the thick capsule and cortex. Preoperatively the assistant is warned of the possibility of a small strand of vitreous following so that he is alerted to help the surgeon either by proper retraction or by handing the surgeon the scissors to cut the strand of vitreous should it follow the capsule. If anticipated, this vitreous loss can be reduced by cutting the attachment of the capsule to the vitreous at the appropriate time. Pains should be taken to prevent adhesions to the wound. However, the opening must not be so small that maneuvers of any of the instruments or the removal of the capsule or the cortex will be impeded. For example, if the operator feels from his preliminary studies that a hard sclerotic cortex is to be anticipated, the opening must be larger.

When using the "French hooks," by carefully turning and lifting the heel of these hooks as the incision or the iris is approached, one can avoid engaging these structures with the point and yet not lose the hold on the capsule and the cortex. The traction on the membrane is slow and from side to side. If the traction seems excessive, I will abandon this procedure and, usually without losing the grip on the membrane, will cut the membrane or create a triangular flap with Vannas, Berens, deWecker or McLean scissors. Ordinarily, I prefer the Vannas.

I routinely have a special table prepared with a wide variety of capsule forceps (usually in pairs) to be used for "hand-over-hand" maneuvers with the capsule. These include the newest Barraquer fragment forceps designed for working through a small opening (Fig. 175, *left*), the Bonaccolto forceps with duck-bill blades and a variety of other capsule forceps (Fig. 175, *right*).

In addition to general anesthesia or supplemental intravenous anesthesia, I routinely use a retrobulbar injection and massage. As a rule, I do not use (as advocated by others) the Flieringa-Bonaccolto ring, carbonic anhydrase inhibitors, urea or alpha-chymotrypsin, nor do I precede my operation with a slanting incision in the lower cornea for injection of air or saline postoperatively. On occasion I have used modifications of the Sato methods.

The question has been asked of me, "How should one handle the capsule in a patient, 7 years of age, who shows a membrane following a linear extraction with a complete iridectomy? Vision is 20/100."

In the case of a 7-year-old patient, because of the possible amblyopia one must first consider whether removal of the capsule is for cosmetic reasons or to help the vision. If I felt that there was a reasonably good chance to improve the vision, the capsule, depending on its thickness, would be handled as already described.

Summary

In the adult, because of the use of new technics and chemical zonulolysis, there is an increase in the number of intracapsular extractions and, consequently, a decrease in the need for capsulotomies and capsulectomies. In congenital and traumatic cataracts in children the problem is essentially the same. It is important to remember that if a membrane is cut or removed, severe push or pull must be avoided. If the surgeon anticipates from the appearance of the membrane that a capsulotomy has been or will probably be unsuccessful, then a capsulectomy or actual removal of part of the membrane is indicated. In removal of the membrane the surgeon must remember that among the dreaded complications, especially be-

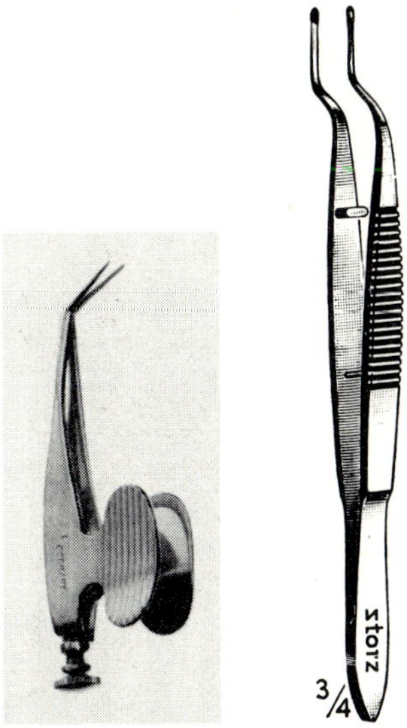

FIG. 175. (*Left*) Barraquer fragment forceps (Storz instrument No. E-1878). (*Right*) Capsule fragment forceps, Guyton-Clark (Storz instrument No. E-2134).

TABLE 2. DOSAGE FOR SYSTEMIC THERAPY IN INTRAOCULAR INFECTION*
(Listed in order of preference)

AGENT	DOSAGE
A. *Effective against gram-positive and gram-negative organisms*	
1. Chloramphenicol	3 gm. priming dose—oral or I.M. 1 gm. every 8 hr.
2. Kanamycin (Kantrex)	3 gm. priming dose—I.M. 1 gm. every 8 hr.
3. Penicillin with streptomycin	1 million units I.M. every 6 hr. (Benemid to enhance level) 1 gm. I.M. every 8 hr.
4. Tetracyclines: demethylchlor—(Declomycin)	2 gm. priming dose—oral 1 gm. every 8 hr.
5. Sulfonamides Sulfadiazine	4 gm. priming dose—oral 1 gm. every 4 hr.
Sulfamethoxypridazine (Kynex, Midicel)	1 gm. priming dose—oral 0.5 gm. every 12 hr.
B. *Primarily effective against gram-positive infections (especially penicillin-resistant Staph.)*	
1. Erythromycin	
—propionate (Ilosone)	2 gm. priming dose—oral 1 gm. every 8 hr.
—succinate (Erythrocin)	100 mg. every 4 hr.—I.M.
2. Oleandomycin: triacetyl—(Cyclamen, TAO)	3 gm. priming dose—oral 1 gm. every 8 hr.
3. Novobiocin (Albamycin, Canthomycin)	2 gm. priming dose—oral 1 gm. every 8 hr.
4. Vancomycin (Vancocin)	2 gm. priming dose—I.V. 1 gm. every 8 hr. ×7 doses 1 gm. every 12 hr.
5. Spiramycin	3 gm. priming dose—oral 1 gm. every 8 hr.

* Leopold, I. H., and Apt, L.: Am. J. Ophthal. *50*:1225.

cause of excessive tugging, are hemorrhage, secondary glaucoma and detachment of the retina.

MACULAR EDEMA AND CYSTS

The cause of macular edema and cysts is usually unknown. It might possibly be an acceleration of an existing process, perhaps related to hypotony or to a low-grade iridocyclitis. Systemic cortisone may be of some help in these cases. Since this is a vascular problem, vasodilators may be indicated.[16]

The poor vision resulting from postoperative macular edema and cysts must be differentiated from condensation of vitreous elements and from spontaneous rupture of the hyaloid membrane. In the case of condensation of vitreous elements,

TABLE 3. DOSAGE FOR SUBCONJUNCTIVAL THERAPY IN INTRAOCULAR INFECTION*

AGENT	DOSE
A. *Listed in order of preference*	
1. Neomycin	100–500 mg.
2. Bacitracin	10,000 units
plus	
Polymyxin B	5.0–10 mg.
3. Erythromycin	2.5 mg.
or	
Novobiocin	15 mg.
plus	
Polymyxin B	5.0–10 mg.
4. Penicillin	500,000 units
plus	
Streptomycin	50 mg.
5. Soframycin	250–500 mg.
B. *Alphabetical listing of additional agents*	
Amphotericin-B	15 μg.
Carbomycin	2.5 mg.
Chloramphenicol	1.25 mg.
Kanamycin	10–20 mg.
Oleandomycin	1.25 mg.
Spiramycin	10–20 mg.
Tetracyclines	2.5 mg.

* Leopold, I. H., and Apt, L.: Am. J. Ophthal. *50*:1225.

as a rule the vitreous contains residual opacities from a previous uveitis. Occasionally at the time of surgery, blood laid down on the vitreous face may explain a reduction in vision. As to the treatment of this condition, if local medications, such as cortisone drops, and the passage of time are not helpful, a small opening with a sharp needle-knife may be tried.

In reference to spontaneous rupture of the hyaloid, vitreous enters the anterior chamber usually a month to a year later (Fig. 176). The exact cause of this is unknown. The initial symptoms may include pain and blurred vision. Under the

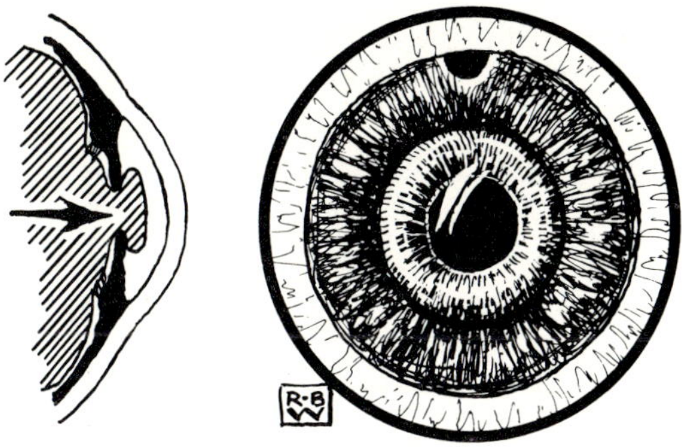

FIG. 176. Intact vitreous protruding through pupil. (Modified from Haik, G. M.: Symposium on Diseases and Surgery of the Lens, St. Louis, Mosby)

slit lamp the vitreous can be seen entering the anterior chamber despite the fact that an intracapsular cataract extraction has been performed. In most cases vision will return spontaneously, and there will be no other complications.

POSTOPERATIVE INFECTIONS

There are no major changes in the treatment of postoperative infection at this time. New drugs appear and changes

TABLE 4. SOLUTIONS FOR INTRACAMERAL INJECTION OR IRRIGATION*

ANTIBIOTIC	CONCENTRATION
	(per ml.)
Amphotericin-B	500 μg.
Bacitracin	500–1000 units
Carbomycin	1–2 mg.
Chloramphenicol	1–2 mg.
Erythromycin	1–2 mg.
Neomycin	2.5 mg.
Penicillin	1000–4000 units
Polymyxin B	0.1 mg.
Streptomycin	0.5–5 mg.
Tetracyclines	2.5–5 mg.

* Leopold, I. H., and Apt, L.: Am. J. Ophthal. *50*:1225.

in bacterial sensitivity alter the program, but, on the whole, the general picture is still the same. Leopold and Apt[14] have summarized nicely the dosages for systemic and subconjunctival therapy in intraocular infection along with solutions for intracameral injection or irrigation (see Tables 2, 3 & 4).

At this time oral chloramphenicol is still the broad-spectrum antibiotic with superior ability to penetrate the ocular tissues. Although the incidence of blood dyscrasia is low, the drug should not be used indiscriminately. Blood studies should be conducted repeatedly during the course of treatment.

Where bacterial and sensitivity studies have been made, the prompt use of the appropriate antibiotic and chemotherapeutic agent and the proper choice of the route of administration are most important. When possible, it is best to use the appropriate drug locally in the form of drops subconjunctivally as well as systemically and in massive doses.

If no improvement is noted within 24 hours, systemic corticosteroid therapy is added. Fungal infection must always be suspected and treated. Medical and bacteriologic consultants should be called in early.

The differential diagnosis of postopertive bacterial infection must include postoperative iridocyclitis (see below) and postoperative fungal infection (see p. 169).

POSTOPERATIVE IRIDOCYCLITIS

The differential diagnosis of postoperative iridocyclitis should include: (1) normal trauma incident to cataract surgery; (2) incarceration of foreign materials in the wound; and (3) lens-induced uveitis. With the use of alpha-chymotrypsin it is felt that there is less "push and pull" in removing the lens and more intracapsular extractions; consequently, there are fewer cases of postoperative iridocyclitis.

Normal Trauma Incident to Cataract Surgery

Postoperative iridocyclitis may be due to the normal reaction to the trauma of uncomplicated cataract surgery. In most cases it subsides without complication, and special treatment is not indicated.

Incarceration of Foreign Materials in the Wound

Incarceration of iris, lens cortex or capsule, vitreous, cilia, metal, suture material, glass, cotton, powder or ointments can cause an iridocyclitis which manifests itself by the usual signs of iridocyclitis. Serious visual disability can follow. In this type of iridocyclitis, prevention is the best treatment. Vitreous strands can lead to retinal detachment, and the cutting of these strands is not without danger. Cilia, glass, cotton, powder and ointments should be watched and removed if the iridocyclitis does not subside. Cilia on the iris may cause a cyst which can be excised. Lens capsule or lens-iris incarceration can lead to wound separation and infection. Severe iris prolapse can lead to sympathetic ophthalmitis. (Treatment of iris prolapse is discussed in Chapter 2; see p. 56.) Lens capsule resists digestion and should be suspected in persistent postoperative nonsuppurative inflammation. Surgical intervention may be necessary if no other cause for the inflammation has been found.

Lens-induced Uveitis

Lens-induced uveitis is assumed to be caused by sensitization to lens protein. Clinically the inflammation resembles that observed in infectious processes. The presence or the absence of a low-grade inflammation has not been ruled out.

Essentially, the treatment consists of opening the wound and irrigating the anterior chamber of its purulent-type exudate and lens substance. This can be done as early as 5 days or as soon as the diagnosis is made. In a true lens-induced uveitis no antibiotics are necessary (see p. 135).

Summary

Postoperative iridocyclitis can result from a normal reaction to surgical trauma, incarceration of foreign substances or lens-induced uveitis. The differential diagnosis between postoperative iridocyclitis, bacterial infection and fungal infection can be difficult.

FUNGAL ENDOPHTHALMITIS FOLLOWING CATARACT EXTRACTION

Fungal infection, an increasingly common complication of cataract extraction, resembles postoperative iridocyclitis of endogenous origin or low-grade bacterial infection. It progresses slowly and is relatively benign; however, most of these infected eyes eventually require enucleation despite the subacute character of the infectious process.

Clinically, as distinguished from postoperative bacterial infection which usually is apparent within 24 to 48 hours after surgery, there is little indication of an abnormality until approximately 2 weeks or longer after surgery, at which time most patients have been discharged from the hospital. However, some cases may show clinical signs on the 8th postoperative day.

Some pain and an increasing redness of the eye are the first signs of trouble. The slit lamp discloses a marked aqueous flare and cellular exudate in the anterior chamber. This is followed in a few days by a minimal hypopyon in the inferior portion of the anterior chamber. The anterior vitreous shows one or more hazy gray-white areas at the margin of the pupil in the anterior vitreous.

The hypopyon often disappears spontaneously whether or not antibiotic treatment is started. The aqueous increases in turbidity, developing stringy gelatinous strands running from the anterior vitreous to the bottom of the anterior chamber. A thick fibrinopurulent exudate may resemble a ball of cotton in the vitreous face next to the lens.

Light perception usually remains good but may, if the process continues, proceed to poor light projection. Enucleation may be necessary in some cases because of actual or threatened perforation of the globe.

Laboratory Diagnosis

Laboratory diagnosis may be made by aspirating the anterior chamber with an Amsler needle. The gram stain may show fungal elements. Hyphae or spores of fungi may be seen by examination in 10 per cent potassium hydroxide. Slants of brain-heart infusion agar are suitable for bacteria, while Sabouraud's dextrose agar, liver-spleen-glucose blood agar and Littman oxgall agar are needed for fungal studies. A negative bacterial culture should alert the surgeon to fungal infection.

Treatment

Only amphotericin B seems to be of value in intraocular fungal infection. One must start with 0.4 mg./Kg. of the amphotericin B dissolved in 500 ml. of 5 per cent glucose in distilled water given at approximately 20 to 30 drops per minute over a 6-hour period. An optimal dose is 1 to 1.2 mg./Kg.

Semiweekly determination of blood urea nitrogen is imperative.

Anterior chamber injections of amphotericin B (35 μg.-40 μg. dissolved in 0.05 ml. of distilled water) have been used but are irritating. Amphotericin B must be dissolved in distilled water, not saline. Solutions for injection are discarded after 24 hours. Eye drops of this solution are discarded after 4 days.

In the presence of a known fungal infection, one should avoid steroids and certain antibiotics, especially the tetracyclines. Streptomycin must not be used, and the closely similar neomycin and kanamycin also should be avoided. However, penicillin, chloramphenicol, bacitracin, erythromycin and the sulfonamides do not appear to stimulate fungal growth.[25]

OPTIC NEURITIS FOLLOWING CATARACT SURGERY

Until recently there has been very little reported in the literature on optic neuritis following cataract surgery.

In 1958, Reese and Carroll[19] reviewed the cases of 17 patients with optic neuritis following cataract extraction; 9 of these patients were observed by Reese and Carroll personally, and the others had been reported to them by colleagues.

The following conditions should be considered in the differential diagnosis of optic neuritis following cataract surgery: (1) ocular hypotony with papilledema; (2) optic neuritis due to uveitis; (3) optic atrophy due to retrobulbar injection; and (4) macular edema with central scotoma and reduced visual acuity such as that described by Nicholls.[17] (The individual with this type of optic neuritis normally does not see well after surgery.) Feeling that this last sentence might be misunderstood, in a recent correspondence, Dr. Nicholls stated,

> In actual fact I have found this condition to be benign for the most part. The vision fails rapidly at the time that the oedema occurs, which as you say may appear shortly or after a considerable period following surgery, and then after a period the oedema goes down and the vision returns to normal. Since the date of writing this article, I collected something like 20 more cases. In three of them a definite cyst developed in the foveal region. In all three cases the cyst subsequently subsided with a full restoration of sight. In one female patient, a cyst developed in each eye. I feel that the only type of case in which there should be a guarded prognosis is in that where there is a marked degree of arteriosclerosis.

Reese and Carroll stated that their patients did not have hypotony, nor did they show any indication of uveitis. In all of these patients the macular zone had been studied thoroughly, but no evidence of change was noted in that area.

Infrequently optic neuritis may appear following uncomplicated intracapsular cataract extraction, usually from the 6th to the 12th week following surgery. After the operation the vision is normal, but during the active phase of the neuritis acuity ranges from 20/70 to 20/200 and is associated with central scotoma. Of the 17 eyes reported by Reese and Carroll, the final vision returned to 20/30 or better in only six eyes and it ranged from 20/40 to hand movements in the remainder, with an average of about 20/50. (Initially the usual findings include edema of the nerve head associated with flame-shaped hemorrhages.) Ultimately there is some pallor of the nerve and an atresia or sclerosis (silver-wire appearance) of one or more of the smaller arterioles around the disc. Three patients who had both eyes operated on suffered the same complication in each eye, but seven other patients had no complications following operation on the second eye.

In those cases described by Nicholls, macular edema occurred at the time of operation in some instances and in others sometime after the operation. It was suggested that "the predisposing cause is a vascular instability in the retina and/or choroid in the macular region, partly at least brought about by cataract extraction."[17] Five of Dr. Nicholls' patients had vascular hypertension to some degree. The precipitating cause, he felt, was "in some cases anxiety, possibly producing vasospasm while in others prolapse of the vitreous through the pupil played a part."[17]

It is important to refract or at least place a pinhole and a +10.00 lens over the operated eye as soon as possible so that should the vision fail at a later date, the patient will understand that it was not, in all probability, the fault of the surgeon. It is felt that few of these cases can be blamed on injury by the needle or by the anesthetic agent given in the retrobulbar anesthetic. Most of these cases are probably unrelated to the surgery per se. However, Dr. Reese reports that he has not used a retrobulbar injection for more than 2 years, and during this period he has not experienced a single case of postoperative optic neuritis.[18] On the other hand, Dr. Edmund Spaeth commented that he "has used retrobulbar injections for many years and has had only one optic nerve neuritis." He feels that other than a possible vascular relationship they are not related. Unfortunately, vitamins, antibiotics and steroids are of no real help.

POSTOPERATIVE CONSIDERATIONS OF CATARACT PATIENTS

Since there are no major changes in postoperative care, no detailed description of modern trends in the postoperative routine will be made. At one extreme some physicians recommend sending the patient home the day of surgery or the day following surgery. Some even recommend cataract extraction as an office procedure. Hospital bed and personnel shortages are the reasons given for this approach.

I agree with Dunnington that I would not want a cataract extraction done on my eye as an office procedure; flat chambers cannot be detected and treated on an outpatient basis. I place enough strong sutures in my cataract closure so that I have no objection to the patient's walking to the bathroom on the day of surgery rather than being catheterized, and I like to have him return to limited activity. If he is in bed, I instruct him "to walk a mile in bed." Because it helps to prevent phlebitis, rubber stockinettes are used routinely on all my cataract patients. Because hyphema occurs on about the 4th or the 5th day, I usually like to wait until the 6th postoperative day before discharging the patient.

Postoperative care today depends somewhat on problems related to nursing and personnel shortages and on whether a patient is in a hospital with or without a section devoted to patients with eye problems.

On discharge from the hospital, the patient and a member of his family are instructed to stop in our office where the eye is again inspected by me and the dressing is changed. The family member who will be responsible for changing the dressing every day is given a slow and careful explanation of this procedure while he observes the actual dressing that day. On going home, written instructions in simple language detailing all the problems are read by the *one* family representative chosen to be responsible for the care of the patient. Questions are answered, and, if necessary, the visiting nursing service is contacted.

We find that this extra time spent in trying to anticipate some of the problems is adequately repaid in better postoperative results.

REFERENCES

1. Barraquer, Joaquin: An. Inst. Barraquer *3*:100, No. 1, 1962.
2. Berliner, M. L.: Biomicroscopy of the Eye, vol. 2, p. 927, New York, Hoeber, 1949.
3. Castroviejo, Ramon: Personal communication.
4. Chandler, P. A.: *In* Callahan, A.: Surgery of the Eye: Diseases, Springfield, Thomas, 1956.
5. Chandler, P. A., and Maumenee, A. E.: A major cause of hypotony, Trans. Am. Acad. Ophthal. Otolaryng., p. 563, July-Aug., 1961.
6. Dunnington, J. H.: Complications of cataract surgery, Lecture, New York Eye and Ear Infirmary Alumni meeting, New York, April 11, 1962.
7. Estrada, W. D.: Personal communication.
8. Galin, M. A.: Intraocular pressure following cataract extraction, A.M.A. Arch. Ophth. *66*:80, 1961.
9. Gundersen, Trygve: Surgical treatment of bullous keratopathy, A.M.A. Arch. Ophth. *64*:260, 1960.
10. Hogan, M. J.: Surgical treatment of epithelial cysts of the anterior chamber, A.M.A. Arch. Ophth. *64*:286, 1960.
11. Hogan, M. J., and Zimmerman, L. E.: Ophthalmic Pathology, p. 156, Philadelphia, Saunders, 1962.
12. Johnson, L. V.: Clinical treatment of bullous keratopathy, Trans. Am. Ophth. Soc. *55*:543, 1957.
13. Kennedy, P. J.: The treatment of cysts of the iris with electrolysis, Eighth Annual Clinical Conference of the Wills Eye Hospital, Philadelphia, Feb. 18, 1956.
14. Leopold, I. H., and Apt, L.: Postoperative intraocular infections, Am. J. Ophthal. *50*:1225, 1960.

14a. McLean, John: Note on epithelial downgrowth, 22nd Clinical Meeting of the Wilmer Residents Assoc., Baltimore, Md., April 25-27, 1963.

15. Maumenee, A. E.: Epithelial invasion of the anterior chamber, Am. J. Ophthal. *41*:929, 1956.
16. Nicholls, J. V. V.: Macular edema in association with cataract extraction, Am. J. Ophthal. *37*:665, 1954.
17. ——: Concurrence of macular edema with cataract extraction, A.M.A. Arch. Ophth. *55*:595, 1956.
18. Reese, A. B.: An appraisal of the current trend in cataract surgery, Montgomery Lecture, Ireland, 1962.
19. Reese, A. B., and Carroll, F. D.: Optic neuritis following cataract extraction, Am. J. Ophthal. *45*:659, 1958.
20. Sato, Tutomu: *In* Holmes, W. (ed.): Geographic Ophthalmology, Springfield, Ill., Thomas, 1959.
21. Stoker, F. W.: *In* Callahan, A.: Surgery of the Eye: Diseases, p. 225, Springfield, Thomas, 1956.
22. Sugar, H. S.: (Lecture) Yale Post Graduate Program, March 11, 1960.
23. ——: Personal communication.
24. Swan, K. C.: Basal iridectomy for prevention and treatment of persistent shallow chamber after cataract extraction, Eye Digest, p. 5, Jan., 1958.
25. Theodore, F. H., *et al.*: The diagnosis and management of fungus endophthalmitis following cataract extraction, A.M.A. Arch. Ophth. *66*:163, 1961.

6

Enzymatic Zonulolysis in Lens Extraction*

Joaquin Barraquer, M.D., *Director, Instituto Barraquer, Barcelona, Spain*

My clinical experience and that of other authors has shown that enzymatic zonulolysis simplifies operative technique and increases the percentage of intracapsular lens extractions. Enzymatic zonulolysis has been adopted by surgeons from all parts of the world since the first report on this subject.[1]

This chapter will stress the *complications* and their prevention.

Several authors[6] mention complications, such as intensive and persistent striate keratitis, massive liberation of iris pigment, hyaloid rupture, secondary glaucoma, retinal detachment, and so forth. Such complications have been exceptional in my series. Experience has shown that they are not connected with the use of α-chymotrypsin and are easily avoided by careful surgical technique. However, a higher incidence of complications resulting from poor wound healing has been observed, namely, (1) delayed re-formation of the anterior chamber; (2) anterior synechiae with hypertension; (3) reopening of the corneal wound; (4) iris prolapse; (5) late loss or flattening of the anterior chamber. The incidence of these complications is higher in the first series of phacoeresis with enzymatic zonulolysis than in classical phacoeresis, especially in elderly patients.

Another complication deserving attention because of its frequency, though it lacks importance, is subconjunctival filtration (Fig. 177). Anterior chamber and ocular tension usually remain normal. Filtration, usually insignificant, disappears spontaneously within a few days. In one case, filtration persisted in the form of a cystic cicatrix; however, ocular tension and chamber depth remained normal.

More pronounced filtration through the corneal wound may cause delayed reformation of the anterior chamber with its inherent complications.

An incision without conjunctival flap

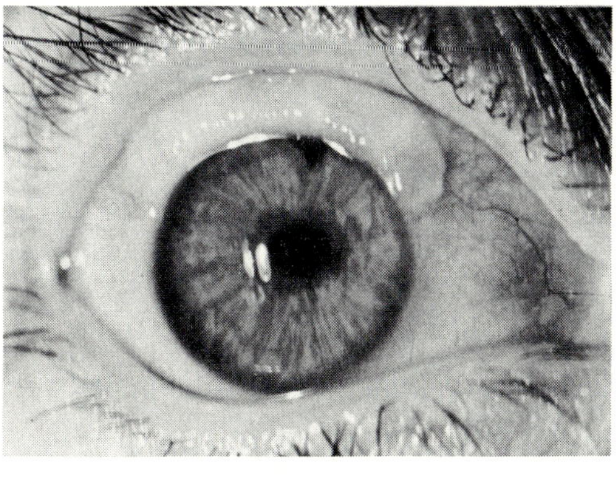

FIGURE 177

(Barraquer, Joaquin: A.M.A. Arch. Ophth. *66*:32)

* Reprinted with permission of the A.M.A. Archives of Ophthalmology, July, 1961, Vol. 66, p. 6-11.

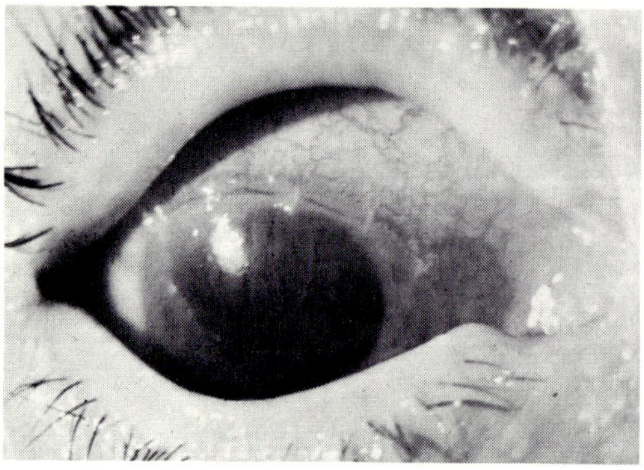

FIGURE 178

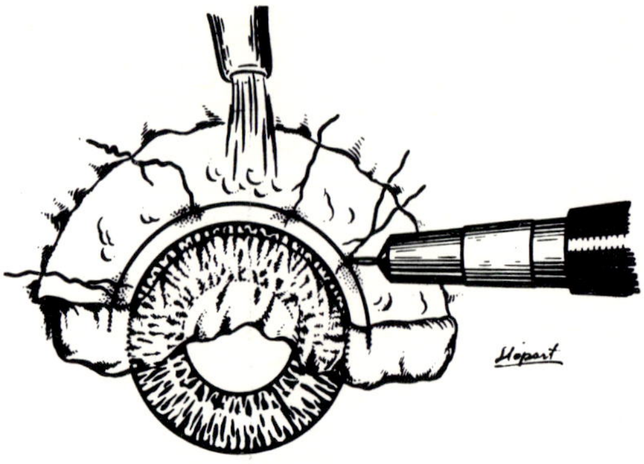

FIGURE 180

increases the risk of reopening of the wound, striate keratitis, etc. (Fig. 178).

These complications also occur with the classical techniques. However, in these series they seem to occur more frequently. This suggested that the enzyme causes delayed corneal wound healing, although Bedrosian's experimental work on rabbits[2] seems to prove that there is no such delay. In an attempt to improve the results, the original technique has been modified as follows:

A. Preparation of the α-chymotrypsin solution.

1. A 1:5,000 α-chymotrypsin solution is prepared. Lower concentrations are not so effective.

2. The solution should be fresh, because the enzyme loses activity after a few hours.

3. The solution should be at room temperature, or near 37° C. The solution is at its very best at body temperature, but it loses its activity more rapidly at that

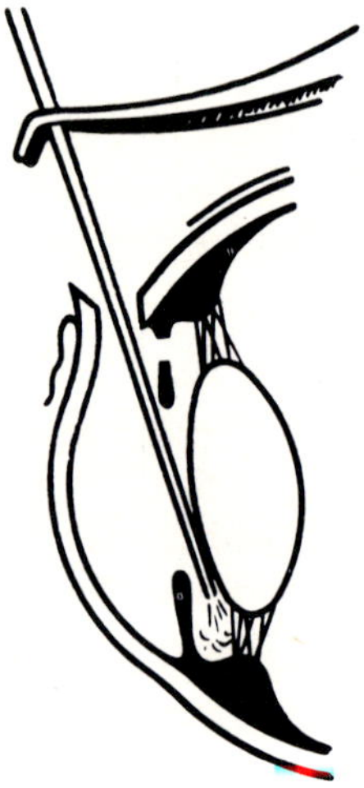

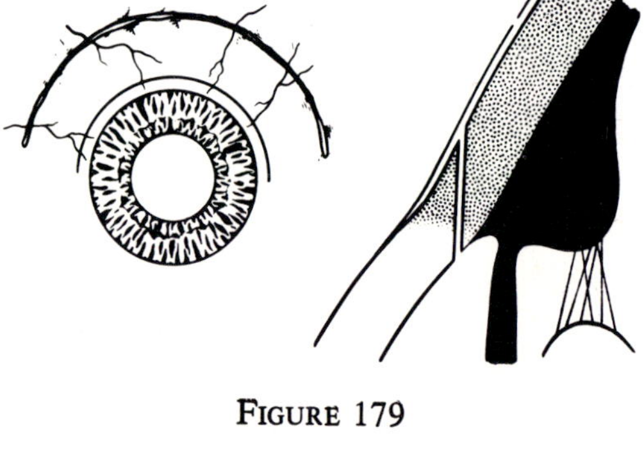

FIGURE 179

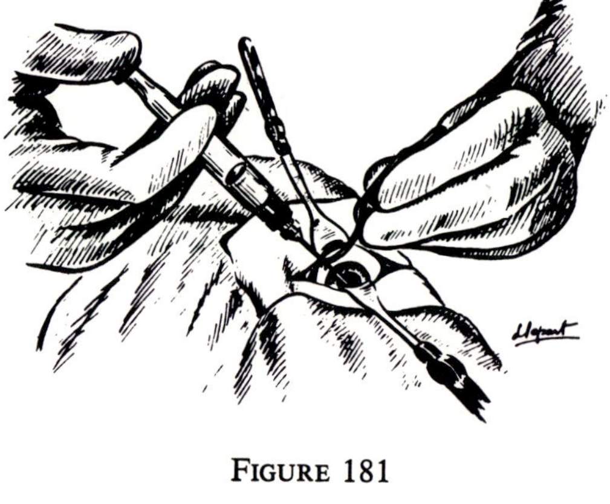

FIGURE 181

level. Therefore, it is preferable to use it at room temperature.

4. The chymotrypsin must be free from calcium, since this increases the stability of the enzyme,[5] which is undesirable.

5. The syringe and cannula should be sterilized with dry heat, because residual alcohol or detergents would inactivate the enzyme.

B. General anesthesia supplemented with curare akinesia.

C. Dilation of the pupil to about 8 mm. with 10% phenylephrine (Neo-Synephrine) hydrochloride. This is important, because of the constricting effect of repeated chamber washings.

D. Corneoscleral conjunctival incision. The essentials of a satisfactory incision are (1) even section lines in the vascular zone (for better coaptation and rapid and safe cicatrization) and (2) a conjunctival flap of sufficient size to cover the incision (imbrication) (Fig. 179).

Because of the site of incision, it is necessary to perform careful hemostatis of the scleral border. The preferred method is by galvanocautery. This is strictly limited to the ends of the bleeding vessels made easily visible by continuous irrigation with saline solution (Fig. 180).

An ample incision (180-200 degrees) facilitates the surgical maneuvers within the eye and prevents trauma to the corneal endothelium.

E. A peripheral iridectomy of medium size. This secures a good communication between anterior and posterior chambers.

F. A corneoscleral suture placed at 12 o'clock. The loops are laid aside so as not to interfere with the opening of the incision.

G. Washing of the anterior chamber. Should any blood appear in the anterior chamber, it must be washed out by means of a saline solution. α-Chymotrypsin has been shown to form a coagulum with blood or plasma elements which interposes between the wound edges, delaying or preventing healing.[3]

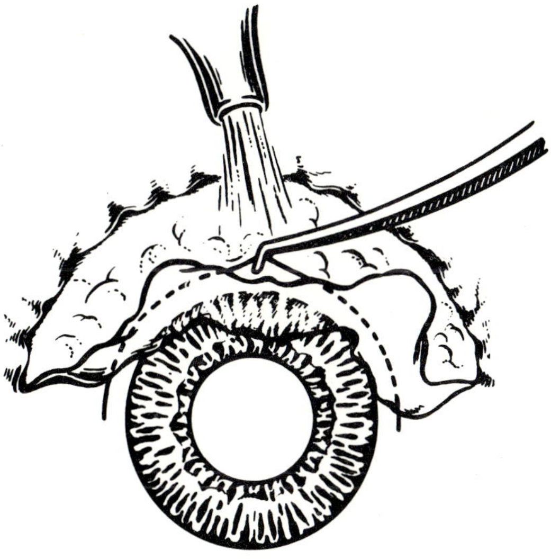

FIGURE 182

H. Irrigation of the posterior chamber.

1. A 1:5,000 α-chymotrypsin solution is injected into the posterior chamber with the use of a precision syringe and a smooth silver cannula.

2. By these means, direct irrigation of the zonule is carried out. It is advisable to press the cannula lightly against the lens in order to avoid trauma to the pigmentary layer of the iris (Fig. 181).

3. One or 2 cubic centimeters of the solution is slowly injected. In young patients, the enzyme is distributed over the 4 quadrants; in elderly patients, it is sufficient to irrigate the inferior quadrants.

4. Immediately afterward the conjunctiva and the incision borders are irrigated with saline solution, the anterior chamber being held closed by means of forceps (Fig. 182). One or 2 minutes later, depending on the patient's age and

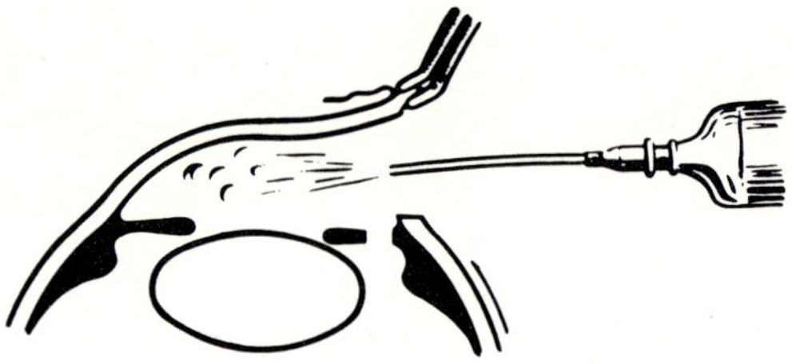

FIGURE 183

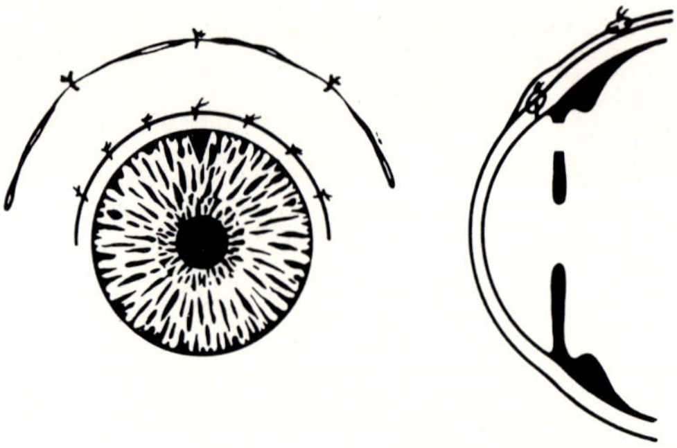

FIGURE 185

type of cataract, the anterior chamber is washed out (Fig. 183).

5. In cases of vitreous degeneration, it is advisable to place a Flieringa ring on the anterior segment to keep the globe from collapsing and the vitreous from escaping during the operative procedure. Zonulolysis will be very difficult if not impossible when vitreous humor is in contact with the zonule. Chymotrypsin must be applied very near to the zonule and in all of the quadrants, but in a small quantity, in order to reduce the possibility of its passing into the vitreous.

I. Lens extraction.

1. The erysiphake is preferable for lens extraction. This allows a firm grasp of the lens without exerting undue pressure on the anterior capsule.

2. Tumbling of the lens facilitates the separation of the posterior capsule from the hyaloid membrane. However, a sliding extraction is advisable in hard and flat lenses.

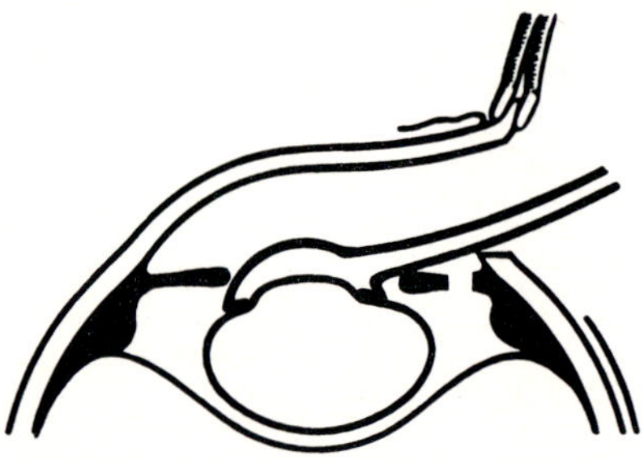

FIGURE 184

3. The incision must be wide open to prevent irritation of the corneal endothelium due to excessive contact during the extraction (Fig. 184). Furthermore, inspection of hyaloid and vitreous is easier.

4. Capsulohyaloid adherences found when tumbling is attempted may be separated with the aid of the endothelial surface of the cornea and external pressure. This maneuver is also helpful when vitreous tends to prolapse.

5. In cases of traumatic cataract or fragile lens capsule, the Smith-Indian method is the technique of choice. A slight pressure, first on the limbus at the 12 o'clock meridian, then 3 mm. outside the limbus at the 6 o'clock meridian, initiates the tumbling of the lens through a well-dilated pupil. Counterpressure is exerted against the cornea until the lens is delivered. If the lens is firmly attached and does not respond to these manipulations, α-chymotrypsin should be reinstilled.

J. Irrigation after extraction.

1. Irrigation with a 1:10,000 acetylcholine solution after the extraction quickly produces constriction of the pupil.

2. Care must be taken during all these irrigation maneuvers not to touch the corneal endothelium, or the iris, with the instruments. This mechanical traumatism

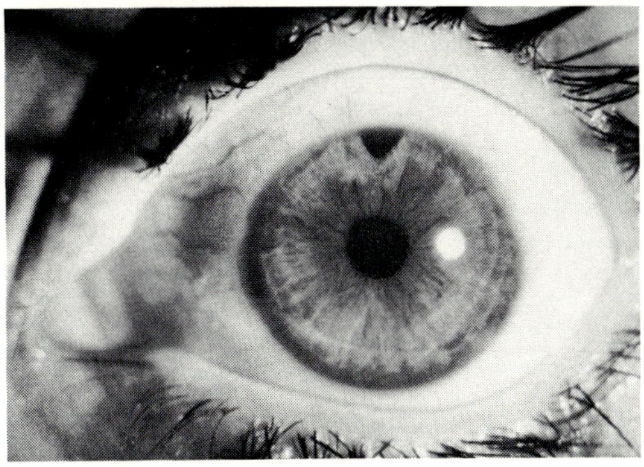

FIGURE 186

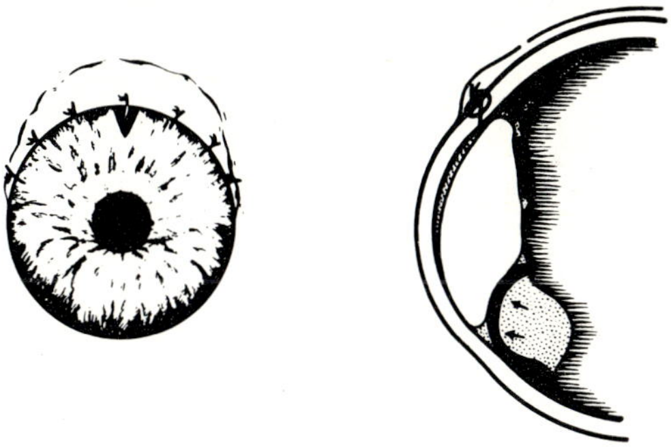

FIGURE 187

could be responsible for many complications otherwise attributed to the enzyme itself.

K. Corneoscleral sutures.

1. Multiple corneoscleral subconjunctival sutures secure a tight, safe, waterproof closure of the wound. The conjunctiva is not included in the corneoscleral suture which facilitates the correct placement of the stitches (radially and in depth) (Fig. 185).

2. No. 8-0 pure silk produces no, or very little, inflammatory foreign body reaction and is well tolerated. Seven or more corneoscleral stitches are inserted, so that the tension is distributed evenly over the entire incision area. The sutures are covered by the conjunctival flap and left in place (Fig. 186). Thus closure in two planes is perfect, since all the corneoscleral stitches are buried, the irritation they could provoke reduced to the minimum and the wound healing faster and safer. The conjunctival flap is fixed with 2 or 3 simple conjunctival sutures.

L. Filling the anterior chamber.

1. The anterior chamber is filled with artificial aqueous humor. In exceptional cases, a small amount of sterile air is injected into the anterior chamber.

2. Systemic air injection is not advisable, as the air may block the peripheral iridectomy and the pupil, and provoke secondary hypertension. The risk is proportional to the amount of air. If too much air is injected, the iris is pushed against the hyaloid and the aqueous humor cannot pass into the anterior chamber (Fig. 187).

3. Air injection is combined with section of the prolapse and reduction of the vitreous fibers by means of a fine cyclodialysis spatula (0.5 mm.) in cases of vitreous loss. The air bubble is injected before applying the spatula for better visual control of the vitreous strands.

M. Subconjunctival injection of cortisone and instillation of pilocarpine ointment.

Summarizing, delayed wound healing may be minimized by observing the following points:

(a) The incision should be made about 1 mm. from the limbus in the scleral vascularized area, with a conjunctival flap.

(b) Suturing should be very carefully done.

(c) The α chymotrypsin should remain the shortest possible time within the eye and should be removed as quickly as possible from the incision area.

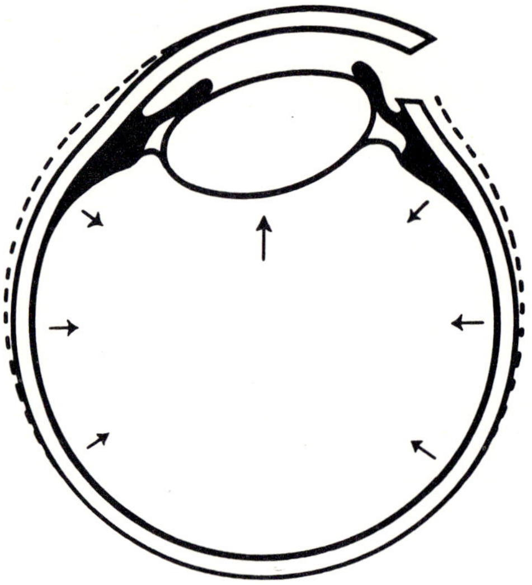

FIGURE 188

This completes the description of complications concerning cicatrization and their management. If the above points are strictly observed, the method gives excellent results in patients over 20 years of age.

The difficulties arising from attempted total extraction in patients under 20 years of age will now be considered. Surgical intervention is difficult due to a marked tendency to vitreous prolapse. If the operation is properly performed, the results can be very satisfactory in individuals from 10 to 20 years of age.

However, in children under 10 years of age, a rather high incidence of serious complications following vitreous loss and delayed formation of the anterior chamber has occurred.

This vitreous loss may be attributed to the difficulty in liberating the capsular ligament. In addition, there is a greater scleral elasticity in children. When an attempt is made to remove the lens, the vitreous is pulled forward due to the persistence of the hyaloid-capsular adherence, and at the same time it is pushed from behind by the elastic sclera. Small orbital volume and problems with anesthesia must also be considered.

α-Chymotrypsin was left longer in the posterior chamber for the purpose of liberating hyaloideocapsular ligament. The consequence was an increase of complications. The lens was pushed forward by the vitreous even before its extraction was attempted (Fig. 188). This phenomenon has also been observed in enucleated children's eyes.[4]

Prolonged action of α-chymotrypsin has a lytic effect not only upon the lens capsule, but also upon the filaments of the same origin which connect the anterior limiting membrane of the vitreous humor to the ciliary body and the ora serrata. The vitreous humor thus liberated easily prolapses because of the greater scleral elasticity in children. This would also explain the delayed information of the anterior chamber with pupillary block and its consequences.

In my first and present series, congenital cataracts were removed without vitreous loss, by limiting the time of action of the enzyme to 2 minutes only for softening the zonule, and completing the operation in the classical way.

The highest incidence of complications in children occurred in my intermediate series and coincided with using an increased time of α-chymotrypsin in the posterior chamber.

Operation *in children* should be considered dangerous and should be limited to experimental cases until a safe technique for total extraction is found. There is a wide field open for investigation on low-pressure anesthesia, intravenous urea acting as an ocular hypotensive, and the Flieringa ring increasing the scleral rigidity. *Extracapsular extraction* in children remains the method of choice in this age group.

REFERENCES

1. Barraquer, J.: Zonulolisis enzimatica: Contribucion a la cirugia del cristaline (Nota Previa), An. Med. Cir. *38*:255, 1958.
2. Bedrossian, R. H.: Alpha-chymotrypsin: its effect on the rabbit zonule, lens capsule, and corneal wound healing, A.M.A. Arch. Ophth. *62*:216, 1959.
3. Fink, A. I., Bernstein, H. N., and Binkhorst, D.: The effect of alpha-chymotrypsin on corneal wound healing, A.M.A. Ophth. *64*:104, 1960.
4. Legrand, J.: Film presented before the 66th Congress of the French Ophthalmological Society, 1959.
5. Schwartz, B., and Schwartz, J. B.: A review of the biochemistry and pharmacology of alpha-chymotrypsin, Trans. Am. Acad. Ophthal. Otolaryng, Jan.-Feb., 1960.
6. Weekers, R., Lavergne, G., and Stassart-Hourlay, C.: Avantages et inconvenients de la zonulolyse enzymatique dans l'extraction du cristallin cataracte, Bull. Soc. Belg. Ophthal. *120*:539, 1958.

7

Anterior Chamber Lenses*

Professor Benedetto Strampelli, *Chief of Ophthalmology, Reunited Hospitals, Docent of Ophthalmology, Eye Clinics and University of Rome, Rome, Italy*

Seven years' experience with acrylic anterior chamber lenses has proved the biological tolerance of the eye to methyl methacrylate, as demonstrated by some of my cases operated on since 1953, in which the lens is still perfectly tolerated.

However, endothelial dystrophy and bullous keratitis may sometimes be caused by friction with the edge of all methyl methacrylate lenses, particularly if the size is inaccurate. Research was undertaken to find a more suitable type of lens and technique.

After the various models of lenses made entirely of acrylic (Strampelli, Baron, Scharf, Schreck, Bietti, Apollonio, Barraquer, Salleras, Ridley, Boberg, and Choyce), the idea was conceived of making the central optic part of the lens of acrylic material and the external portion of flexible loops, so as to act as a spring (in Supramid† or other similar material), as first advocated by Dannheim and later adopted by Lieb and Guerry.

But even with this method it was found to be difficult to judge the exact size and position of the lens in the anterior chamber, and there was still occurrence of the complication described above.

Definitive results have not yet been ascertained with a new type of elastic support as designed by Joaquin Barraquer.

In order to avoid contact with the cornea at the iridocorneal angle, first Sourdille,* and then Epstein in South Africa, suggested the use of a groove-edged lens to fit like a stud into the iris collarette, since contact with the iris is to be considered unimportant.

A similar means of avoiding contact with the iridocorneal angle was adopted by Binkhorst, using acrylic lenses fixed with 4 acrylic clips to the pupil; as a rule this results in a pupillary block which is counteracted by means of a basal iridectomy. However, this lens is not suitable for all cases because of its pupillary position. Discission would be extremely difficult, and insertion after intracapsular extraction harmful to the hyaloid; if the anterior chamber becomes flattened postoperatively corneal contact may occur, and the lens is not suitable in any case when the crystalline lens is still *in situ*.

The best way at the moment is, in my opinion, to suspend the lens in the center of the anterior chamber without letting it touch any part of the chamber wall. This is achieved by keeping the lens in place with threads which pass through the corneoscleral wall and which are fixed to its external surface.

This solution was proposed by me in

* Reprinted with permission of the A.M.A. Archives of Ophthalmology, July, 1961, Vol. 66, p. 12-17.

† Synthetic nonabsorbable suture material.

* Personal communication.

1956 at the Congress of Ophthalmology in Madrid, and later, in 1957 at the meeting of the Italian Society at Milan, I described some of my cases operated on with this method.

A transscleral attachment with a totally rigid acrylic lens was proposed by Apollonio. Later Parry demonstrated a lens which was acrylic in the optical section and of tantalum in the external part, which was fixed by protruding points perforating the sclera. This rigid scleral-perforating attachment could, however, cause mechanical difficulties (perforation of the overlying conjunctiva), which I believe is possible to avoid by use of Supramid threads for the scleral attachment.

This new solution is based on my personal surgical experience of the tolerance of Supramid traction thread in cyclodialysis in several hundred cases of glaucoma since 1955. In these cases, although the thread perforates the corneoscleral wall near the limbus, passing from the anterior chamber onto the external surface of the sclera, I have not, up to the present, observed bullous keratitis due to the presence of this perforating thread.

This new technique of anterior chamber implant may be adopted in all those cases in which my original all-acrylic lens was applicable, i.e., in aphakia after intra- or extracapsular extraction, as well as in the presence of the crystalline lens in high ametropia.

The results so far obtained by this method of Supramid fixation of the lens in the anterior chamber appear to confirm my expectations. At the present time I use lenses in which the optical part is acrylic and the attachment made of Supramid. It remains to be seen whether quartz or silicate glass may be more suitable for the optical portion.

Intracameral lenses similar to my original all-acrylic model have been made en-

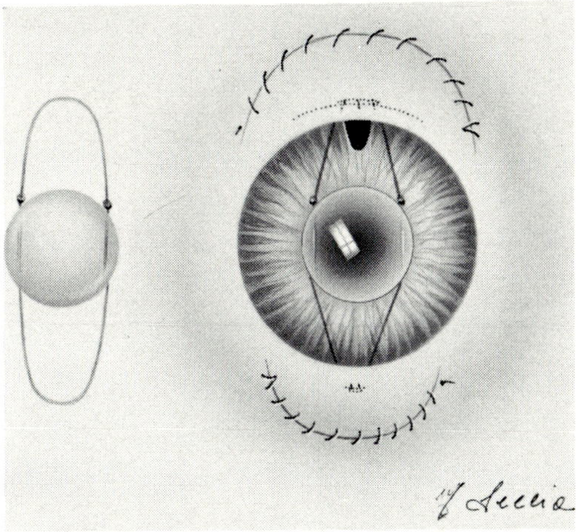

FIG. 189. Acrylic lens held in position by a Supramid thread placed so as to form an ellipse 14 mm. long.

tirely of silicate glass by Zeiss, according to instructions by Emmrich.

I have now ordered the preparation by Zeiss of disc-shaped quartz lenses with lateral holes to allow optical fixation with Supramid loops. I am not yet able to give precise information on the advantages of silicate glass over acrylic material. So far the only practical advantages are the absence of postoperative deposits on the lens and the facility of sterilization, since the quartz and Supramid lens may be boiled, whereas the acrylic and Supramid lens must be sterilized in a solution of quartamonium 1%, or with ultraviolet rays, or by humanization (Strampelli, Apollonio) by leaving it for a few months in the subcutaneous tissue.

The present type of lens, to which I refer in this chapter, has a disc-shaped or lenticular optical part of 5 mm. diameter made of acrylic material (biconvex, biconcave, planoconvex, planoconcave, or meniscus) and has 2 lateral canals as in the lenses of Dannheim and Lieb. A Supramid thread passes through these canals to form an ellipse; this thread is soldered so that it cannot become de-

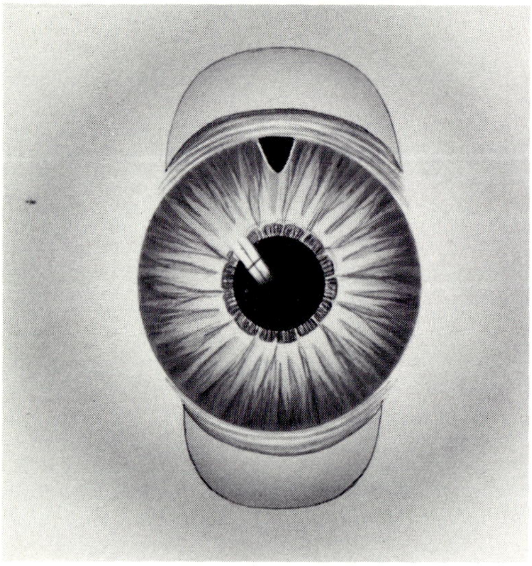

FIG. 190. The conjunctiva is detached above and below.

tached with traction or permit displacement of the lens. The average total length of the ellipse (superior loop, lens, and inferior loop) is about 14 mm. These lenses are manufactured by Morcher of Stoccarda.*

The operation is performed as follows:

* Kurt Morcher, 91 Reinsburgstrasse, Stuttgart W. Germany.

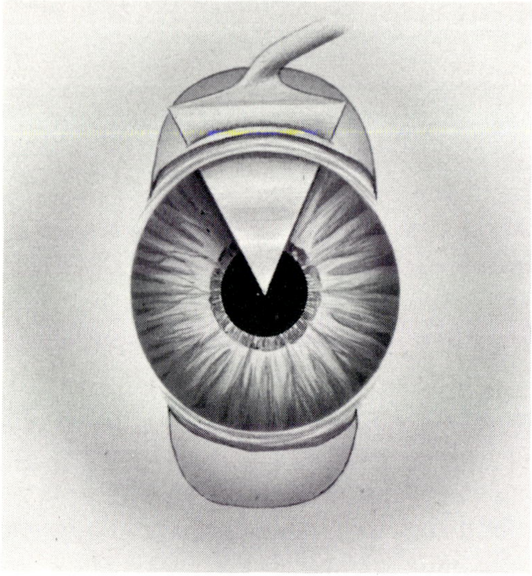

FIG. 191. The anterior chamber is opened above.

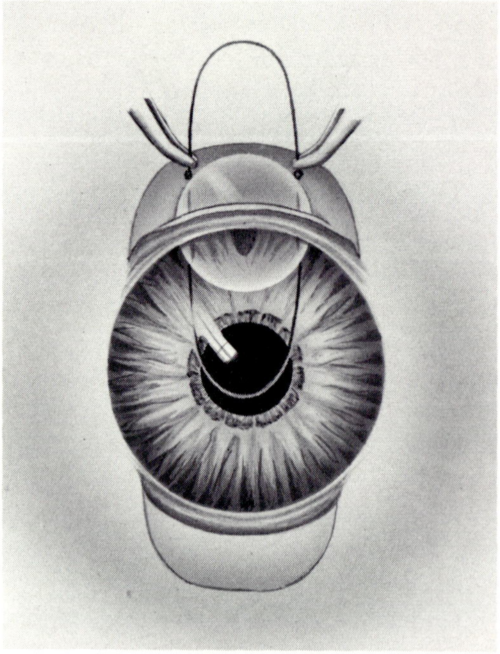

FIG. 192. The acrylic lens is introduced into the anterior chamber.

The bulbar conjunctiva is detached at 12 and at 6 o'clock, the anterior chamber is penetrated at 12 o'clock with a keratome, and the lens is inserted leaving the su-

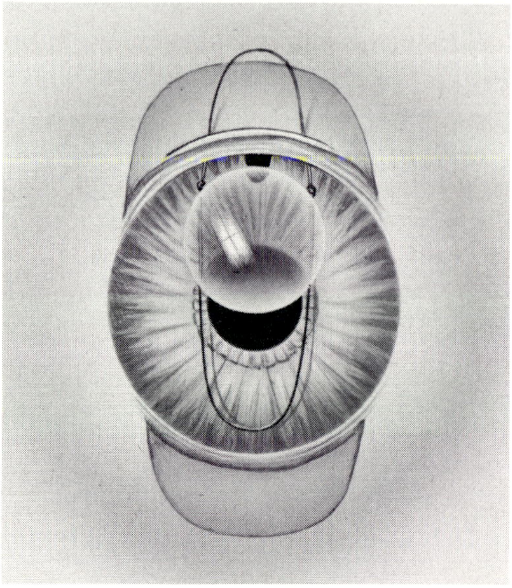

FIG. 193. The superior loop of Supramid protrudes from the sclera.

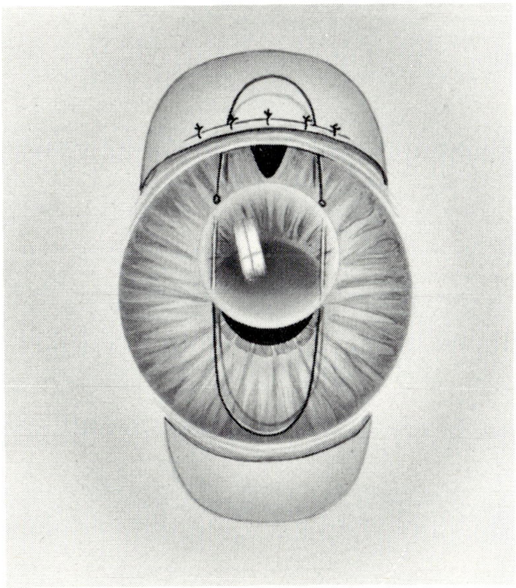

FIG. 194. The sclera is sutured with pure silk leaving the Supramid loop protruding.

perior loop outside. The scleral incision is closed with pure silk sutures and the loop recovered with conjunctiva. A very small keratome is then introduced into the anterior chamber at 6 o'clock and the in-

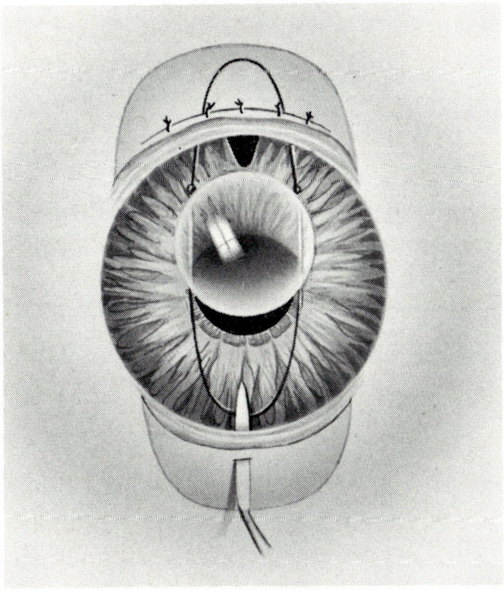

FIG. 195. The anterior chamber is opened below.

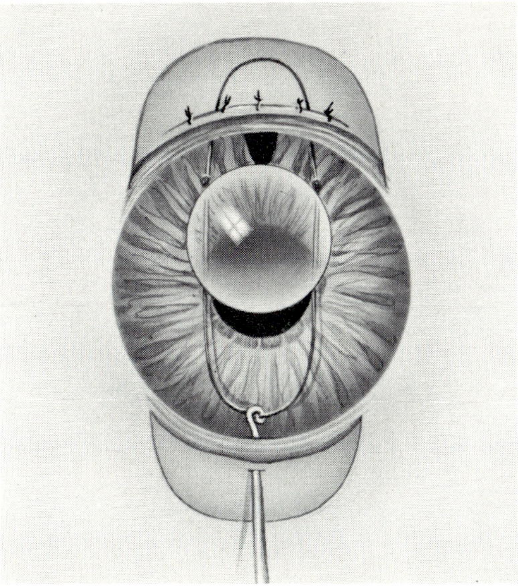

FIG. 196. A hook holds the inferior loop of Supramid.

ferior loop is taken with a special hook and withdrawn to the external surface where it is sutured to the sclera with pure silk and then re-covered with conjunctiva.

(The pure entire operation is facilitated if the anterior chamber is kept constantly full of air, which should be introduced with a special pneumatizor).

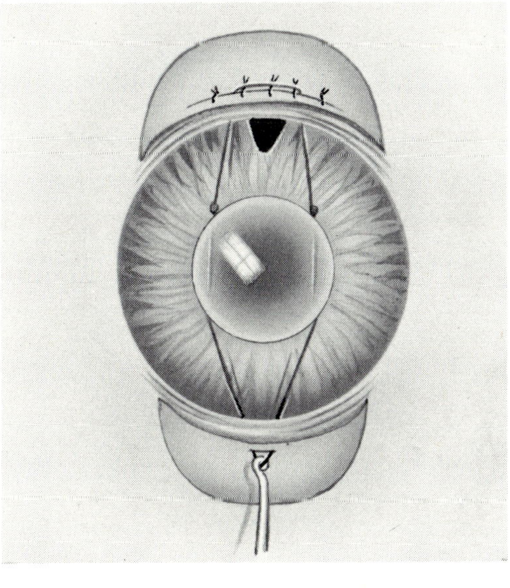

FIG. 197. The inferior loop protrudes from the sclera.

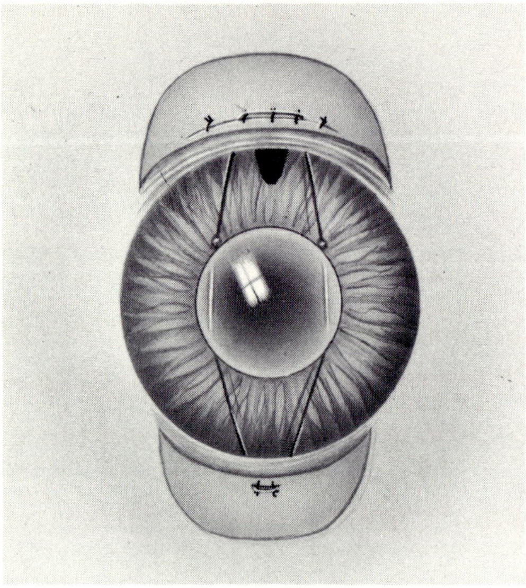

FIG. 198. The inferior loop is sutured to the sclera with pure silk.

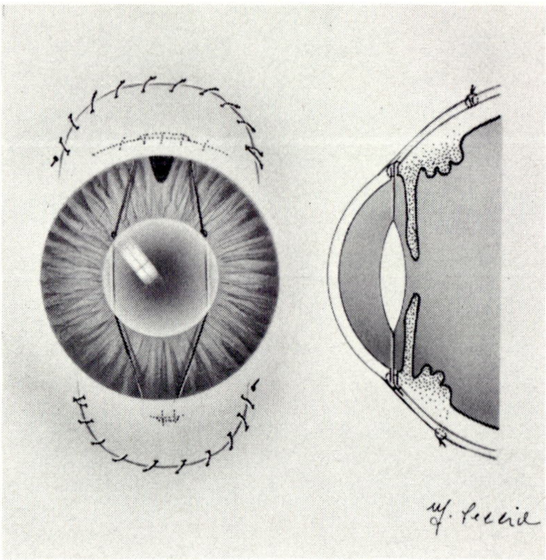

FIG. 200. The lens in anterior chamber; frontal view and section of the eye.

It is advisable to perform the usual iridectomy or basal iridotomy in the upper part.

If so desired, introduction of the lens by this method can take place at the time of extraction of the cataract, either extra- or intracapsular. In the latter case, the anterior chamber must be full of air when the lens is introduced. It is usually preferable, however, to perform the operation in 2 steps.

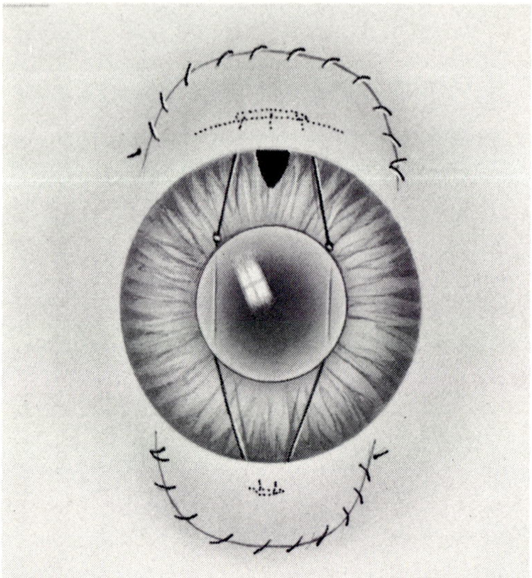

FIG. 199. The conjunctiva is sutured.

So far in 4 years' experience none of the cases treated by this method have suffered from bullous keratitis, though the cases are not numerous enough to give a definitive opinion.

In conclusion, although results are extremely encouraging up to now, it must of course be remembered that the method is still in the experimental stage and must be practiced with prudence.

At the present time the indications for performing the implant should be restricted to cases of unilateral aphakia (particularly after traumatic cataract), where a contact lens is not tolerated, or when fusion with the contact lens proves difficult to maintain and it can be hoped to develop good fusional amplitude with the intracameral lens.

8

Light Coagulation in the Treatment and the Prevention of Complications After Cataract Surgery

Gerd Meyer-Schwickerath, M.D., *Professor of Ophthalmology, University of Bonn, Head of the Eye Department, Municipal Eye Clinic, Essen, Germany*
Wolfgang Höpping, M.D., *Facharzt für Augenkrankheiten, Essen, Germany*

In the treatment of complications arising from cataract surgery, there exist three general areas of indications for light coagulation:

1. Light coagulation of iris prolapses
2. The treatment of updrawn pupil or pupillary membrane
3. Prophylaxis of aphakic detachment

LIGHT COAGULATION OF IRIS PROLAPSE

Because of the improved and safer technics of modern cataract surgery, postoperative iris prolapse has become a rare occurrence. Occasionally, however, even the most experienced surgeons will encounter it, whether it be due to an inadequately placed corneoscleral suture, a sudden rise of intraocular tension or other accidents such as those related to cerebral arteriosclerosis. In the case of fresh iris prolapse, the surgical reposition and careful placement of additional sutures is possible. However, with this technic, it is not always possible to avoid loss of bulging vitreous. Thus, a secondary operation may be more difficult than the entire primary cataract extraction. In the case of an iris prolapse of long standing, reposition is no longer possible. However, when possible the prevention or the surgical repair of a cystic scar is desirable, since a chronic hypotony or a continuous irritation may jeopardize the eye. In these cases treatment with cautery and a conjunctival flap has been recommended. Blaskowicz recommends a "cicatricectomy"; that is, the surgical excision of the cystic scar followed by a conjunctival flap covering. However, all these measures, carry with them the risk of a second operative procedure. Following a personal communication from Dr. Paul Wetzig from Colorado Springs we have been treating postoperative iris prolapses with light coagulation in order to avoid the disadvantages of a second more complicated operative procedure.

TECHNIC

As for the technic used in the management of iris prolapses, it is unimportant whether one is dealing with a fresh post-

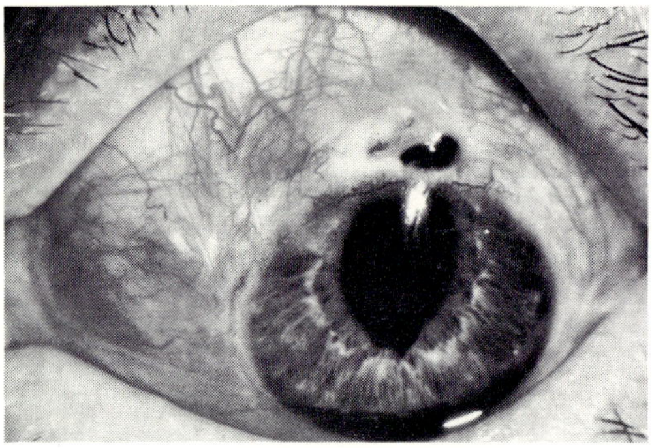

FIG. 201. Iris prolapse immediately after light coagulation.

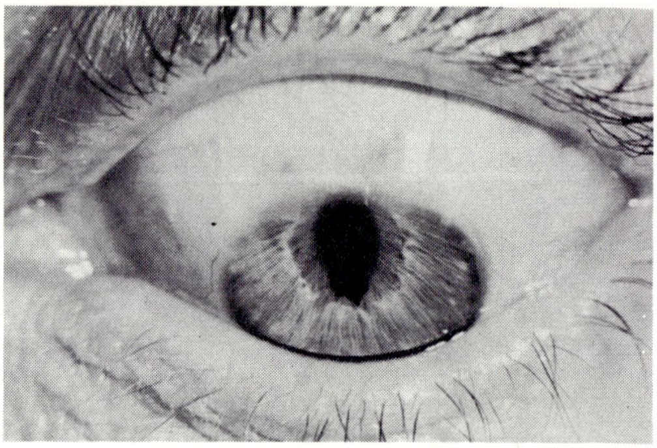

FIG. 203. Iris prolapse 2 months after light coagulation.

operative iris prolapse or one which has persisted for months or years. In the case of a fresh iris prolapse, the surgeon may wait 1 or 2 days until the irritation of the eye has receded somewhat. In two cases we have treated the iris prolapse on the following day with good results. The eye is anesthetized with a retrobulbar injection and with topical anesthesia. For the coagulation, the auxiliary apparatus for surface coagulation of the iris or the skin is used. Depending on the size of the iris prolapse, one may use an image-field diaphragm opening of 3.0 or 4.5. With a change in the diaphragm opening the distance between the electrodes also must be altered. In iris coagulation, the plastic ring constructed for this procedure usually is placed between the lids and is filled with water in order to protect the cornea from overheating. However, this is not necessary in coagulation of an iris prolapse. Since the prolapsed iris lies directly under the conjunctiva, with proper focusing the cornea will remain outside the beam of light. Therefore, an ordinary speculum may be used. Then the bundle of light should be focused on the iris prolapse and with "normal load" I (the green scale on the control panel), and with the intensity diaphragm open (position 0 on the optical beam director) coagulation may be carried out. Very few coagulations (5 to 10) of about ¾ second duration are sufficient. The entire area of prolapsed iris is thus coagulated. Since the conjunctiva absorbs a small amount of light, minimal reaction to the coagulation is noted on the conjunctiva. On the other hand, coagulated iris tissue shows a shrinkage reaction; its structure becomes hazy and the color is somewhat lightened. In three of our cases so treated, we noticed that during the coagulation, the iris within the anterior chamber and the pupil were pulled toward the prolapsed area. At first we considered this occurrence to be a definite disadvantage of the method. However, the postoperative course has proved that even in these cases no higher

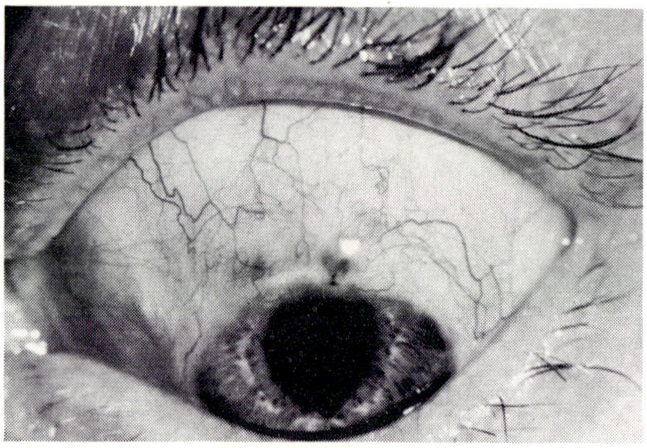

FIG. 202. Iris prolapse 12 days after light coagulation.

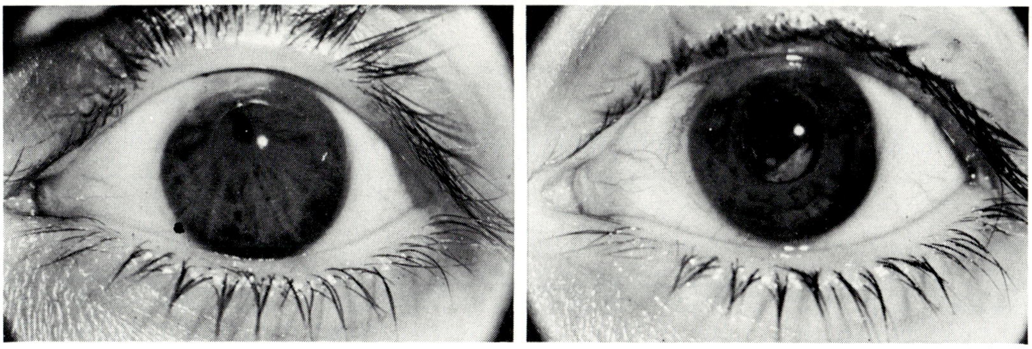

FIG. 204. (*Left*) An updrawn pupil after cataract extraction. (*Right*) The same case after light coagulation.

position of the pupil developed than that observed after surgical correction of the condition. As the coagulated iris dissolves, the pupil drops proportionately toward its original position again. The procedure, which lasts only a few minutes, is completed by the application of cortisone and antibiotic ointment; the eye is then bandaged. In the first postoperative days there is usually a slightly increased irritation of the eye; the conjunctiva is strongly hyperemic in the area of coagulation and is somewhat milky in color (Fig. 201). The coagulated iris dissolves slowly. On the 5th to the 10th day, the area appears as a glassy staphyloma. All these changes disappear during the second to the third week (Fig. 202). At that time a smooth nonirritated scar with a few pigment rests remains (Fig. 203). In those cases in which larger pieces of iris are left, which might give rise to another cystoid scar, light coagulation can always be repeated.

THE TREATMENT OF UPDRAWN PUPIL OR PUPILLARY MEMBRANE

When as a complication of cataract operation the pupil is updrawn or when the postoperative infection causes a pupillary membrane, it is possible to attempt light coagulation in order to form a new pupil (Figs. 204-206).

TECHNIC

The procedure is as follows. A retro-

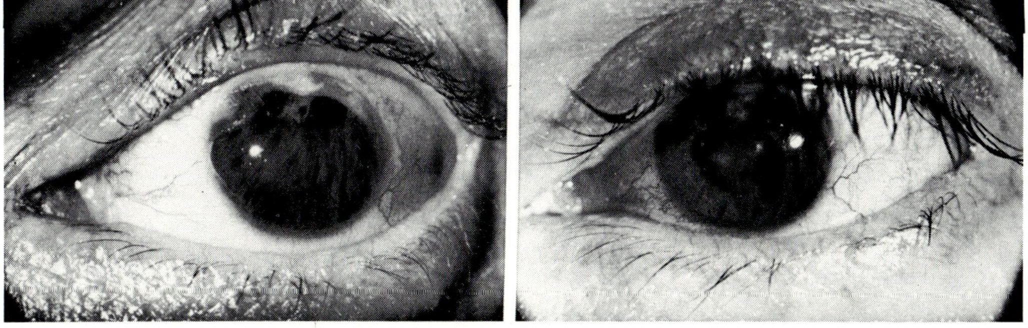

FIG. 205. (*Left*) An updrawn pupil after cataract extraction. (*Right*) The same case after light coagulation.

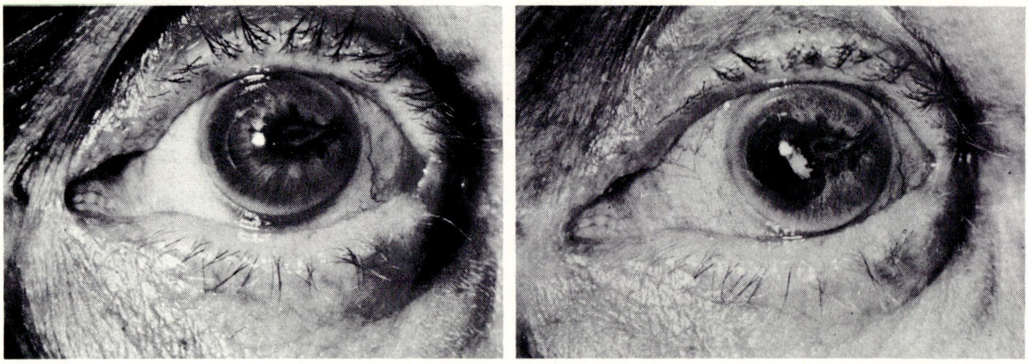

FIG. 206. (*Left*) A pupillary membrane before light coagulation. (*Right*) The same case after light coagulation.

bulbar injection is given in order to ensure complete akinesia of the globe. To keep the cornea as clear as possible, topical anesthetic drops are no longer used. A lid speculum is not used; instead, the lids are held open with a plastic ring which is filled with Ringer's solution so that the cornea is well covered with fluid. Coagulation follows with "normal load" III (position 3 on the green scale). Settings up to overload III (position 3 on the red scale) may be used. One should begin with the lesser intensity according to the reaction one obtains. The intensity diaphragm remains fully open (position 0 on the optical beam director) and the image-field diaphragm remains at 4½. The results when an artificial pupil is made by the use of light coagulation depend on well-pigmented iris tissue. The best results are obtained when one is dealing with an updrawn pupil in which the iris is of normal structure. In these cases, one can either coagulate the lower pupillary border and thus enlarge the existing pupil in a downward direction or one may attempt to make an entirely new pupil below the updrawn pupil. Either may be obtained without any great difficulty. It is somewhat more difficult to burn a hole in a pupillary membrane caused by a postoperative infection, since in these cases the iris tissue is atrophied and contains little pigment. If a white "after-cataract" is present behind the pupil, success will only be obtained by burning a hole through this also. This will occur if during the iris coagulation, there is an explosive type of reaction by which the "after-cataract" is torn open. In general, however, this explosive type of primary reaction in iris coagulation, which results in immediate formation of a new pupil, occurs only when the iris is well pigmented and of normal structure before coagulation. In the case of pupillary membranes which have followed infection and which may even be attached to "after-cataracts" with synechiae, this is hardly ever the case. In the latter type, the primary coagulation reaction is seen only as a shrinking and a dehydration of the coagulated iris tissue. During the immediate postoperative course, the coagulated area becomes more and more atrophic, and the iris tissue may completely resorb so that a hole is formed. In case only partial resorption is obtained, a second or a third course of light coagulation may always be tried. If because of a whitish secondary membrane behind the pupil, a total pupillary opening is not obtained by light coagulation, nevertheless the surgical treatment of the membrane now is less risky, since the operative site is better exposed and the danger of hemorrhage is less. D. Vörösmarthy in Hungary describes his experiences in burning a hole through the "after-cataract" by light coagulation. One drop of the patient's own blood (from an arm vein) which has been prevented from clotting with sodium citrate (the ratio of sodium citrate to venous blood is 1:5) is placed just anterior to the surface of the secondary membrane in the anterior chamber following a careful puncture using a fine needle. Then a low dose of light coagulation is aimed directly at the blood in order to "glue" it to the anterior surface of the "after-cataract." When this blood turns brown, the actual therapeutic light coagulation follows. We ourselves have had no experience with this procedure.

In the cases of rubeosis iridis, the risk of bleeding with the iridectomy is especially great. In two such cases we have prepared the field for cataract surgery by preliminary light coagulation. First, we coagulated the iris section between 10:30 and 1:30 o'clock. Four weeks later, it was possible to do a total iridectomy without hemorrhage.

When one gets an explosion during iris coagulation, one coagulation may suffice to form a pupil. In other cases, we coagulate 5 to 10 times from ¼ to 1 second in duration until a definite shrinkage reaction is visible. After all light coagulations on the anterior chamber, it is absolutely necessary to use local steroid therapy. The severity of the inflammatory reaction depends on the size of the coagulated area. For 1 or 2 weeks postoperatively, one may see cells and flare in the anterior chamber. These particles deposit themselves in the chamber angle. For this reason, these eyes show a tendency toward increased intraocular pressure. This is particularly true when a chronic glaucoma is present preoperatively. In the latter cases, a prophylactic dose of acetazolamide (Diamox) is recommended.

In very flat chambers, despite the utilization of a moist chamber on the cornea, postoperative corneal clouding may follow. In such cases, by means of the injection of air or a physiologic balanced salt solution, it is possible to deepen the anterior chamber preoperatively.

PROPHYLAXIS OF APHAKIC DETACHMENT

We do not give any special treatment to prevent retinal detachment in aphakia. We operate following the same principles used in phakic eyes which are detachment prone, and in those cases where we feel that prophylactic light coagulation of the retina is indicated (see *Light Coagulation* by G. Meyer-Schwickerath, Mosby, 1960). In order to study all retinal changes properly, 8 weeks after cataract surgery we subject the patient to a careful retinal examination including the most peripheral retina with scleral indentation.

Eyes with aphakic detachment of the retina frequently show a particularly intensive inflammatory response postoperatively. Frequently there are posterior synechiae between the pupil and the anterior surface of the vitreous. A bound-down pupil is the result. This prevents the careful examination and the proper treatment of the eye with detachment. In many of these cases, by means of light coagulation on the bound-down pupillary edge we have succeeded in widening the pupil and thus creating a larger opening for the examination and the therapy of the retinal detachment. Especially in those cases where the fellow eye became totally blind after cataracts and retinal detachments, the second eye is examined very carefully. If there are areas of equatorial degeneration present, these are then treated with light coagulation. In the case of nuclear cataracts, coagulation is frequently possible even before cataract surgery. In other cases, the prophylactic coagulation is carried out 4 to 6 weeks after cataract surgery. If no areas of equatorial degeneration are apparent, light coagulation is limited to those areas which seemed in retrospect to have been the cause of the difficulty in the fellow eye.

SUMMARY

Light coagulation may be used to treat certain complications of cataract extraction such as iris prolapses, updrawn pupils or pupillary membranes, and in the prophylaxis of aphakic detachment.

9

Cataract Extraction by Application of Low Temperature

Tadeusz Krwawicz, M.D., *Professor of Ophthalmology, Director of Ophthalmological Clinic, Medical Academy, Lublin, Poland*

INTRODUCTION

The operative treatment of cataract, even in its modern form, has a very long tradition. Nevertheless, we are still far from ultimate answers in this field. Of course, there are some universally accepted principles, but the risk of failure remains considerable, and it has been justly said that while the patient, fully relaxed and sedated, serenely awaits the beginning of the operation, the surgeon takes the knife with apprehension. One of the most beautiful of the ophthalmologic operations is often marred by the deplorably great part which chance plays in its performance.

The technical improvements recently introduced into cataract surgery, and especially the possibility of applying enzymatic zonulolysis, have created conditions that make it easier and safer to extract the cataractous lens. However, there remain certain difficulties which potentially endanger the smooth and uneventful course of the operation. Zonulolysis alone is not a safeguard against accidents during a proposed intracapsular cataract extraction; equally important is the condition of the lens capsule, which can be thin because of degenerative changes or excessively tight. Numerous reports show that rupture of the lens capsule is not a rare accident during operations combined with zonulolysis. It would seem then that zonulolysis will not solve the problem so long as the technic of handling the capsule remains imperfect. From this one may conclude that to assure consistently good results, more attention should be paid to the method of grasping the capsule.

The idea of applying low temperature to cataract extraction occurred to us during our laboratory investigations on the possibility of preserving tissues by freezing. Some experiments with frozen-dried animal lenses made it necessary to develop a method by which the lens could be extracted undamaged from the eye. This proved to be quite a problem, as it was usually the capsule that broke first. Then we used for the first time a copper wire (soldered to a piece of metal) which was chilled in a mixture of dry ice and methyl alcohol. The exposed lens was touched with the refrigerated wire, and the effect was so striking that we decided to study more closely the possibilities suggested by this phenomenon. In the course of further experiments on animals and on enucleated human eyes we developed a technic, of which the essential points are as follows.

METHOD

Our method consists in the use of a pencil-shaped instrument, for which we have suggested the name cryoextractor (Fig. 207). It is made of copper, which is a good conductor of heat, and has a small ball at its end. The whole instrument is nickel-plated and mounted in a plastic holder, which protects the operator's hand against cold. A cotton glove should be worn as an additional precaution. To minimize the possibility of accidentally touching the cornea or the iris with the cold metal, the tapering end of the cryoextractor is insulated with a silk thread, so that only the ball-shaped end

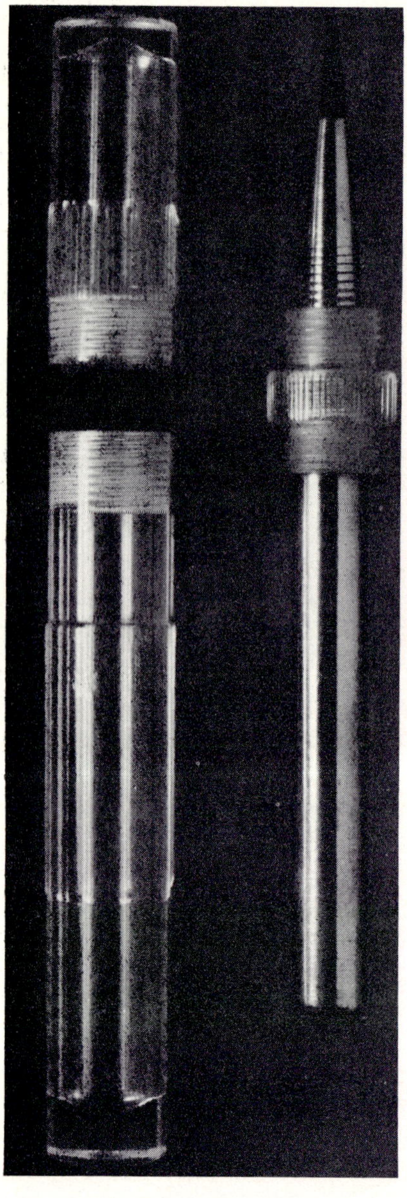

FIG. 207. Cryoextractor (actual size).

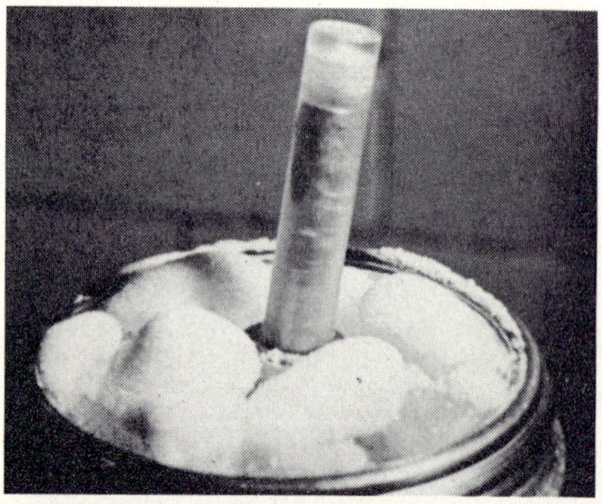

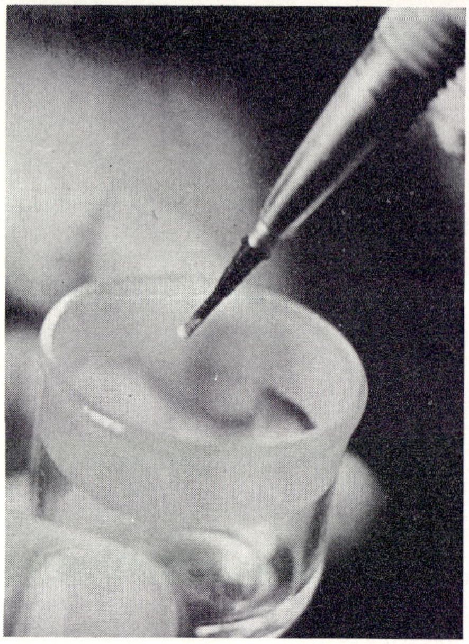

FIG. 208. Chilling of sterile cryoextractor.

FIG. 209. The ball-shaped end of the cryoextractor is coated with a thin layer of ice.

is left bare. In the latest model of the instrument the end is divided into two or three steps. Since minor variations in the shape and the size do not influence the performance of the cryoextractor, it does not seem necessary to give its exact dimensions.

The refrigeration of the cryoextractor occurs in a mixture of dry ice and *methyl* alcohol in which the temperature −79° C. can be obtained. To ensure asepsis, the sterile cryoextractor does not come into direct contact with the refrigerating mixture but is chilled in a silver vessel filled with *ethyl* alcohol. The vessel, which is shown in Figure 208, is then placed in a larger container with the refrigerating mixture. If required, it can be placed in a deep-freeze provided with an alcohol thermostat. Before application, the tip of the instrument is wiped with a sterile napkin to remove the remaining alcohol. It was found that the action of the cryoextractor is greatly enhanced when its tip is coated with a thin layer of ice. Therefore, it is our routine practice to dip the ball-shaped end into distilled water before its application to the lens (see Fig. 209).

The initial stages of the operation do not differ from those of the conventional methods, except that the section is a little wider than is usual (Fig. 210). The corneoscleral suture should be laid with special care, so that it can be used for lifting the corneal flap to expose the lens. Iridotomy is carried out, and the iris is pulled upward with a retractor. Pressure is exerted on the lower part of the cornea, so that the upper part of the lens inclines toward the operative wound. It is then that the ball shaped end of the cryoextractor is applied to the exposed lens at 12 o'clock near the equator (Fig. 211). Care should be taken to see that the surface of the lens is neither too wet—the

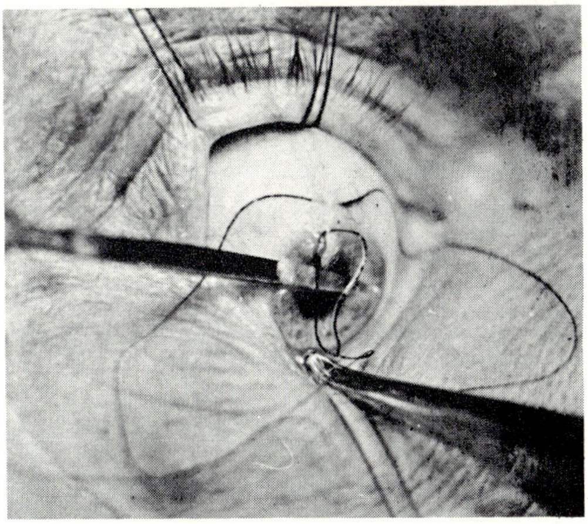

FIG. 210. The section is carried out, wider than usual.

excess of the aqueous should be removed before the application of the instrument, nor too dry from long exposure. Immediately after application, the part of the capsule which is in contact with the metal, and the underlying cataractous masses are frozen and adhere firmly to the instrument, so that it is possible to manipulate the lens freely. Figure 212 shows that part of the procedure in which the zonular fibers are broken by rotating movements to the right and the left. Figure 213 shows the lens almost completely freed from the zonular fibers. In Figure 214 the cataract is completely delivered, and it will now require some effort to separate it from the cryoextractor. The further stages of the operation need no special description, since they are identical to those of the routine procedure.

ENZYMATIC ZONULOLYSIS

Cataract extraction by application of low temperature can be combined with enzymatic zonulolysis. It is used in cases in which an increased resistance of the zonular fibers is expected, mostly in patients between 30 and 60 years of age. A

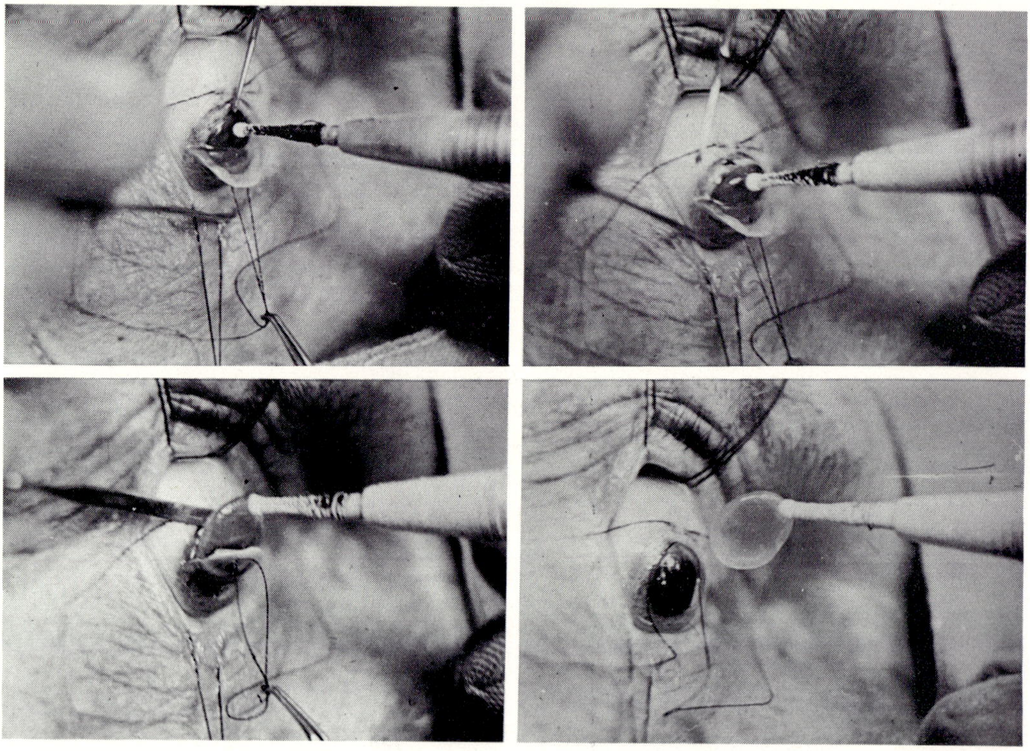

FIG. 211. (*Top, Left*) The cryoextractor is applied to the lens at 12 o'clock near the equator.

FIG. 212. (*Top, Right*) The zonular fibers are broken with rotating movements.

FIG. 213. (*Bottom, Left*) The lens is almost completely freed from the zonular fibers.

FIG. 214. (*Bottom, Right*) The delivered cataract adhering firmly to the cryoextractor.

smooth course of the operation then is almost invariably assured.

The modern methods of obtaining hypotony through anesthesia and akinesia make it possible to minimize the risk of vitreous loss.

Our method has been devised as a safeguard against accidents which force the operator to end the planned intracapsular operation and shift to an extracapsular extraction, with the risk of leaving fragments of the capsule or cortical masses in the anterior chamber. Initially we limited the application of the present method to cases of intumescent cataract only, but it was soon found that it can be used for the extraction of all other types of cataract, including complicated cataracts. Accordingly, the use of the cryoextractor has become a routine practice with us in all cataract operations.

MANAGEMENT OF COMPLICATIONS

Mention should be made of the possible complications which may be attributed to the application of cryoextraction, and especially of capsular complications, which may occur in patients with greatly thinned or tightened capsules. In about 2.28 per cent of 660 operations performed so far, the capsule showed a tendency to rupture in its lower part during the final stage of the operation, with occasional escape of a part of the cataractous mass. The probable cause of the rupture of the capsule is its excessive shrinking in the area where the cryoextractor is applied and its consequent inability to withstand the pressure of the liquid masses. It is also possible that a too-narrow section, through which the cataract is occasionally delivered, may contribute to the occurrence of this accident. The rupture of the capsule is an infrequent and comparatively harmless complication and has practically no influence on the completion of the intracapsular extraction. No case has been noted so far in which the capsule has detached itself from the cryoextractor or has broken; it always could be removed as a whole.

Another operative complication which may result from the application of the present method of cataract extraction is accidental touching of the cornea or the iris with the tip of the cryoextractor. Prompt separation of the adhering tissue with a spatula makes it possible to proceed with the operation without further difficulties. No harmful sequelae of this complication have been observed.

Care should be taken not to break the continuity of the lens capsule when iridotomy is carried out, or when the iris is pulled upward with a retractor. When the capsule has been damaged, it is still possible to perform the operation by applying the cryoextractor to the point of the injury; this may prove to be difficult when the breach is extensive or when there is some escape of the cortical masses.

SUMMARY

Clinical experience shows that the use of the cryoextractor can afford a reliable protection against the risk of incomplete removal of the capsule. There is no more room for chance in grasping the capsule, and the intended intracapsular extraction is carried out without difficulty.

BIBLIOGRAPHY

Krwawicz, T.: Brit. J. Ophthal. *45*:279, 1961.
——: Klin. Oczna *31*:201, 1961.
——: Brit. J. Ophthal., in press.
——: Biul. Lub. Tow. Nauk., in press.

10

The Management of the Dislocated Lens

F. Phinizy Calhoun, Jr., M.D., *Professor of Ophthalmology, Chairman of the Department and Director of Montgomery Laboratory of Ocular Pathology (Emory), Atlanta, Ga.*

INTRODUCTION

The removal of a subluxated or completely dislocated lens should be a carefully planned procedure and ordinarily is not considered to be an operative complication. The present discussion will deal mainly with such planned procedures, but a brief mention should be made first about the *unexpected* dislocation of a lens during cataract surgery, when the management becomes that of a true surgical complication.

In such cases the surgeon is surprised to find, after retrobulbar injection and wide pupillary dilatation, that the lens has tilted or has even fallen posteriorly into the vitreous. Sometimes this may not occur until after the eye is opened, or after zonulolysis, or when there occurs a copious loss of fluid or solid vitreous. Such cases should be diagnosed or suspected preoperatively in patients with glaucoma or high myopia by careful slit-lamp and gonioscopic examination and wide pupillary dilatation and by looking for iridodonesis and signs of fluid vitreous or formed vitreous in the anterior chamber. Many cases of atypical open-angle glaucoma are associated with inconspicuous subluxated cataracts, although the mechanism of the glaucoma is not clear.

The management of this unexpected complication during cataract surgery is discussed in Chapter 2. If subluxation or posterior luxation is apparent before the eye is opened, then the surgeon may proceed as outlined in the appropriate sections below. If the dislocation occurs after the eye is opened, the lens usually cannot be grasped with forceps or the erisophake unless it can be supported by a lens spoon or loop. If the dislocated lens is accessible, one must do an immediate complete iridectomy and loop extraction. If the vitreous is very fluid and permits the lens to fall posteriorly "out of sight," then removal by irrigation (see below) is indicated. Obviously, once the eye is opened, the double-needle operation for lens support cannot be done, but occasionally such a lens is accessible for double transfixion by two separate needles.

INDICATIONS FOR PLANNED REMOVAL OF DISLOCATED LENSES

The extremely high incidence of severe complications associated with the extraction of dislocated lenses, as described in most textbooks and articles on the subject, has made most surgeons hesitate to operate in such cases. However, recent advances in technic (to be described below) should lessen the general pessimism about operating such cases and help us to more clearly define the indications for operation.

Luxations into the Anterior Chamber

Indications for Operation. Operative removal of the lens is always indicated in such cases when there is uveitis, glaucoma or intermittent impairment of vision. The glaucoma in such cases usually is due to the pupillary block produced by a large lens overlying the pupil. The controversial cases are those in which a very small lens floats in and out of the pupil, making it difficult to trap and remove the lens, and those traumatic cases in which a large clear lens lies in the anterior chamber with blood, and glaucoma may not yet be present due to the hypotony of trauma. I have found that these latter cases have a stormy postoperative course if operated early and recommend waiting until the eye has recovered somewhat or until glaucoma develops.

Technic. Although attempts should be made to contract the pupil behind the lens with miotics, the presence of formed vitreous sometimes interferes. In my opinion, strong miotics such as DFP,* Humorsol,† etc., should not be used in such cases because of the tendency toward retinal detachment. Even though a lens may appear to be trapped in the anterior cham-

* Diisopropyl fluorophosphate.

† Decamethylene bis-(m-dimethylaminophenyl-N-methylcarbamate) dimethobromide.

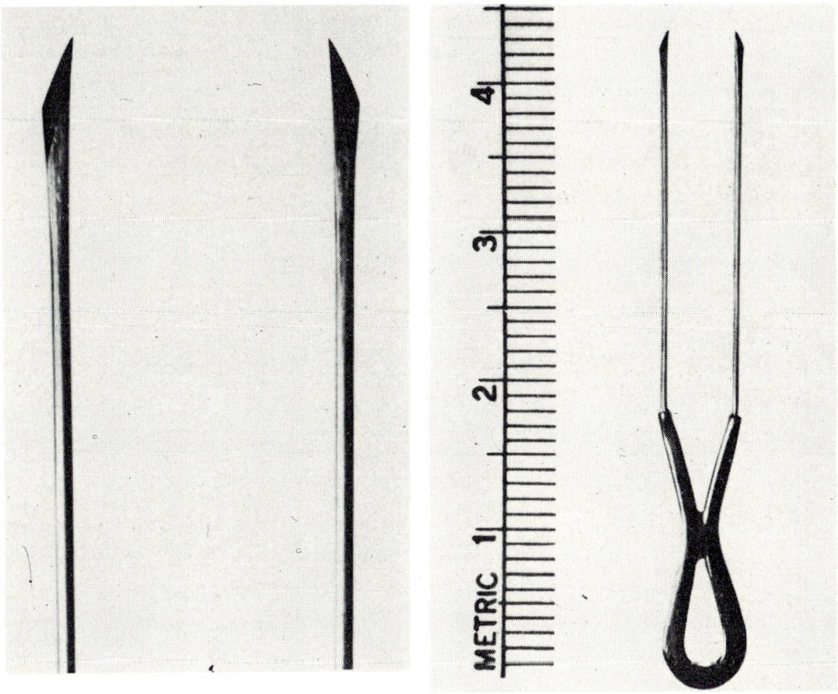

FIG. 215. The Calhoun-Hagler cutting edge double needle. (Reproduced with permission of the American Ophthalmological Society)

ber before operation, on giving a retrobulbar injection and opening the anterior chamber, conditions change completely. Not only may the lens drop back into the vitreous, but, also, vitreous presentation and loss are likely.

Ideally, the lens in such cases should have secure support of some kind so that it will remain in an accessible position. One way to do this is to transfix the lens with one or more knife-needles passed into the anterior chamber just behind the limbus before the eye is opened. With the lens thus prevented from falling posteriorly, the eye is opened and the lens is trapped for removal by passing a lens spoon or loop behind it.

A most important consideration in the surgical removal of any type of dislocated lens is the prevention of vitreous loss and collapse of the globe. Of great help in this regard is a Flieringa wire ring which is sewn to the sclera around the cornea before the eye is opened. The *scleral support* thus provided helps to prevent collapse of the scleral coat and loss of vitreous.

Another method of trapping and supporting a lens which is either luxated into the anterior chamber or subluxated, which has the advantage of providing excellent scleral support as well, is the double-needle operation described by Barraquer[1] and by Calhoun and Hagler.[3] In this operation a double needle or bident is passed through the pars plana, directed behind the subluxated or anteriorly luxated lens, and out the opposite pars plana and sclera (Figs. 215 and 216).

The two needles of the instruments used by these authors are 4 mm. apart, which is satisfactory for the average sized lens. Because small lenses may tilt and slip through or around the double needle, Barraquer has recently designed an instrument with three blades or needles.

I believe that a complete iridectomy should be performed in every operation for removal of a dislocated lens because it helps to prevent an updrawn pupil and pupillary block and makes easier the visualization and the management of retinal detachment should it develop later.

Subluxations

Indications for Operation. In general, a subluxated lens should be removed if it is a mature or hypermature cataract, if there is evidence of a lens-induced uveitis, for optical reasons such as high lenticular myopia or astigmatism or troublesome monocular diplopia, or if complete luxation seems imminent.

Associated glaucoma may sometimes be relieved by removing the subluxated lens but sometimes will be made worse or will be produced where it was not present before operation. Therefore, the presence of glaucoma is an uncertain indication for lens removal because the mechanism of the glaucoma associated with a subluxated lens is usually not understood. If the vision is fairly good, then it is best to be conservative and to treat the glaucoma medically or by glaucoma surgery.

The controversial cases are the children with congenital subluxation of the lens. Operation cannot be approached lightly because of the high incidence of complications such as vitreous loss and retinal detachment. I recommend conservatism in the surgical treatment of this condition in children.

Technic. This is essentially the same as that used in anterior chamber luxations in that lens support by means of transfixion or a double needle passed behind the lens is necessary, and also that scleral

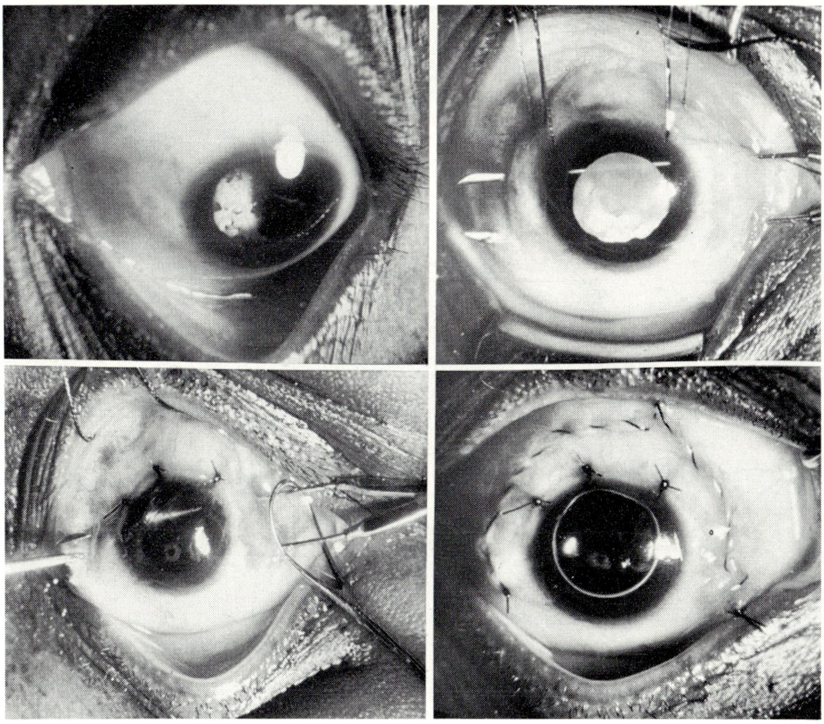

FIG. 216. A case with a shrunken cataract luxated into the vitreous illustrating the use of the Calhoun-Hagler double needle. (A) Prior to operation. (B) Lens (6.5 mm. in diameter) has been trapped in pupillary area by using the author's needle with patient in prone position. (C) After the cataract is removed and the sutures tied, the sclera is fixed at needle exit sites, and slight counterpressure is applied around the exit sites with a lens loop prior to withdrawal of the needle. (D) At completion of the operation showing air bubble in the anterior chamber. (Reproduced with permission of the Transactions of the American Ophthalmological Society)

support by means of a Flieringa ring or a double needle is desirable. I believe that the double-needle operation is the best for providing support of both lens and sclera.

In adults the lens may be removed in capsule. In children it is best to do a needling of the lens rather than try to remove the lens in capsule. A complete iridectomy should be done in all cases except those treated by discission.

Luxations into the Vitreous

Indications for Operation. With the advent of a better operation than blind fishing in the vitreous with a loop, I recommend removal of those luxations into the vitreous when the cataract is mature or hypermature, or when there is lens-induced uveitis, but only when the lens can be made to settle into the pupillary area with the patient in a prone position. In time the hypermature cataract in the vitreous tends to fragment, produce a severe uveitis and become fixed to the retina. It is important to remove such cataracts before these complications develop. Many cases with a lens in the vitreous and a quiet eye have glaucoma, and some have retinal detachment. The mechanism of the glaucoma in such cases is not clear when pupillary block and hypersecretion can be ruled out and when the filtration angle is normal gonioscopically. Therefore, glaucoma is not a constant indication for operation, but, in my experience, in most cases, removal of the lens from the lower vitreous will benefit the glaucoma. Chandler[4] disagrees and believes that pupillary block causes the glaucoma; he advocates iridectomy or transfixion of the iris.

If a retinal detachment co-exists with the dislocated lens, the lens should be removed first.

Technic. Even though a posteriorly dislocated lens can be made to settle into the pupillary area with the patient in the prone position, usually it cannot be made to get far enough into the anterior chamber to be trapped by miotics, because the pupil in such cases neither dilates nor constricts too well and because some collection of formed vitreous remains between the lens and the cornea in the prone position, preventing complete access of the lens to the anterior chamber.

Since the vitreous is very fluid in most cases of complete posterior lens luxation, Verhoeff[6] has introduced a method of floating the lens into the pupillary space by irrigating the vitreous with a stream of normal saline. Iliff[5] uses two erisophakes in a similar method based on the same principle. A valuable adjunct to the method of irrigating the lens from the vitreous is to have an assistant follow the movements and the position of the lens by observing it with indirect ophthalmoscopy during the irrigation.

Another method of removing a lens in the vitreous is by the use of the double needle described previously[1, 3] in which the lens is trapped by placing the patient in a prone position, floating the lens into the pupillary space and passing the double needle through the pars plana on both sides. With the needle in place, the patient is then turned into a supine position and the lens is removed in the usual manner.

ADVANTAGES OF THE DOUBLE-NEEDLE OPERATION

1. The same double needle and technic can be used for operations on the subluxated as well as the luxated lens in all age groups.
2. Vitreous loss is greatly reduced in frequency and amount because the needle furnishes excellent scleral support, and the lens is supported in an accessible position in front of the vitreous.
3. Except when needling is indicated, it permits an intracapsular extraction in all cases as opposed to operations in which the lens is deliberately transfixed for removal.
4. The incidence of serious postoperative complications is lower than with other methods.

COMPLICATIONS OF THE DOUBLE-NEEDLE OPERATION

1. The lens may be displaced or lacerated by the sharp edges of the double-needle unless the instrument is directed posteriorly at first. This may result in an extracapsular extraction.
2. Vitreous bleeding may occur if the double-needle tips are dragged across the opposite ciliary processes or are withdrawn and introduced repeatedly into the opposite pars plana. Once the plane and the direction of counterpuncture is determined, it should be continued and not changed.
3. Should a trapped lens be rather small and begin to slide either between or

around the blades of the double needle, a single needle or a small knife of any type can be inserted at right angles to the double needle to prevent the lens from falling back.

4. Firm scleral fixation at points of both entrance and exit of the double-needle are necessary on withdrawing it at the end of the operation to prevent compression of the globe and extrusion of vitreous into the sutured incision (Fig. 216).

5. Postoperative vitreous hemorrhage of some degree was present in 10 of the 60 cases in which the author has used the double needle[2] and is more likely to occur in eyes having recent trauma and when performing the operation with the patient in the prone position.

6. Postoperative retinal detachment has occurred in 6 of the author's cases, but in no case have the retinal breaks been related to the double-needle entrance and exit sites in the pars plana, which can usually be identified by indirect ophthalmoscopy.

SUMMARY AND CONCLUSIONS

The diagnosis of a subluxated or luxated lens should be made before lens surgery, so that its management may be carefully planned before operation. Complications are more likely during and after operations on a dislocated lens than they are with usual cataract operations. An attempt has been made to give the indications for operation and the surgical technics, which, in my opinion, are the most effective for the different surgical situations involving a dislocated lens. Lens support and scleral support in removing a dislocated lens are important. The use of the double needle is a preferred substitute for a planned loop extraction.

REFERENCES

1. Barraquer, J. I.: Surgical treatment of the lens displacements, Arch. Soc. Am. Oftal. Opt. *1*:30-38, 1958.
2. Calhoun, F. P., Jr.: Unpublished cases.
3. Calhoun, F. P., Jr., and Hagler, W. S.: Experience with the José Barraquer method of extracting a dislocated lens, Trans. Am. Ophth. Soc. *57*:221-241, 1959.
4. Chandler, P. A.: Surgery of the lens in infancy and childhood, A.M.A. Arch. Ophth. *27*:725, 1942.
5. Iliff, C.: Subluxation of lens, Am. J. Ophthal. *43*:126, 1957.
6. Verhoeff, F. A.: A simple and safe method for removing a cataract from fluid vitreous, Am. J. Ophthal. *25*:725, 1942.

11

A Summation

The basic philosophy that has guided me throughout this book is the question, "Would I want to have this operation done on me or some member of my own family?" The surgeon who does cataract surgery should be guided not by what may look best cosmetically or by anatomic reconstruction but rather by the functional results. Each patient should be treated as if he were the first private patient and each eye as if it were the patient's only eye. In selecting the preoperative steps, the surgeon should consider the problems peculiar to this eye and try to anticipate the pitfalls and possible complications. He should outline mentally beforehand a safe course and possible solutions to problems that may arise. Obviously, this is not always possible. Although these procedures are the correct ones to follow, some surgeons may have to make exceptions. Sometimes the individual functional results may have to be sacrificed, as in the case of mass eye surgery.

My thinking has been influenced by the fact that I cannot gracefully face the patient or the family to report serious complications and that with very few exceptions the management of these complications falls to me. The surgeon finds little joy in his labors when a complication such as a retinal separation occurs in his patient following cataract surgery. He must then spend hours searching for the holes and repairing the retina, whether it be with the light coagulator or with a scleral buckling procedure. The patient and the surgeon find little comfort in knowing that this or that complication would not have occurred if some new instrument had been available or if a new technic had been employed. Both are interested only in the best possible result.

With regard to anesthesia, my preference is local anesthesia; at present I favor 2 per cent Xylocaine, usually without Adrenalin but supplemented with hyaluronidase. During the procedure, the local anesthesia is supplemented with intravenous barbiturates and Demerol given in graduated doses, preferably by an anesthetist. Local anesthesia and retrobulbar injections are preferred in all cases combined with massage until the pressure, recorded with a sterile tonometer, indicates that the eye may be opened safely. The surgeon must not rely on massaging for a certain number of minutes. A recent suggestion has been made that additional injections be made to paralyze the superior oblique muscle by injections above and nasal to the trochlear nerve. Additional injections of each rectus muscle also have been advised. Recently, Reese and Jones suggested injections between the rectus muscles and avoidance of a retrobulbar anesthesia. Kirby, Barraquer and others agree that supplemental akinesia "enables the surgeon to do operations with a finesse which would not be possible without it."[1]

At present my preference with regard

to sutures is a minimum of 5 postplaced sutures, preferably 6-0 colored, mild chromic. Because of the sharpness of today's needles, with few exceptions, the preplacement of sutures is found to be a little more troublesome. However, the advantages of the preplaced suture can be obtained by postplacing 2 or 3 sutures as the wound is enlarged. Actually, it does not matter whether the sutures are preplaced or postplaced. The important consideration is that they are placed correctly. The new colored mild chromic suture material handles almost as easily as silk and is easily visible. By covering this corneoscleral suture with a limbus-based flap, the small suture abscesses that have been reported by others have not been noted, and the patient has not complained too much. The annoyance of removal of suture material as is necessary with the use of silk is avoided. Some of those who prefer silk have felt that the use of multiple 8-0 silk causes minimal irritation if these are covered with conjunctiva or, especially, if drops incorporating methylcellulose are used when no conjunctival flap is used. Where methylcellulose has been used, it has been reported that the sutures are well tolerated for as long as 3 to 4 months, even in the cornea, without a conjunctival covering. It is not too time consuming to add more sutures at the time of surgery, since it gives the surgeon more peace of mind to have 5 or more corneoscleral sutures.

As to sliding or tumbling, my preference has changed from an almost routine sliding technic to a tumbling technic in most cases; when carefully performed it seems easier and produces no greater incidence of complications. Results with forceps or with the erisophake are perhaps about the same. The erisophake is the instrument of choice in many intumescent lenses. Most North American surgeons, especially since the advent of alphachymotrypsin, strongly advise the use of capsule forceps in a sliding technic. A strong supporter of tumbling is Dr. Joaquin Barraquer, who has had the greatest experience with chemical zonulolysis; he still continues to use the erisophake and to tumble unless he encounters a hard or a flat lens, in which case he prefers to slide. The precautions outlined by Dr. Barraquer are followed. To avoid corneal damage, I apply the erisophake before complete zonulolysis has taken place. In cases of known Fuchs' dystrophy, in hard or flat lenses or where the upper pole of the lens seems to favor a sliding maneuver, the capsule forceps is used and the lens slid out. In selected cases, such as in an intumescent lens with a fragile capsule, an iridectomy will be performed and alpha-chymotrypsin used. Here, neither the capsule forceps nor the erisophake will be used, but the lens will be gently expressed by a loop or equivalent instrument from below. This technic is different from the classic Smith-Indian procedure, and it can be dangerous. In reference to management of the iris, except for selected cases where two or three small peripheral iridectomies will be performed, I no longer use iridotomies. In most cases, a vertical iridotomy is preferred to a sector iridectomy, not only because the cosmetic appearance is good, but chiefly because there are fewer complications postoperatively.

Although I prefer the intracapsular extraction in practically all adult cases, one should pause to reflect on the number of fine results one can have in a routine well-planned extracapsular extraction. One should consider the statement of a respected surgeon who has performed some of the most daring of modern operations when he, in all seriousness, says that he would want "a well-planned extracapsular extraction" on his own eye. However, I continue to favor intracapsular cataract extractions using alpha-chymotrypsin, especially in individuals in the 20 to 50 age group or where there may be a resistant zonule.

Although at one time I did a series of cases with direct zonular stripping and although on occasion lenses were removed with the cornea completely folded downward (Dr. Barraquer's "open-sky" maneuver) at present I prefer a "middle-of-the-road" course to a direct visualization of every step of the cataract extraction. Also in terms of modern instrumentation, I do not like doing cataract extractions under the operative microscope. This instrument has been used in the operating room, but I feel that its disadvantages exceed its advantages.

In summary, my clinical impressions on the round pupil as opposed to a sector iridectomy (as a rule I prefer a vertical iridotomy—a modification of a sector iridectomy) seems to be borne out by the conclusions reached by C. Dwight Townes in a series of 360 operations for senile cataracts. Townes conclusions, to which I subscribe, were as follows:

1. This study appears to bear out the impression that eyes operated upon with complete iridectomy in cataract extraction suffer fewer complications and progress through quieter convalescent periods than do eyes upon which peripheral iridectomy is done.
2. There is no statistically significant difference in visual results obtained by the two types of iridectomy.[3]

In reference to round pupils and some of my impressions on cataract extractions reported elsewhere, it is interesting to note and compare more recent and independent conclusions drawn from a summary from Greece of clinical observations on 1,000 cases of operations for cataract in 1961. The operative technic included corneal or limbal incisions without a conjunctival flap, five corneal or limbal sutures, sector iridectomy or two peripheral iridotomies. Extraction of the lens was made with an Arruga forceps applied at the upper pole or, in cases with an intumescent cataract, either with the erisophake or by a Smith-Indian method. Alpha-chymotrypsin was used in a number of cases, and acetylcholine (1:10,000) was instilled to obtain miosis.

The work of the author, Dr. Polychoronakos, was summarized as follows:

1. The type of incision plays an important role in the success of the operation. A very scleral incision is as dangerous as a very corneal one.
2. With peripheral iridotomy or iridectomy the following complications are more frequent than with complete iridectomy: rupture of the capsule, iris prolapse, deformation of the pupil, postoperative glaucoma. The optical results are similar either after complete iridectomy or after peripheral iridectomy or iridotomy. He is therefore in favour of complete iridectomy, in spite of the better cosmetic results of the other two methods.
3. The use of alpha-chymotrypsin in cases of senile and symptomatic cataracts facilitates intracapsular extraction and does not give rise to more complications.
4. In seventy-seven cases in which acetylcholine was used no case of iris prolapse was observed.
5. Instillation of Phenylephrine starting from the fifth day after the operation helps prevent posterior synechiae.
6. Hyphemia was rarely observed which was attributed to the type of incision and sutures used.
7. In cases of delayed restoration of the anterior chamber secondary glaucoma was rare (only one case among fourteen).
8. In cases of very corneal incisions secondary glaucoma is more frequent.[2]

The combination of glaucoma and cataracts presents a difficult problem. In the case of cataract in which miotic controlled angle-closure glaucoma is present (i.e., without angle block) lens extraction cures both the cataract and the potential angle-closure glaucoma. This is not true in acute angle closure with angle block.

In open-angle glaucoma, some surgeons will always operate the glaucoma first if there is a cataract and the ocular pressure is not controlled by the medications, systemic and local, given frequently and in the highest concentrations possible. I feel that if the glaucoma can be controlled with 1 per cent pilocarpine alone, and if there is a cataract, very often an iridectomy and removal of the lens will be sufficient. Some surgeons prefer to combine simultaneous glaucoma surgery, such as an iris inclusion or sclerectomy, with the extraction of the lens.

While the use of acrylic lenses after cataract extraction is not advocated by me in this text, those pioneers who have sought to perfect the material and the technic for anterior chamber implants must be admired. For this reason Prof. Strampelli's chapter on the use of acrylic lenses has been included. As stated previously, my choice is an intracapsular cataract extraction with the use of a contact lens if the patient desires and can tolerate it.

As to complications, I have been fortunate in having a minimum of flat chambers even when alpha-chymotrypsin was used. Part of this success may be related to the small amount of alpha-chymotrypsin used when it was used, and also possibly because of the precautions of carefully irrigating the wound edge and then removing the alpha-chymotrypsin excess from the anterior chamber. It is to be remembered that only enough alpha-chymotrypsin is needed to weaken the zonules, not to dissolve them. Other contributory factors to the success of the procedure may be the proper placing of 5 or more sutures, usually with a conjunctival flap to cover them. In addition, the use of pilocarpine at the time of surgery and 10 per cent Neo-Synephrine and a cycloplegic such as scopolamine or atropine starting on the first postoperative day is also of help. If 10 per cent Neo-Synephrine and mydriatics are helpful in restoring flat chambers because they break the pupillary block, it seems logical to use them in the postoperative routine. In avoiding one of the most dreaded complications, loss of vitreous, retrobulbar anesthesia supplemented with intravenous anesthesia has been found to be very helpful. A limited amount of retrobulbar solution carefully injected, followed by massage, and a recorded tonometric pressure have always been good guides as to whether or not the eye can be entered. In addition, the appearance of the cornea and the eye itself should guide the surgeon as to the problems he may expect. If there is a retrobulbar hemorrhage or one cannot reduce the pressure to safe limits, then the surgeon should not hesitate to postpone the operation until another day. Despite today's modern advances, if when the eye is opened there is a threat of vitreous loss or damage to the eye, the surgeon should choose the technic of lens extraction which offers the greatest safety in his hands under the circumstances. It is these modern advances which now permit him a greater choice. I am not immune to the loss of vitreous or other complications and again express the hope here, as I did in a previous book, that someday we will speak no longer of the management of complications of eye surgery but only of their avoidance.

ADDENDA

Since this book was submitted for publication, there have been a number of valuable contributions to the literature on eye surgery. We can cite only a very few of the most important of these.

Swan (A.M.A. Arch. Ophth. *69*:191, 1963) has made the suggestion that the order of treatment for shallow chamber without demonstrable wound leak should be as follows:

1. Medical—intensive mydriatic therapy, sometimes alternated with miotics to mobilize the pupil
2. Mechanical (about 8 days postoperatively)—point pressure on the iris through the cornea to mechanically disrupt iris adhesions to the vitreous face
3. Surgical—(a) peripheral iridectomy and (b) other surgical procedures, rupture of the vitreous face, sclerotomy.

Stocker *et al.* (Am. J. Ophthal. *55*:547, 1963) have reported that they feel that there is no contraindication to the use of alpha-chymotrypsin in early cases of Fuchs' dystrophy. On the contrary, they feel that it is possible to remove the lens with minimal trauma to the endothelium if the technic is adapted properly.

Chandler and Grant (A.M.A. Arch. Ophth. *68*:353, 1962) have shown that mydriatic-cycloplegic treatment may be of some help in some cases of malignant glaucoma. The reader is also referred to the editorial in the *A.M.A. Archives of Ophthalmology* (*69*:421, 1963) for a discussion of glaucoma following injury.

REFERENCES

1. Kirby, D. B.: Advanced Surgery of Cataract, Philadelphia, Lippincott, 1955.
2. Polychronakos, D.: Clinical observations on one thousand cases of operations for cataract, Arch. Soc. Ophth. Grèce du Nord *10*:202, 1961.
3. Townes, C. D.: Complete or peripheral iridectomy in cataract surgery, Trans. Am. Ophth. Soc. *56*:145, 1958.

Index